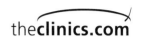

DENTAL CLINICS
OF NORTH AMERICA

Temporomandibular Disorders
and Orofacial Pain

GUEST EDITOR
Henry A. Gremillion, DDS

January 2007 • Volume 51 • Number 1

An Imprint of Elsevier, Inc.
PHILADELPHIA LONDON TORONTO MONTREAL SYDNEY TOKYO

W.B. SAUNDERS COMPANY
A Division of Elsevier Inc.

Elsevier Inc. • 1600 John F. Kennedy Boulevard • Suite 1800 • Philadelphia, Pennsylvania 19103-2899

http://www.dental.theclinics.com

DENTAL CLINICS OF NORTH AMERICA   Volume 51, Number 1
January 2007   ISSN 0011-8532
Editor: John Vassallo; j.vassallo@elsevier.com   ISBN-13: 978-1-4160-4302-7
                                                                     ISBN-10: 1-4160-4302-0

The ideas and opinions expressed in *The Dental Clinics of North America* do not necessarily reflect those of the Publisher. The Publisher does not assume any responsibility for any injury and/or damage to persons or property arising out of or related to any use of the material contained in this periodical. The reader is advised to check the appropriate medical literature and the product information currently provided by the manufacturer of each drug to be administered to verify the dosage, the method and duration of administration, or contraindications. It is the responsibility of the treating physician or other health care professional, relying on independent experience and knowledge of the patient, to determine drug dosages and the best treatment for the patient. Mention of any product in this issue should not be construed as endorsement by the contributors, editors, or the Publisher of the product or manufacturers' claims.

Dental Clinics of North America (ISSN 0011-8532) is published quarterly by Elsevier Inc., 360 Park Avenue South, New York, NY 10010-1710. Months of issue are January, April, July, and October. Business and Editorial Offices: 1600 John F. Kennedy Boulevard, Suite 1800, Philadelphia, PA 19103-2899. Customer Service Office: 6277 Sea Harbor Drive, Orlando, FL 32887-4800. Periodicals postage paid at New York, NY and additional mailing offices. Subscription prices are $171.00 per year (US individuals), $281.00 per year (US institutions), $83.00 per year (US students), $204.00 per year (Canadian individuals), $347.00 per year (Canadian institutions), $116.00 per year (Canadian students), $231.00 per year (international individuals), $347.00 per year (international institutions), and $116.00 per year (international students). International air speed delivery is included in all *Clinics* subscription prices. All prices are subject to change without notice. **POSTMASTER:** Send address changes to *Dental Clinics of North America*, Elsevier Periodicals Customer Service, 6277 Sea Harbor Drive, Orlando, FL 32887–4800. Customer Service: 1-800-654-2452 (US). From outside of the US, call 1-407-345-4000.

The Dental Clinics of North America is covered in *Index Medicus, Current Contents/Clinical Medicine, ISI/BIOMED* and *Clinahl.*

Printed in the United States of America.

GUEST EDITOR

HENRY A. GREMILLION, DDS, Professor, Department of Orthodontics, and Director, Parker E. Mahan Facial Pain Center, University of Florida College of Dentistry, Gainesville, Florida

CONTRIBUTORS

RONALD C. AUVENSHINE, DDS, PhD, Director, Orofacial Pain Clinic, Michael E. DeBakey VA Hospital; Associate Clinical Professor, The University of Texas Dental Branch, Houston, Texas

GLENN T. CLARK, DDS, MS, Director and Professor, Department of Diagnostic Sciences, Orofacial Pain and Oral Medicine Center, University of Southern California School of Dentistry, Los Angeles, California

CHARLES R. CARLSON, PhD, ABPP, Professor and Chair, Department of Psychology, and Professor, Department of Oral Health Science, University of Kentucky, Lexington, Kentucky

M. FRANKLIN DOLWICK, DMD, PhD, Professor and Associate Chairman, Division of Oral and Maxillofacial Surgery, University of Florida College of Dentistry, Gainesville, Florida

ROGER B. FILLINGIM, PhD, Professor, Department of Community Dentistry and Behavioral Science, College of Dentistry, University of Florida; North Florida/South Georgia Veterans Health System, Malcolm Randall VA Medical Center, Gainesville, Florida

JAMES FRICTON, DDS, MS, Professor, Diagnostic and Biological Sciences, University of Minnesota School of Dentistry, Minneapolis, Minnesota

STEVEN B. GRAFF-RADFORD, DDS, Co-Director, The Pain Center, Cedars-Sinai Medical Center, Los Angeles, California

HENRY A. GREMILLION, DDS, Professor, Department of Orthodontics, and Director, Parker E. Mahan Facial Pain Center, University of Florida College of Dentistry, Gainesville, Florida

SHELDON G. GROSS, DDS, Clinical Associate Professor, University of Connecticut Health Center, Farmington, Connecticut

KENNETH M. HARGREAVES, DDS, PhD, Professor of Endodontics, University of Texas Health Science Center at San Antonio School of Dentistry, San Antonio, Texas

MICHAEL A. HENRY, DDS, PhD, Professor of Endodontics, University of Texas Health Science Center at San Antonio School of Dentistry, San Antonio, Texas

STEVE KRAUS, PT, OCS, MTC, Clinical Associate of Rehabilitation Medicine, Emory University School of Medicine, Atlanta, Georgia

LARRY Z. LOCKERMAN, DDS, Instructor of Surgery, Temporomandibular Joint/Headache Center, University of Massachusetts Memorial Medical Center, University of Massachusetts Medical School, Worcester, Massachusetts

ROBERT L. MERRILL, DDS, MS, Adjunct Professor and Director, Graduate Orofacial Pain Program, UCLA School of Dentistry, Los Angeles, California

CYNTHIA D. MYERS, PhD, LMT, Director of Integrative Medicine Program, H. Lee Moffitt Cancer Center & Research Institute; Assistant Professor, Department of Interdisciplinary Oncology, College of Medicine, University of South Florida, Tampa, Florida

JEFFREY P. OKESON, DMD, Professor and Chair, Department of Oral Health Science, and Director of the Orofacial Pain Program, University of Kentucky College of Dentistry, Lexington, Kentucky

SARAVANAN RAM, BDS, MDS, Assistant Clinical Professor, Department of Diagnostic Sciences, Orofacial Pain and Oral Medicine Center, University of Southern California School of Dentistry, Los Angeles, California

RENÉ M. SHINAL, PhD, Postdoctoral Associate, Department of Community Dentistry and Behavioral Science, College of Dentistry, University of Florida, Gainesville, Florida

CHRISTOPHER J. SPENCER, DDS, Associate Clinical Professor, Department of Orthodontics, Parker E. Mahan Facial Pain Center, University of Florida College of Dentistry, Gainesville, Florida

ALAN STILES, DMD, Facial Pain Management, Oral and Maxillofacial Surgery Department, Thomas Jefferson University, Philadelphia, Pennsylvania

CONTENTS

Preface   xi
Henry A. Gremillion

**Overview of Orofacial Pain: Epidemiology and Gender
Differences in Orofacial Pain**   1
René M. Shinal and Roger B. Fillingim

> Chronic orofacial pain is a prevalent problem that encompasses
> numerous disorders with diverse causes and presenting symp-
> toms. Compared with men, women of reproductive age seek treat-
> ment for orofacial pain conditions, as well as other chronic pain
> disorders more frequently. Important issues have been raised
> regarding gender and sex differences in genetic, neurophysiologic,
> and psychosocial aspects of pain sensitivity and analgesia. Efforts
> to improve our understanding of qualitative sex differences in pain
> modulation signify a promising step toward developing more
> tailored approaches to pain management.

Peripheral Mechanisms of Odontogenic Pain   19
Michael A. Henry and Kenneth M. Hargreaves

> In this article, we review the key basic mechanisms associated with
> this phenomena and more recently identified mechanisms that are
> current areas of interest. Although many of these pain mechanisms
> apply throughout the body, we attempt to describe these mechan-
> isms in the context of trigeminal pain.

Central Mechanisms of Orofacial Pain   45
Robert L. Merrill

> The orofacial pain clinician must understand the difference
> between peripheral and central mechanisms of pain. Particularly,
> one has to understand the process of central sensitization as it
> relates to the various orofacial pain conditions to understand
> orofacial pain. Understanding leads to more effective treatment.

Myogenous Temporomandibular Disorders: Diagnostic and Management Considerations 61
James Fricton

Myogenous temporomandibular disorders (or masticatory myalgia) are characterized by pain and dysfunction that arise from pathologic and functional processes in the masticatory muscles. There are several distinct muscle disorder subtypes in the masticatory system, including myofascial pain, myositis, muscle spasm, and muscle contracture. The major characteristics of masticatory myalgia include pain, muscle tenderness, limited range of motion, and other symptoms (eg, fatigability, stiffness, subjective weakness). Comorbid conditions and complicating factors also are common and are discussed. Management follows with stretching, posture, and relaxation exercises, physical therapy, reduction of contributing factors, and as necessary, muscle injections.

Joint Intracapsular Disorders: Diagnostic and Nonsurgical Management Considerations 85
Jeffrey P. Okeson

This article reviews common intracapsular temporomandibular disorders encountered in the dental practice. It begins with a brief review of normal temporomandibular joint anatomy and function followed by a description of the common types of disorders known as internal derangements. The etiology, history, and clinical presentation of each are reviewed. Nonsurgical management is presented based on current long-term scientific evidence.

Temporomandibular Disorders: Associated Features 105
Ronald C. Auvenshine

Temporomandibular disorder (TMD) encompasses a number of clinical problems involving the masticatory muscles or the temporomandibular joints. These disorders are a major cause of nondental pain in the orofacial region, and are considered to be a subclassification of musculoskeletal disorders. Orofacial pain and TMD can be associated with pathologic conditions or disorders related to somatic and neurologic structures. When patients present to the dental office with a chief complaint of pain or headaches, it is vital for the practitioner to understand the cause of the complaint and to perform a thorough examination that will lead to the correct diagnosis and appropriate treatment. A complete understanding of the associated medical conditions with symptomology common to TMD and orofacial pain is necessary for a proper diagnosis.

Temporomandibular Disorders and Headache 129
Steven B. Graff-Radford

Headache is a common symptom, but when severe, it may be extremely disabling. It is assumed that patients who present to dentists with headache often are diagnosed with a temporomandibular disorder (TMD), although many may have migraine. TMD as a collective term may include several clinical entities, including myogenous and arthrogenous components. Because headache and TMD are so common they may be integrated or separate entities. Nevertheless, the temporomandibular joint (TMJ) and associated orofacial structures should be considered as triggering or perpetuating factors for migraine. This article discusses the relationship between the TMJ, muscles, or other orofacial structures and headache.

Psychological Factors Associated with Orofacial Pains   145
Charles R. Carlson

This article develops the case for why trigeminal pain is a unique and challenging problem for clinicians and patients alike, and provides the reader with insights for effective trigeminal pain management based on an understanding of the interplay between psychologic and physiologic systems. There is no greater sensory experience for the brain to manage than unremitting pain in trigeminally mediated areas. Such pain overwhelms conscious experience and focuses the suffering individual like few other sensory events. Trigeminal pain often motivates a search for relief that can drain financial and emotional resources. In some instances, the search is rewarded by a treatment that immediately addresses an identifiable source of pain; in other cases, it can stimulate never-ending pilgrimages from one health provider to another.

Temporomandibular Disorders, Head and Orofacial Pain: Cervical Spine Considerations   161
Steve Kraus

Head and orofacial pain originates from dental, neurologic, musculoskeletal, otolaryngologic, vascular, metaplastic, or infectious disease. It is treated by many health care practitioners, such as dentists, oral surgeons, and physicians. The article focuses on the nonpathologic involvement of the musculoskeletal system as a source of head and orofacial pain. The areas of the musculoskeletal system that are reviewed include the temporomandibular joint and muscles of mastication—collectively referred to as temporomandibular disorders (TMDs) and cervical spine disorders. The first part of the article highlights the role of physical therapy in the treatment of TMDs. The second part discusses cervical spine considerations in the management of TMDs and head and orofacial symptoms. It concludes with an overview of the evaluation and treatment of the cervical spine.

Temporomandibular Joint Surgery for Internal Derangement   195
M. Franklin Dolwick

Surgery of the temporomandibular joint (TMJ) plays a small, but important, role in the management of patients who have temporomandibular disorders (TMDs). There is a spectrum of surgical procedures for the treatment of TMD that ranges from simple arthrocentesis and lavage to more complex open joint surgical procedures. It is important to recognize that surgical treatment rarely is performed alone; generally, it is supported by nonsurgical treatment before and after surgery. Each surgical procedure should have strict criteria for which cases are most appropriate. Recognizing that scientifically proven criteria are lacking, this article discusses the suggested criteria for each procedure, ranging from arthrocentesis to complex open joint surgery. The discussion includes indications, brief descriptions of techniques, outcomes, and complications for each procedure.

Neuropathic Orofacial Pain: Proposed Mechanisms, Diagnosis, and Treatment Considerations 209
Christopher J. Spencer and Henry A. Gremillion

The most common reason patients seek medical or dental care in the United States is due to pain or dysfunction. The orofacial region is plagued by a number of acute, chronic, and recurrent painful maladies. Pain involving the teeth and the periodontium is the most common presenting concern in dental practice. Non-odontogenic pain conditions also occur frequently. Recent scientific investigation has provided an explosion of knowledge regarding pain mechanisms and pathways and an enhanced understanding of the complexities of the many ramifications of the total pain experience. Therefore, it is mandatory for the dental professional to develop the necessary clinical and scientific expertise on which he/she may base diagnostic and management approaches. Optimum management can be achieved only by determining an accurate and complete diagnosis and identifying all of the factors associated with the underlying pathosis on a case-specific basis. A thorough understanding of the epidemiologic and etiologic aspects of dental, musculoskeletal, neurovascular, and neuropathic orofacial pain conditions is essential to the practice of evidence-based dentistry/medicine.

Four Oral Motor Disorders: Bruxism, Dystonia, Dyskinesia and Drug-Induced Dystonic Extrapyramidal Reactions 225
Glenn T. Clark and Saravanan Ram

This article reviews four of the involuntary hyperkinetic motor disorders that affect the orofacial region: bruxism, orofacial dystonia, oromandibular dyskinesia, and medication-induced extrapyramidal syndrome–dystonic reactions. It discusses and contrasts the clinical features and management strategies for spontaneous, primary, and drug-induced motor disorders in the orofacial region. The article provides a list of medications that have been reported to cause drug-related extrapyramidal motor activity, and discusses briefly the genetic and traumatic events that are associated with spontaneous dystonia. Finally, it presents an approach for management of the orofacial motor disorders. The contraindications, side effects, and usual approach for medications and injections are covered. An overview of the indications, contraindications, and complications of using botulinum toxin as a therapeutic modality is discussed briefly.

A Critical Review of the Use of Botulinum Toxin in Orofacial Pain Disorders   245

Glenn T. Clark, Alan Stiles, Larry Z. Lockerman, and Sheldon G. Gross

This article reviews the appropriate use, cautions, and contraindication for botulinum neurotoxin (BoNT) and reviews the peer-reviewed literature that describes its efficacy for treatment of various chronic orofacial pain disorders. The literature has long suggested that BoNT is of value for orofacial hyperactivity and more recently for some orofacial pain disorders; however, the results are not as promising for orofacial pain. The available data from randomized, double-blind, placebo-controlled trials (RBCTs) do not support the use of BoNT as a substantially better therapy than what is being used already. The one exception is that BoNT has reasonable RBCT data to support its use as a migraine prophylaxis therapy. The major caveat is that the use of BoNT in chronic orofacial pain is "off-label".

Complementary and Alternative Medicine for Persistent Facial Pain   263

Cynthia D. Myers

This article discusses complementary and alternative medicine (CAM), reviews literature on the prevalence of use of CAM by the general adult population in the United States and by patients with persistent facial pain, and summarizes published, peer-reviewed reports of clinical trials assessing the effects of CAM therapies for persistent facial pain. Results indicate that many patients use CAM for musculoskeletal pain, including persistent facial pain. Preliminary work on selected complementary therapies such as biofeedback, relaxation, and acupuncture seems promising; however, there are more unanswered than answered questions about cost-effectiveness, efficacy, and mechanisms of action of CAM for persistent facial pain.

Index   275

FORTHCOMING ISSUES

April 2007

    Esthetic Design, Materials and Methods
    John R. Calamia, DDS, Mark Wolff, DDS, PhD,
    and Richard J. Simonsen, DDS, MS, *Guest Editors*

July 2007

    Dental Materials
    Lyle Zardiackas, PhD, Tracy Dellinger, DDS, MS,
    and Mark Livingston, DDS, *Guest Editors*

October 2007

    Dentistry's Role in Disaster Response
    Michael D. Colvard, DDS, MTS, MS, *Guest Editor*

RECENT ISSUES

October 2006

    Medical Conditions and Their Impact on Dental Care
    James R. Hupp, DMD, MD, JD, MBA, *Guest Editor*

July 2006

    Implantology
    Mark V. Thomas, DMD, *Guest Editor*

April 2006

    Tissue Engineering
    Franklin García-Godoy, DDS, MS, *Guest Editor*

THE DENTAL
CLINICS
OF NORTH AMERICA

Dent Clin N Am 51 (2007) xi–xii

Preface

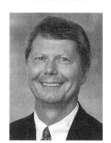

Henry A. Gremillion, DDS
Guest Editor

Since the last issue on temporomandibular (TMD) disorders and orofacial pain presented in the *Dental Clinics of North America* (April 1997), there has been an explosion of scientific, technologic, and procedural advances in this complex field. The amalgamation of the science with the art of dentistry has resulted from an enhanced appreciation for and the ability to provide evidence-based diagnosis and care.

Pain and compromised function are the most common reasons for which people seek health care. Historically, dentistry has been most effective regarding the diagnosis and management of acute pain conditions. However, more than one in four Americans, approximately 75 million people, live in chronic pain. Many of these individuals experience pain in the orofacial region. Our role as diagnosticians, becoming physicians of the masticatory system and orofacial area, is more important than ever. We must develop an increased clinical awareness of pain and its many facets. For example, we now appreciate that diagnosis of painful conditions involving the head and neck is frequently complicated by referred pain or co-existing conditions that may lead the practitioner down a path of well-intentioned but misdirected care.

Our profession is at the forefront in the establishment of a new and expanded mind-set reflected in the clinician/scientist model. Dentistry must assume the role of leader in the field of diagnosis and management of pain and dysfunction in the most complexly innervated area of the human body, the stomatognathic system and its contiguous structures.

As guest editor, I wanted to provide a forum in which the many facets of orofacial pain would be presented. The broad scope and depth of information contained in this issue is testimony to the rapidly and ever-expanding body of clinically relevant information in the field of TMD and orofacial pain. I wish to thank the authors for their excellent effort and cooperation in putting this volume together. I am especially grateful to John Vassallo, editor of the *Dental Clinics of North America*, for his patience, support, and guidance.

Henry A. Gremillion, DDS
Department of Orthodontics
Parker E. Mahan Facial Pain Center
University of Florida College of Dentistry
PO Box 100437
Gainesville, FL 32610-0437, USA

E-mail address: hgremillion@dental.ufl.edu

ELSEVIER
SAUNDERS

THE DENTAL
CLINICS
OF NORTH AMERICA

Dent Clin N Am 51 (2007) 1–18

Overview of Orofacial Pain: Epidemiology and Gender Differences in Orofacial Pain

René M. Shinal, PhD[a], Roger B. Fillingim, PhD[a,b],*

[a]Department of Community Dentistry and Behavioral Science, College of Dentistry, University of Florida, P.O. Box 103628 Gainesville, FL 32610-3628, USA
[b]North Florida/South Georgia Veterans Health System, Malcolm Randall VA Medical Center, 1601 SW Archer Road, Gainesville, FL 32608-1197, USA

Pain is the number one reason people seek health care; it is deemed the "fifth vital sign," to mark its importance as health status indicator [1]. The most widely used definition of pain is an "unpleasant sensory and emotional experience associated with actual or potential tissue damage, or described in terms of such damage" [2]. Pain is a personal experience that reflects the totality of genetic, physiologic, and psychosocial contributions. An area that is receiving considerable attention is the influence of biologic sex and gender role identity on the experience of pain. This article provides an overview of current findings regarding sex and gender differences in clinical and experimental pain responses, with particular attention to findings pertaining to orofacial pain. Evidence is presented from human and nonhuman animal studies that address sex differences in pain sensitivity, pain tolerance, and analgesia. The potential mechanisms involved, as well as implications for future research and clinical practice, are discussed.

Epidemiology of orofacial pain

Orofacial pain refers to a large group of disorders, including temporomandibular disorders (TMDs), headaches, neuralgia, pain arising from dental or mucosal origins, and idiopathic pain [3,4]. The classification and epidemiology of orofacial pain presents challenges because of the many anatomic structures involved, diverse causes, unpredictable pain referral

---

* Corresponding author. Department of Community Dentistry and Behavioral Science, College of Dentistry, University of Florida, P.O. Box 103628 Gainesville, FL 32610-3628.
E-mail address: rfilling@ufl.edu (R.B. Fillingim).

0011-8532/07/$ - see front matter © 2007 Elsevier Inc. All rights reserved.
doi:10.1016/j.cden.2006.09.004
dental.theclinics.com

patterns and presenting symptoms, and a lack of consensus regarding differential diagnostic criteria [5,6]. Despite these obstacles, several investigators and professional associations have made progress in developing diagnostic criteria [7–9]. For example, the International Association for the Study of Pain and the International Headache Society have developed widely used orofacial pain diagnostic criteria [10,11]. Similarly, Dworkin and LeResche [12] have proposed Research Diagnostic Criteria for TMD, including a dual axis system for classifying patients according to the predominant pain source (eg, muscle pain, disk displacement, joint condition) and any associated psychosocial features (eg, disability, depression, somatization). The often weak association between pain and observable tissue pathology has prompted researchers and clinicians to use a multidimensional approach for studying this widespread problem [13].

Chronic orofacial pain affects approximately 10% of adults and up to 50% of the elderly [4]. There is evidence that sex differences in masticatory muscle pain and tenderness emerge as early as 19 years of age [14]. Women of reproductive age, with a concentration of women in their 40s, seek treatment for orofacial pain more frequently compared to men by a 2:1 ratio [15–17]. Moreover, a greater proportion of women seek treatment for other pain conditions, such as migraine and tension-type headaches, fibromyalgia, autoimmune rheumatic disorders, chronic fatigue, orthopedic problems, and irritable bowel syndrome [16,18,19]. Women are more likely to seek medical care for pain; however, they also report more pain for which they do not seek treatment [20,21]. This holds true for all bodily symptoms, and for those with unknown etiology [22–24]. Women also experience more symptom recurrences and more intense pain. These differences persist when apparent confounding factors, such as sex differences in the prevalence rates of medical conditions and gynecologic pain, are controlled statistically [22].

Kohlmann [17] noted that, among patients who presented with orofacial pain lasting at least a week, more than 90% complained of pain in other body areas as well. Patients who have orofacial pain share many similarities with other patients who have chronic pain, such as a moderate correlation between reported symptoms and objective pathologic findings, maladaptive behaviors (eg, parafunctions), social and psychologic distress, impairment of daily activities, occupational disability, and higher rates of health care use [16,25,26]. The result is a diminished quality of life that is constrained by pain experiences.

Numerous factors with varying degrees of empiric support have been posited to explain sex differences in pain prevalence. These include differences in descending central nervous system pathways that modulate pain signal transmission [27–29], genetics [30], and the effects of gonadal hormones [31–34]. Also, a vast literature addresses psychosocial sex differences in symptom appraisal, socialization and gender roles, abuse and trauma, depression and anxiety, gender bias in research and clinical practice, and race and ethnicity [22,35].

Sex differences in responses to experimental pain

Although numerous factors inevitably contribute to sex differences in the prevalence and severity of clinical pain, the senior author and colleague [28] previously suggested that sex differences in the processing of pain-related information could play an important role. That is, a higher level of pain sensitivity among women may serve as a risk factor for developing certain pain disorders, including chronic orofacial pain. A robust and expanding literature that addresses sex differences in experimental pain sensitivity is available, and these findings are discussed below.

Nonhuman animal research

Considerable research with nonhuman animals (primarily rodents) has examined whether males and females differ regarding responses to noxious stimuli [24,28,36] and analgesia [37–39]. Rodent studies have yielded mixed information concerning sex differences in pain perception and analgesia (called "nociception" and "antinociception," respectively, when referring to nonhuman animals). A comprehensive meta-analysis by Mogil and colleagues [39] found that female rats were more sensitive to electrical shock and chemically-induced inflammatory nociception (eg, abdominal constriction, formalin tests) in most studies; however, results using thermal assays were equivocal. Of the 23 studies reviewed, 17 reported no significant sex differences; in the remainder, females exhibited more sensitivity to the hot plate test than did males. With regard to radiant heat and hot water immersion, most studies reported no sex differences, with 8 reporting increased sensitivity in male rats and 2 reporting increased sensitivity in female mice. To clarify discrepancies, the investigators conducted additional nociceptive testing and morphine antinociception experiments using a variety of outbred mice and rats. Regarding nociception and morphine antinociception, there was a significant interaction between sex and genotype (ie, strain) of rodents. To complicate matters, strain differences can be relevant for one sex, but not the other, and vary according to the pain assay. Female nociception and antinociception also change across the estrous cycle; however, when female mice were tested as a randomly mixed group (ie, estrous and diestrus), sex differences tended to diminish. The investigators noted that males and females might use qualitatively distinct neurochemical mechanisms to modulate nociception. They also suggested that the organizing effects of early hormone exposure during development might have more impact than do adult gonadal hormone fluctuations.

Human research

Laboratory pain research in humans suggests that women are more sensitive to several forms of laboratory pain compared with men. Consistent with rodent research, there is considerable variability in the magnitude and direction of sex differences [24,28,36]. A meta-analysis conducted by Riley and colleagues [40] found that women generally show lower pain thresholds and tolerances than do men to a variety of noxious laboratory stimuli. Effect sizes for pain threshold and tolerance ranged from large to moderate, and varied according to pain assay. Pressure pain and electrical stimulation demonstrated the largest effects for the 22 studies reviewed, whereas thermal pain yielded inconsistent results. The investigators concluded that small sample sizes contributed to inadequate statistical power and inconsistent results. Regarding cold pressor stimulation, studies show that men generally display higher pain thresholds and tolerance, and lower pain ratings than do women [41]; however, Logan & Gedney [42] noted a significant sex-by-session interaction such that women anticipated and reported more pain than did men after a second session of forehead cold pressor testing. There were no sex differences during the initial cold pressor session, however. This indicates that previous experience with pain can affect subsequent pain perception and modulation in a sex-dependent fashion.

Several studies have examined laboratory models of orofacial pain. For example, Karibe and colleagues [43] noted that healthy female controls experienced more masticatory muscle pain during 6 minutes of gum chewing than did men, and had more pain (compared with pretest measures) an hour after chewing. Similarly, Plesh and colleagues [44] assessed jaw pain tolerance in healthy subjects during and after bite force tasks. Both sexes had increased pain during bite tasks; however, postclenching pain lasted longer for women. Notably, women reported significantly more baseline pain upon jaw movement on the second day of testing, whereas men did not report an increase in baseline pain 24 hours later. The investigators ruled out muscular microtrauma because there were no significant differences in postexertion pressure pain tolerance or threshold. Instead, they suggested that neuronal hypersensitivity might play a role in postexertion hyperalgesia.

Injection of algesic substances into the facial and cervical muscles also has been used as an experimental model that mimics head and neck pain of muscular origin [45]. Injections of hypertonic saline or glutamate solutions into the trapezius muscle produced significantly more pain among women relative to men [46,47]. Similarly, pain induced by glutamate injections into the masseter muscle was more intense, larger in area, and longer lasting in women [48]. Thus, sex differences in pain perception extend to experimental models of particular relevance for clinical orofacial pain.

Another experimental pain model that may be of significant clinical relevance is temporal summation of pain. Temporal summation refers to a perceived increase in pain that is generated by rapidly repeated noxious stimulation [49]. This phenomenon is believed to be the perceptual correlate that occurs when high-frequency stimulation of C-fibers (C polymodal nociceptive afferents) amplifies second-order neuronal activity in the spinal cord dorsal horn (ie, windup). This series of events involves N-methyl-D-aspartate [NMDA] glutamate receptors [50,51]. Temporal summation is thought to reflect central neural mechanisms similar to those that are responsible for the hyperalgesia and allodynia that characterize many forms of clinical pain [51–57]. Healthy women exhibit more robust temporal summation than do men in response to thermal, electrical, and mechanical stimulation [29,58,59]. Staud and colleagues [60] showed that patients who had fibromyalgia exhibited greater temporal summation of heat pain and heightened after-sensations compared with healthy controls. Similarly, patients who had TMDs showed greater temporal summation of thermal and mechanical pain compared with pain-free controls [61,62]. Such findings invite speculation that individuals who display exaggerated temporal summation of pain might be at greater risk for developing central sensitization of pain pathways, which may reflect a predisposition for developing chronic pain syndromes [29]. There is a need for prospective longitudinal studies to determine whether enhanced temporal summation of pain precedes chronic pain, or is a consequence thereof.

Brain imaging studies

A rapidly expanding body of research uses functional brain imaging in an attempt to identify cerebral responses that are associated with the experience of pain [27,63–66]. Several brain regions have emerged consistently as areas that are activated during acute exposure to noxious stimuli. Acute painful events often elicit activity in the primary and secondary somatosensory cortices, insular cortex, anterior cingulate, and prefrontal cortices [27]. Bilateral thalamic and brain stem activation have been associated with general arousal (eg, attention) in response to noxious stimuli [65], whereas limbic system components (eg, anterior cingulate, medial prefrontal, insular cortices) are believed to reflect emotional aspects of pain anticipation and processing [27,65,67]. The periaqueductal gray, regions of the anterior cingulate, and the orbitofrontal cortex are implicated in endogenous pain modulation [27].

A small body of evidence addresses sex differences in brain activation patterns in the contralateral insula, thalamus, and prefrontal cortex in response to experimentally evoked pain. For example, in response to a painful thermal stimulus, patterns of pain-related brain activation showed similarity between the sexes; however, women showed greater activation in the contralateral prefrontal cortex, contralateral insular and anterior cingulate cortex, and cerebellar vermis compared with men [68]. In contrast, Derbyshire and colleagues [69] reported greater heat pain–related activation among men versus women in bilateral parietal cortex, and in contralateral primary and secondary somatosensory, prefrontal, and insular cortices. Women showed greater activation in ipsilateral perigenual cortex. This conflicting pattern of results likely reflects differences in stimulus characteristics. Specifically, Paulson and colleagues [68] used an identical (50°C) contact heat stimulus, which was rated as more painful by women, whereas Derbyshire and colleagues [69] adjusted the intensity of their laser stimulus to be equally painful across sexes.

Several studies have examined sex differences in cerebral responses to stimuli delivered to deep abdominal body tissues (ie, visceral stimulation). Berman and colleagues [70] found that, compared with women who had irritable bowel syndrome (IBS), men who had IBS showed greater bilateral insular cortex activation to rectal pressure. These investigators subsequently showed that rectal distention produces greater activation in ventromedial prefrontal and right anterior cingulate cortex, and left amygdala among women who had IBS, whereas men who had IBS showed greater activation in right dorsolateral prefrontal cortex, insula, and periaqueductal gray [71]. In contrast, Hobson and colleagues [72] found no sex differences in cortical activity evoked from esophageal stimuli in healthy subjects.

Thus, these findings involving somatic and visceral stimuli indicate substantial overlap in brain areas that are involved in acute pain processing between men and women. The variable sex differences that have emerged across studies likely depend upon the stimulus properties and population characteristics.

Sex differences in analgesic systems

Many organisms, including humans, possess natural pain control mechanisms (ie, endogenous systems). Nonhuman animal studies have revealed sex differences for at least one form of endogenous pain modulation: stress-induced analgesia (SIA). In rodents, mildly stressful events (eg, brief swims in tepid water) recruit endogenous opiate systems, whereas intensely stressful events (eg, forced cold-water swims) recruit nonopioid systems (eg, NMDA glutamate receptors) more heavily [24,73]. Given the same stressor, female rodents usually have equal or less SIA than do males. Blocking opioid or NMDA receptors reverses SIA in male and ovariectomized female mice, but not in intact female mice. This suggests that the neurochemical and hormonal mechanisms that support SIA might differ for female and male animals [74,75].

Methods for investigating endogenous pain inhibition also are available in humans. One frequently used method is assessment of diffuse noxious inhibitory controls (DNIC). DNIC, or counterirritation, refers to the process whereby one noxious stimulus inhibits the perception of a second painful stimulus. This phenomenon is believed to reflect descending inhibition of pain signals [76,77]. DNIC is presumed to operate through activation of descending supraspinal inhibitory pathways that are initiated by release of endogenous opioids [78–81]. Several studies have investigated sex differences in the efficacy of DNIC, with mixed results. France and Suchowiecki [82] reported that ischemic arm pain produced equal reductions in the nociceptive flexion reflex (NFR, a pain-related reflex in the biceps femoris in response to electrical stimulation of the lower extremity) activity in women and men, which indicated no differences in DNIC. Serrao and colleagues [29] recorded the NFR and pain intensity for 36 healthy adults randomized to a baseline, nonpainful control or a painful cold pressor DNIC condition. As expected, women, on average, had lower NFR temporal summation thresholds than did men. The cold pressor produced greater increases in the stimulus intensity at which temporal summation elicited a reflex in men compared with women, which indicated greater DNIC among men. In contrast, Baad-Hansen and colleagues [83] found no sex differences in the ability of an ice-water DNIC to modulate intraoral pain that was induced by the application of a topical irritant (ie, capsaicin) in healthy participants.

Responses to analgesic medication (ie, exogenous analgesia) also might differ as a function of sex, although the findings are far from consistent. For example, clinical studies have indicated greater morphine analgesia among women [84], among men [85], and others have reported no sex differences in morphine analgesia [86,87]. Consistent sex differences have been reported in the analgesic effects of mixed action opioids (eg, pentazocine, butorphanol, nalbuphine), which produce analgesia, in part, by binding of κ-receptors [88]. This class of medications also has partial agonist action at δ-receptors and antagonist action at μ-receptors, which complicates the side effect profile [89]. Among patients who experienced postoperative pain after third molar extraction, Gear and colleagues [89] demonstrated that pentazocine and butorphanol produced greater and longer-lasting analgesia among women versus men. Subsequently, these investigators found that a 5-mg dose of nalbuphine had paradoxic antianalgesic effects on men [90]. To obtain analgesia, men required higher doses (20 mg) than did women (10 mg). This trend persisted when body weight was included as a covariate. Men also had more pain by the end of the study protocol, whereas women, on average, did not return to their baseline pain levels. This study demonstrates that subtle sex differences exist in response to κ-opioids.

Experimental pain models also have been used to explore sex differences in opioid analgesia. With an electrical pain assay, women have shown greater analgesic potency but slower onset and offset of morphine analgesia than did men [91], although these investigators failed to include a placebo condition and subsequently observed no sex differences in analgesic responses to morphine-6-glucuronide, an active metabolite of morphine [92]. Zacny [93] reported that μ-opioid agonists (eg, morphine, meperidine, hydromorphone) produced greater analgesic responses among women using cold pressor pain, but no sex differences in analgesia emerged for pressure pain. The authors' group [94] found no sex differences in morphine analgesia using pressure, heat, and ischemic pain. Regarding mixed action opioids, Zacny and Beckman [95] reported that men experienced slightly, though not significantly, greater analgesia in response to butorphanol. The authors and colleagues [96] reported no sex differences in pentazocine analgesia;

however, the melanocortin-1-receptor genotype (*MC1R*) was associated with pentazocine analgesia in a sex-dependent manner [30]. Specifically, women with two variant *MC1R* alleles, associated with red hair and fair skin, reported significantly greater analgesia with the κ-opioid pentazocine during thermal and ischemic pain testing compared with women with one or no variant *MC1R* allele; *MC1R* genotype was not associated with analgesic responses among men.

In summary, evidence from clinical and experimental pain models present a mixed picture of sex differences in response to opioids, and the presence of sex differences likely depends on multiple factors, including the specific opioid agonist and dose used, the pain model tested, and the timing of postdrug assessments. Moreover, human and nonhuman animal data suggests that sex-by-genotype interactions may influence the findings of such studies.

Clinical relevance of experimental pain responses

It has not been determined whether common mechanisms underlie sex differences in the epidemiology of clinical pain and sensitivity to experimental pain; however, this possibility is supported by increasing evidence that experimental pain sensitivity predicts clinical pain responses [97]. Indeed, patients who have certain chronic pain disorders, such as TMD [56,61], IBS [98], headache pain [99], and fibromyalgia [57], exhibit increased sensitivity to a variety of experimental pain stimuli. Moreover, some evidence suggests that within populations that have chronic pain, greater experimental pain sensitivity is associated with greater severity of clinical symptoms [100–103].

Fillingim and colleagues [104] investigated the relationship between heat pain tolerance and threshold in healthy adults, and reports of daily pain in the month preceding pain testing. Consistent with previous studies, women reported more pain sites (but not more pain episodes) and greater health care use in the month preceding experimental testing. Women also displayed increased sensitivity to thermal pain after adjusting for baseline sensitivities in warmth detection. Women who reported higher levels of clinical pain during the month preceding testing exhibited lower thermal pain thresholds and tolerances than did those who reported less clinical pain; however, men showed no significant relationship between clinical and experimental pain.

Growing evidence also suggests that experimental pain sensitivity may predict future pain severity and response to treatment. Indeed, several studies now indicate that laboratory pain sensitivity that is assessed presurgically predicts severity of postsurgical pain [105–107]. Also, pretreatment ischemic pain tolerance predicted pain reductions following multidisciplinary treatment among women, but not among men, who had chronic pain [101]. More recently, pretreatment heat pain thresholds predicted the effectiveness of opioids for neuropathic pain [108]. Taken together, these findings support the clinical relevance of experimental pain assessment, which implies that sex differences in experimental pain sensitivity are related to sex differences in clinical pain.

Responses to nonpharmacologic treatment

Women and men may respond differently to pharmacologic pain treatment, but little is known about sex differences in the effectiveness of nonpharmacologic interventions for pain. In a study of orofacial pain, women who had TMD showed significant decreases in pain 2 years after multidisciplinary treatment, whereas pain reports among men who had TMD remained unchanged [109]. In the experimental setting, a cognitive intervention encouraging a sensory focus aimed at pain reduction significantly attenuated pain intensity among men but not women [110]. Also, exercising on a treadmill reduced cold pressor pain ratings in women but not men, whereas playing video games decreased pain in men but not women [111]. In the clinical setting, conventional physical therapy was more effective for men who had back pain, whereas intensive dynamic back exercises produced greater pain reduction among women [112]. In another study, women who had back pain showed significant improvements in health-related quality of life with cognitive behavioral treatment and the combination of cognitive behavioral treatment plus physical therapy, whereas men showed no benefit [113]. Other recent findings indicate similar treatment gains for women and men following active rehabilitation for chronic low back pain [114], and one study reported better outcomes from multidisciplinary treatment among men [115]. Thus, these findings are mixed, but, on balance, they suggest greater treatment responses for women, especially when treatments are multimodal.

Mechanisms underlying sex differences in pain perception

Several mechanisms have been proposed to explain gender differences, including "biologic" factors, such as genetic and hormonal influences as well as sex differences in endogenous pain modulation. In addition, "psychosocial" processes have been suggested, including gender roles and other cognitive/affective influences. Before discussing these putative explanatory mechanisms, it is worth noting that this distinction between "psychosocial" and "biologic" contributions is artificial, because psychosocial variables can reflect or alter the underlying biologic processes that are involved in the modulation of pain. In addition, sex differences in pain inevitably are driven by multiple mechanisms; therefore, reductionistic attempts to identify the reason for sex differences likely will be unsuccessful.

Gonadal hormones may contribute to sex differences in pain modulation and opioid analgesia. Experimental pain perception varies across the menstrual cycle in healthy women, with the greatest pain sensitivity occurring perimenstrually [116]. The severity of some pain disorders fluctuates with the menstrual cycle [117–119]. For example, in patients who have TMD, peak pain occurs perimenstrually and at the time of ovulation [120]. It is hypothesized that rapidly dropping estrogen levels may be associated with heightened symptoms in this population. Hormone replacement therapy also has been associated with an increased risk for developing TMDs [121] and back pain [122,123], and women who were using exogenous hormones reported more severe orofacial pain compared with women who were not using hormones [124]. Furthermore, postmenopausal women who were taking hormone replacement showed lower pain thresholds and tolerances compared with women who were not taking hormone replacement and men [125,126]. Thus, endogenous and exogenous hormonal events affect clinical and experimental pain responses.

Psychosocial factors also contribute to sex differences in responses to pain. Psychologic distress is common among patients who have orofacial pain [127]. Several studies indicate that psychologic factors play a larger role when TMD pain is myogenic (as opposed to arthrogenic), perhaps because of more parafunctional behaviors in the former group [128–130]. Regarding emotion, two dimensions seem to be especially important for pain modulation: valence—whether an emotion is positive or negative, and arousal—how intensely the emotion is experienced [131]. Although negative and positive emotions can influence pain, more research has addressed the effect of negative emotions. For example, fear is a high-intensity negative emotion that is associated with threat or perception of imminent harm. The fear response is characterized by autonomic arousal and temporary pain attenuation (ie, "fight, flight, or freeze"). Fear-based analgesia is not studied readily in humans because of ethical considerations. In comparison, anxiety is a lower-intensity negative emotion that often heightens pain sensitivity [131]. Thus, an emotional stimulus can attenuate or amplify pain depending upon how it is perceived.

Aggregate findings suggest that, given the same negative stimuli (eg, upsetting photographs, startling noise), women display more intense affective reactions compared with men. In addition, women report higher base rates of depression and anxiety than do men, which often are associated with increased pain and other physical symptoms [132,133]. These negative affective states generally predict greater sensitivity pain in the laboratory [134]. Thus, higher levels of affective distress might account for some of the increased pain sensitivity among women. Robinson and colleagues [135] found that sex differences in temporal summation of heat pain became nonsignificant after controlling for anxiety, indicating that anxiety mediates gender differences. Several studies suggest that anxiety more strongly predicts experimental pain responses in men than in women, however [136–138]. Similar results have been reported for clinical pain [139]. Thus, it seems that anxiety more strongly predicts clinical and experimental pain among men. Clearly, more investigation is warranted concerning the role of negative emotions during pain processing.

In addition to emotional factors, cognitive variables, such as self-efficacy, anticipation, expectancies, perceived ability to control pain, and coping strategies, can contribute to gender differences in pain perception and treatment outcomes [16,140]. Orofacial patients who have positive pretreatment expectations, and who use adaptive cognitive coping strategies, report better treatment satisfaction [141,142]. Relative to men, women report more worry and catastrophizing in laboratory and clinical pain settings [143,144]. Turner and colleagues [145] found that a catastrophizing coping style was associated with extraoral muscle and joint palpation pain, activity interference, and higher health care use in patients who had TMDs. Despite a greater tendency to catastrophize, Unruh and colleagues [146] found that women use a broader repertoire of coping strategies. Furthermore, men and women seem to derive differential benefits from coping skills training, which highlights the importance of tailoring treatments to meet individual needs [140].

Stereotypic gender roles also should be considered because traditional Western feminine roles may enable reporting pain, whereas masculine roles discourage such complaints. Among men, masculinity has been associated with higher pain thresholds [147]. One study found that men reported less pain to an attractive female experimenter than to a male experimenter, whereas experimenter gender did not influence women's pain reports [148]. Two studies that used standardized measures of gender role demonstrated that gender roles are associated with experimental pain responses, but gender role measures did not account for sex differences in pain [147,149]. More recently, a subscale that assesses willingness to report pain was found to mediate sex differences partially in temporal summation of heat pain [135]. Also, feminine gender role and threat appraisal mediated sex differences in cold pressor pain [140,150]. Thus, gender roles seem to contribute to sex differences in pain sensitivity.

Summary and future directions

Considerable clinical and experimental evidence demonstrates gender and sex differences in the epidemiology, etiology, and manifestation of orofacial pain. Experimental studies in humans consistently indicate greater pain sensitivity among women, although the magnitude of the sex difference varies across studies. Some evidence suggests sex differences in responses to pharmacologic and nonpharmacologic treatments for pain; however, conflicting findings abound. The mechanisms that underlie these sex differences in clinical and experimental pain responses are not understood fully; however, several biopsychosocial factors are believed to contribute, including gonadal hormones, genetics, cognitive/affective processes, and stereotypic gender roles.

A clinically relevant area for future research involves identifying sex-related markers that distinguish individuals who are at risk for developing chronic pain from those who are comparatively resistant. The relative contributions of genetic, anatomic, neurochemical, and hormonal factors remain unknown, although, they all seem to influence the pain experience. It also is important to consider that psychosocial factors exert powerful effects on pain modulation, and the neurobiology of these processes requires further investigation. Most research has focused on the magnitude of sex differences in responses to pain and its treatment; however, a potentially more important issue is identifying sex-specific determinants of pain and treatment outcome. Because pain involves multifactorial and redundant systems, it is unlikely that a single medication or treatment will suit all patients' needs [151]. Thus, increased efforts to elucidate qualitative sex differences may be informative for developing new analgesic agents and multidimensional therapeutic techniques. The advancement of knowledge regarding sex, gender, and pain signifies a promising step toward designing targeted diagnostic techniques and treatment methods.

References

[1] Lanser P, Gesell S. Pain management: the fifth vital sign. Healthc Benchmarks 2001;8(6): 68–70.
[2] International Association for the Study of Pain. Subcommittee on taxonomy of pain teams: a list with definitions and notes on usage. Pain 1979;6:249–52.
[3] Agostoni E, Frigerio R, Santoro P. Atypical facial pain: clinical considerations and differential diagnosis. Neurol Sci 2005;26(Suppl 2):S71–4.
[4] Madland G, Newton-John T, Feinmann C. Chronic idiopathic orofacial pain: I: What is the evidence base? Br Dent J 2001;191(1):22–4.
[5] Esposito CJ. Considerations in the diagnosis of orofacial pain and headache. J Ky Med Assoc 2001;99(10):430–6.
[6] Gremillion HA. Multidisciplinary diagnosis and management of orofacial pain. Gen Dent 2002;50(2):178–86.
[7] Hapak L, Gordon A, Locker D, et al. Differentiation between musculoligamentous, dentoalveolar, and neurologically based craniofacial pain with a diagnostic questionnaire J Orofac Pain 1994;8(4):357–68.
[8] Siddall PJ, Cousins MJ. Pain mechanisms and management: an update. Clin Exp Pharmacol Physiol 1995;22(10):679–88.
[9] Woda A, Tubert-Jeannin S, Bouhassira D, et al. Towards a new taxonomy of idiopathic orofacial pain. Pain 2005;116(3):396–406.
[10] Headache Classification Subcommittee of the International Headache Society. International classification of headache disorders. Cephalalgia 2004;24(Suppl 1):1–151.
[11] Merskey H, Bogduk N. Classification of chronic pain. 2nd ed. Seattle (WA): IASP Press; 1994.
[12] Dworkin SF, LeResche L. Research diagnostic criteria for temporomandibular disorders. J Craniomandib Disord 1992;6:302–55.
[13] Madland G, Feinmann C. Chronic facial pain: a multidisciplinary problem. J Neurol Neurosurg Psychiatry 2001;71(6):716–9.
[14] Krogstad BS, Dahl BL, Eckersberg T, et al. Sex differences in signs and symptoms from masticatory and other muscles in 19-year-old individuals. J Oral Rehabil 1992;19(5): 435–40.
[15] Dao TT, LeResche L. Gender differences in pain. J Orofac Pain 2000;14(3):169–84.

[16] Fillingim RB. Sex, gender and pain: women and men really are different. Curr Rev Pain 2000;4:24–30.

[17] Kohlmann T. [Epidemiology of orofacial pain]. Schmerz 2002;16(5):339–45 [in German].

[18] Buckwalter JA, Lappin DR. The disproportionate impact of chronic arthralgia and arthritis among women. Clin Orthop 2000;372:159–68.

[19] Rollman GB, Lautenbacher S. Sex differences in musculoskeletal pain. Clin J Pain 2001; 17(1):20–4.

[20] Gran JT. The epidemiology of chronic generalized musculoskeletal pain. Best Pract Res Clin Rheumatol 2003;17(4):547–61.

[21] White KP, Harth M. Classification, epidemiology, and natural history of fibromyalgia. Curr Pain Headache Rep 2001;5(4):320–9.

[22] Barsky AJ, Peekna HM, Borus JF. Somatic symptom reporting in women and men. J Gen Intern Med 2001;16(4):266–75.

[23] Unruh AM. Gender variations in clinical pain experience. Pain 1996;65(2–3):123–67.

[24] Wiesenfeld-Hallin Z. Sex differences in pain perception. Gend Med 2005;2(3):137–45.

[25] Dworkin SF. Temporomandibular disorders: a problem in oral health. In: Gatchel RJ, Turk DC, editors. Psychosocial factors in pain. New York: Guilford Press; 1999. p. 213–26.

[26] Warren MP, Fried JL. Temporomandibular disorders and hormones in women. Cells Tissues Organs 2001;169(3):187–92.

[27] Apkarian AV, Bushnell MC, Treede RD, et al. Human brain mechanisms of pain perception and regulation in health and disease. Eur J Pain 2005;9(4):463–84.

[28] Fillingim RB, Maixner W. Gender differences in the responses to noxious stimuli. Pain Forum 1995;4(4):209–21.

[29] Serrao M, Rossi P, Sandrini G, et al. Effects of diffuse noxious inhibitory controls on temporal summation of the RIII reflex in humans. Pain 2004;112(3):353–60.

[30] Mogil JS, Wilson SG, Chesler EJ, et al. The melanocortin-1 receptor gene mediates female-specific mechanisms of analgesia in mice and humans. Proc Natl Acad Sci U S A 2003;100: 4867–72.

[31] Allen AL, McCarson KE. Estrogen increases nociception-evoked brain-derived neurotrophic factor gene expression in the female rat. Neuroendocrinol 2005;81(3):193–9.

[32] Blacklock AD, Johnson MS, Krizsan-Agbas D, et al. Estrogen increases sensory nociceptor neuritogenesis in vitro by a direct, nerve growth factor-independent mechanism. Eur J Neurosci 2005;21(9):2320–8.

[33] Flake NM, Bonebreak DB, Gold MS. Estrogen and inflammation increase the excitability of rat temporomandibular joint afferent neurons. J Neurophysiol 2005;93(3):1585–97.

[34] Kuba T, Kemen LM, Quinones-Jenab V. Estradiol administration mediates the inflammatory response to formalin in female rats. Brain Res 2005;1047(1):119–22.

[35] Robinson ME, Riley JL III, Myers CD. Psychosocial contributions to sex-related differences in pain responses. In: Fillingim RB, editor. Sex, gender, and pain. Seattle (WA): IASP Press; 2000. p. 41–68.

[36] Berkley KJ. Sex differences in pain. Behav Brain Sci 1997;20:371–80.

[37] Averbuch M, Katzper M. A search for sex differences in response to analgesia. Arch Intern Med 2000;160(22):3424–8.

[38] Kest B, Sarton E, Dahan A. Gender differences in opioid-mediated analgesia: animal and human studies. Anesthesiology 2000;93(2):539–47.

[39] Mogil JS, Chesler EJ, Wilson SG, et al. Sex differences in thermal nociception and morphine antinociception in rodents depend on genotype. Neurosci Biobehav Rev 2000;24(3):375–89.

[40] Riley JL, Robinson ME, Wise EA, et al. Sex differences in the perception of noxious experimental stimuli: a meta-analysis. Pain 1998;74:181–7.

[41] Lowery D, Fillingim RB, Wright RA. Sex differences and incentive effects on perceptual and cardiovascular responses to cold pressor pain. Psychosom Med 2003;65(2):284–91.

[42] Logan HL, Gedney JJ. Sex differences in the long-term stability of forehead cold pressor pain. J Pain 2004;5(7):406–12.

[43] Karibe H, Goddard G, Gear RW. Sex differences in masticatory muscle pain after chewing. J Dent Res 2003;82(2):112–6.
[44] Plesh O, Curtis DA, Hall LJ, et al. Gender difference in jaw pain induced by clenching. J Oral Rehabil 1998;25(4):258–63.
[45] Stohler CS, Kowalski CJ. Spatial and temporal summation of sensory and affective dimensions of deep somatic pain. Pain 1999;79(2–3):165–73.
[46] Ge HY, Madeleine P, Arendt-Nielsen L. Sex differences in temporal characteristics of descending inhibitory control: an evaluation using repeated bilateral experimental induction of muscle pain. Pain 2004;110(1–2):72–8.
[47] Ge HY, Madeleine P, Arendt-Nielsen L. Gender differences in pain modulation evoked by repeated injections of glutamate into the human trapezius muscle. Pain 2005;113(1–2): 134–40.
[48] Cairns BE, Hu JW, Arendt-Nielsen L, et al. Sex-related differences in human pain and rat afferent discharge evoked by injection of glutamate into the masseter muscle. J Neurophysiol 2001;86(2):782–91.
[49] Price DD, Hu JW, Dubner R, et al. Peripheral suppression of first pain and central summation of second pain evoked by noxious heat pulses. Pain 1977;3:57–68.
[50] Price DD, Mao J, Mayer DJ. Central neural mechanisms of normal and abnormal pain states. In: Fields HL, Liebeskind JC, editors. Progress in pain research and management. Seattle (WA): IASP Press; 1994. p. 61–84.
[51] Price DD, Mao J, Frenk H, et al. The N-methyl-D-aspartate receptor antagonist dextromethorphan selectively reduces temporal summation of second pain in man. Pain 1994;59: 165–74.
[52] Bendtsen L. Central sensitization in tension-type headache—possible pathophysiological mechanisms. Cephalalgia 2000;20(5):486–508.
[53] Eide PK. Wind-up and the NMDA receptor complex from a clinical perspective. Eur J Pain 2000;4(1):5–15.
[54] Katz WA, Rothenberg R. Section 3: The nature of pain: pathophysiology. J Clin Rheumatol 2005;11(2 Suppl):S11–5.
[55] Sarlani E, Greenspan JD. Gender differences in temporal summation of mechanically evoked pain. Pain 2002;97(1–2):163–9.
[56] Sarlani E, Greenspan JD. Evidence for generalized hyperalgesia in temporomandibular disorders patients. Pain 2003;102(3):221–6.
[57] Staud R. New evidence for central sensitization in patients with fibromyalgia. Curr Rheumatol Rep 2004;6(4):259.
[58] Fillingim RB, Maixner W, Kincaid S, et al. Sex differences in temporal summation but not sensory-discriminative processing of thermal pain. Pain 1998;75(1):121–7.
[59] Sarlani E, Grace EG, Reynolds MA, et al. Sex differences in temporal summation of pain and aftersensations following repetitive noxious mechanical stimulation. Pain 2004; 109(1–2):115–23.
[60] Staud R, Vierck CJ, Cannon RL, et al. Abnormal sensitization and temporal summation of second pain (wind-up) in patients with fibromyalgia syndrome. Pain 2001;91(1–2): 165–75.
[61] Maixner W, Fillingim R, Sigurdsson A, et al. Sensitivity of patients with temporomandibular disorders to experimentally evoked pain: evidence for altered temporal summation of pain. Pain 1998;76:71–81.
[62] Sarlani E, Grace EG, Reynolds MA, et al. Evidence for up-regulated central nociceptive processing in patients with masticatory myofascial pain. J Orofac Pain 2004; 18(1):41–55.
[63] Borsook D, Burstein R, Becerra L. Functional imaging of the human trigeminal system: opportunities for new insights into pain processing in health and disease. J Neurobiol 2004; 61(1):107–25.

[64] Brooks J, Tracey I. From nociception to pain perception: imaging the spinal and supraspinal pathways. J Anat 2005;207(1):19–33.
[65] Peyron R, Laurent B, Garcia-Larrea L. Functional imaging of brain responses to pain. A review and meta-analysis (2000). Neurophysiol Clin 2000;30(5):263–88.
[66] Porro CA. Functional imaging and pain: behavior, perception, and modulation. Neuroscientist 2003;9(5):354–69.
[67] Rainville P, Duncan GH, Price DD, et al. Pain affect encoded in human anterior cingulate but not somatosensory cortex. Science 1997;277(5328):968–71.
[68] Paulson PE, Minoshima S, Morrow TJ, et al. Gender differences in pain perception and patterns of cerebral activation during noxious heat stimulation in humans. Pain 1998;76(1–2):223–9.
[69] Derbyshire SW, Nichols T, Firestone L, et al. Gender differences in patterns of cerebral activation during equal experience of painful laser stimulation. J Pain 2002;3:401–11.
[70] Berman S, Munakata J, Naliboff BD, et al. Gender differences in regional brain response to visceral pressure in IBS patients. Eur J Pain 2000;4(2):157–72.
[71] Naliboff BD, Berman S, Chang L, et al. Sex-related differences in IBS patients: central processing of visceral stimuli. Gastroenterology 2003;124(7):1738–47.
[72] Hobson AR, Furlong PL, Worthen SF, et al. Real-time imaging of human cortical activity evoked by painful esophageal stimulation. Gastroenterology 2005;128(3):610–9.
[73] Vaccarino AL, Kastin AJ. Endogenous opiates: 1999. Peptides 2000;21(12):1975–2034.
[74] Kavaliers M, Choleris E. Sex differences in N-methyl-D-aspartate involvement in kappa opioid and non-opioid predator-induced analgesia in mice. Brain Res 1997;768(1–2):30–6.
[75] Mogil JS, Sternberg WF, Kest B, et al. Sex differences in the antagonism of stress-induced analgesia: effects of gonadectomy and estrogen replacement. Pain 1993;53:17–25.
[76] Price DD, McHaffie JG. Effects of heterotopic conditioning stimuli on first and second pain: a psychophysical evaluation in humans. Pain 1988;34:245–52.
[77] Le Bars D, Dickenson AH, Besson JM. Diffuse noxious inhibitory controls (DNIC). I. Effects on dorsal horn convergent neurones in the rat. Pain 1979;6(3):283–304.
[78] De Broucker T, Cesaro P, Willer JC, et al. Diffuse noxious inhibitory controls in man. Involvement of the spinoreticular tract. Brain 1990;113:1223–34.
[79] Kraus E, Le Bars D, Besson JM. Behavioral confirmation of "diffuse noxious inhibitory controls" (DNIC) and evidence for a role of endogenous opiates. Brain Res 1981;206(2):495–9.
[80] Le Bars D, Dickenson AH, Besson JM. Diffuse noxious inhibitory controls (DNIC). II. Lack of effect on non-convergent neurones, supraspinal involvement and theoretical implications. Pain 1979;6(3):305–27.
[81] Roby-Brami A, Bussel B, Willer JC, et al. An electrophysiological investigation into the pain-relieving effects of heterotopic nociceptive stimuli. Brain 1987;110:1497–508.
[82] France CR, Suchowiecki S. A comparison of diffuse noxious inhibitory controls in men and women. Pain 1999;81(1–2):77–84.
[83] Baad-Hansen L, Poulsen HF, Jensen HM, et al. Lack of sex differences in modulation of experimental intraoral pain by diffuse noxious inhibitory controls (DNIC). Pain 2005;116(3):359–65.
[84] Chia YY, Chow LH, Hung CC, et al. Gender and pain upon movement are associated with the requirements for postoperative patient-controlled iv analgesia: a prospective survey of 2,298 Chinese patients. Can J Anaesth 2002;49(3):249–55.
[85] Cepeda MS, Carr DB. Women experience more pain and require more morphine than men to achieve a similar degree of analgesia. Anesth Analg 2003;97(5):1464–8.
[86] Gordon NC, Gear RW, Heller PH, et al. Enhancement of morphine analgesia by the GABAB agonist baclofen. Neuroscience 1995;69(2):345–9.
[87] Kaiko RF, Wallenstein SL, Rogers AG, et al. Sources of variation in analgesic responses in cancer patients with chronic pain receiving morphine. Pain 1983;15(2):191–200.

[88] Fillingim RB, Gear RW. Sex differences in opioid analgesia: clinical and experimental find-
     ings. Eur J Pain 2004;8:413–25.
[89] Gear RW, Miaskowski C, Gordon NC, et al. Kappa-opioids produce significantly greater
     analgesia in women than in men. Nat Med 1996;2(11):1248–50.
[90] Gear RW, Miaskowski C, Gordon NC, et al. The kappa opioid nalbuphine produces gen-
     der- and dose-dependent analgesia and antianalgesia in patients with postoperative pain.
     Pain 1999;83(2):339–45.
[91] Sarton E, Olofsen E, Romberg R, et al. Sex differences in morphine analgesia: an experi-
     mental study in healthy volunteers. Anesthesiology 2000;93(5):1245–54.
[92] Romberg R, Olofsen E, Sarton E, et al. Pharmacokinetic-pharmacodynamic modeling of
     morphine-6-glucuronide-induced analgesia in healthy volunteers: absence of sex differ-
     ences. Anesthesiology 2004;100(1):120–33.
[93] Zacny JP. Gender differences in opioid analgesia in human volunteers: cold pressor and
     mechanical pain (CPDD abstract). NIDA Res Monogr 2002;182:22–3.
[94] Fillingim RB, Ness TJ, Glover TL, et al. Morphine responses and experimental pain: sex
     differences in side effects and cardiovascular responses but not analgesia. J Pain 2005;
     6(2):116–24.
[95] Zacny JP, Beckman NJ. The effects of a cold-water stimulus on butorphanol effects in males
     and females. Pharmacol Biochem Behav 2004;78(4):653–9.
[96] Fillingim RB, Ness TJ, Glover TL, et al. Experimental pain models reveal no sex differences
     in pentazocine analgesia in humans. Anesthesiology 2004;100:1263–70.
[97] Edwards RR, Sarlani E, Wesselmann U, et al. Quantitative assessment of experimental pain
     perception: multiple domains of clinical relevance. Pain 2005;114(3):315–9.
[98] Drewes AM, Petersen P, Rossel P, et al. Sensitivity and distensibility of the rectum and sig-
     moid colon in patients with irritable bowel syndrome. Scand J Gastroenterol 2001;36(8):
     827–32.
[99] Bendtsen L, Jensen R, Olesen J. Decreased pain detection and tolerance thresholds in
     chronic tension-type headache. Arch Neurol 1996;53(4):373–6.
[100] Clauw DJ, Williams D, Lauerman W, et al. Pain sensitivity as a correlate of clinical status in
      individuals with chronic low back pain. Spine 1999;24(19):2035–41.
[101] Edwards RR, Doleys DM, Lowery D, et al. Pain tolerance as a predictor of outcome fol-
      lowing multidisciplinary treatment for chronic pain: differential effects as a function of
      sex. Pain 2003;106(3):419–26.
[102] Fillingim RB, Maixner W, Kincaid S, et al. Pain sensitivity in patients with temporomandib-
      ular disorders: relationship to clinical and psychosocial factors. Clin J Pain 1996;12:260–9.
[103] Staud R, Cannon RC, Mauderli AP, et al. Temporal summation of pain from mechanical
      stimulation of muscle tissue in normal controls and subjects with fibromyalgia syndrome.
      Pain 2003;102(1–2):87–95.
[104] Fillingim RB, Edwards RR, Powell T. The relationship of sex and clinical pain to
      experimental pain responses. Pain 1999;83:419–25.
[105] Bisgaard T, Kehlet H, Rosenberg J. Pain and convalescence after laparoscopic cholecystec-
      tomy. Eur J Surg 2001;167(2):84–96.
[106] Granot M, Lowenstein L, Yarnitsky D, et al. Postcesarean section pain prediction by
      preoperative experimental pain assessment. Anesthesiology 2003;98(6):1422–6.
[107] Werner MU, Duun P, Kehlet H. Prediction of postoperative pain by preoperative
      nociceptive responses to heat stimulation. Anesthesiology 2004;100(1):115–9.
[108] Edwards RR, Haythornthwaite J, Tella P, et al. Basal heat pain thresholds predict opioid
      analgesia in patients with post-herpetic neuralgia. Anesthesiology 2006;104(6):1243–8.
[109] Krogstad BS, Jokstad A, Dahl BL, et al. The reporting of pain, somatic complaints, and
      anxiety in a group of patients with TMD before and 2 years after treatment: sex differences.
      J Orofacial Pain 1996;10(3):263–9.
[110] Keogh E, Hatton K, Ellery D. Avoidance versus focused attention and the perception of
      pain: differential effects for men and women. Pain 2000;85(1–2):225–30.

[111] Sternberg WF, Bokat C, Kass L, et al. Sex-dependent components of the analgesia produced by athletic competition. J Pain 2001;2:65–74.

[112] Hansen FR, Bendix T, Skov P, et al. Intensive, dynamic back-muscle exercises, conventional physiotherapy, or placebo-control treatment of low-back pain. A randomized, observer-blind trial. Spine 1993;18(1):98–108.

[113] Jensen IB, Bergstrom G, Ljungquist T, et al. A randomized controlled component analysis of a behavioral medicine rehabilitation program for chronic spinal pain: are the effects dependent on gender? Pain 2001;91(1–2):65–78.

[114] Mannion AF, Muntener M, Taimela S, et al. Comparison of three active therapies for chronic low back pain: results of a randomized clinical trial with one-year follow-up. Rheumatology (Oxford) 2001;40(7):772–8.

[115] Keogh E, McCracken LM, Eccleston C. Do men and women differ in their response to interdisciplinary chronic pain management? Pain 2005;114(1–2):37–46.

[116] Fillingim RB, Ness TJ. Sex-related hormonal influences on pain and analgesic responses. Neurosci Biobehav Rev 2000;24:485–501.

[117] Anderberg UM, Marteinsdottir I, Hallman J, et al. Symptom perception in relation to hormonal status in female fibromyalgia syndrome patients. Journal of Musculoskeletal Pain 1999;7:21–38.

[118] Heitkemper MM, Jarrett M. Pattern of gastrointestinal and somatic symptoms across the menstrual cycle. Gastroenterology 1992;102:505–13.

[119] Keenan PA, Lindamer LA. Non-migraine headache across the menstrual cycle in women with and without premenstrual syndrome. Cephalalgia 1992;12(6):356–9.

[120] LeResche L, Mancl L, Sherman JJ, et al. Changes in temporomandibular pain and other symptoms across the menstrual cycle. Pain 2003;106(3):253–61.

[121] LeResche L, Saunders K, Von Korff MR, et al. Use of exogenous hormones and risk of temporomandibular disorder pain. Pain 1997;69(1–2):153–60.

[122] Brynhildsen JO, Bjors E, Skarsgard C, et al. Is hormone replacement therapy a risk factor for low back pain among postmenopausal women? Spine 1998;23(7):809–13.

[123] Musgrave DS, Vogt MT, Nevitt MC, et al. Back problems among postmenopausal women taking estrogen replacement therapy. Spine 2001;26:1606–12.

[124] Wise EA, Riley JLI, Robinson ME. Clinical pain perception and hormone replacement therapy in post-menopausal females experiencing orofacial pain. Clin J Pain 2000;16: 121–6.

[125] Fillingim RB, Edwards RR. The association of hormone replacement therapy with experimental pain responses in postmenopausal women. Pain 2001;92:229–34.

[126] Riley JLI, Robinson ME, Wise EA, et al. A meta-analytic review of pain perception across the menstrual cycle. Pain 1999;81:225–35.

[127] DeLeeuw R, Bertoli E, Schmidt JE, et al. Prevalence of post-traumatic stress disorder symptoms in orofacial pain patients. Oral Surg Oral Med Oral Pathol Oral Radiol Endod 2005; 99(5):558–68.

[128] Auerbach SM, Laskin DM, Frantsve LM, et al. Depression, pain, exposure to stressful life events, and long-term outcomes in temporomandibular disorder patients. J Oral Maxillofac Surg 2001;59(6):628–33.

[129] Glaros AG, Williams K, Lausten L. The role of parafunctions, emotions and stress in predicting facial pain. J Am Dent Assoc 2005;136(4):451–8.

[130] Yap AU, Chua EK, Dworkin SF, et al. Multiple pains and psychosocial functioning/psychologic distress in TMD patients. Int J Prosthodont 2002;15(5):461–6.

[131] Rhudy JL, Williams AE. Gender differences in pain: do emotions play a role? Gend Med 2005;2(4):208–26.

[132] Kroenke K, Spitzer RL. Gender differences in the reporting of physical and somatoform symptoms. Psychosom Med 1998;60(2):150–5.

[133] Moldin SO, Scheftner WA, Rice JP, et al. Association between major depressive disorder and physical illness. Psychol Med 1993;23:755–61.

[134] Rajala U, Keinanen-Kiukaanniemi S, Uusimaki A, et al. Musculoskeletal pains and depression in a middle-aged Finnish population. Pain 1995;61(3):451–7.

[135] Robinson ME, Wise EA, Gagnon C, et al. Influences of gender role and anxiety on sex differences in temporal summation of pain. J Pain 2004;5(2):77–82.

[136] Fillingim RB, Keefe FJ, Light KC, et al. The influence of gender and psychological factors on pain perception. J Gend Cult Health 1996;1:21–36.

[137] Jones A, Zachariae R. Investigation of the interactive effects of gender and psychological factors on pain response. Br J Health Psychol 2004;9(Pt 3):405–18.

[138] Robinson ME, Dannecker EA, George SZ, et al. Sex differences in the associations among psychological factors and pain report: a novel psychophysical study of patients with chronic low back pain. J Pain 2005;6(7):463–70.

[139] Edwards RR, Augustson E, Fillingim RB. Differential relationships between anxiety and treatment-associated pain reduction among male and female chronic pain patients. Clin J Pain 2003;19:208–16.

[140] Keogh E, Herdenfeldt M. Gender, coping and the perception of pain. Pain 2002;97(3): 195–201.

[141] Goossens ME, Vlaeyen JW, Hidding A, et al. Treatment expectancy affects the outcome of cognitive-behavioral interventions in chronic pain. Clin J Pain 2005;21(1):18–26.

[142] Riley JL III, Myers CD, Robinson ME, et al. Factors predicting orofacial pain patient satisfaction with improvement. J Orofac Pain 2001;15(1):29–35.

[143] Fillingim RB, Wilkinson CS, Powell T. Self-reported abuse history and pain complaints among healthy young adults. Clin J Pain 1999;15:85–91.

[144] Roth RS, Geisser ME, Theisen-Goodvich M, et al. Cognitive complaints are associated with depression, fatigue, female sex, and pain catastrophizing in patients with chronic pain. Arch Phys Med Rehabil 2005;86(6):1147–54.

[145] Turner JA, Brister H, Huggins K, et al. Catastrophizing is associated with clinical examination findings, activity interference, and health care use among patients with temporomandibular disorders. J Orofac Pain 2005;19(4):291–300.

[146] Unruh AM, Ritchie J, Merskey H. Does gender affect appraisal of pain and pain coping strategies? Clin J Pain 1999;15(1):31–40.

[147] Otto MW, Dougher MJ. Sex differences and personality factors in responsivity to pain. Percept Mot Skills 1985;61:383–90.

[148] Levine FM, De Simone LL. The effects of experimenter gender on pain report in male and female subjects. Pain 1991;44:69–72.

[149] Myers CD, Robinson ME, Riley JL III, et al. Sex, gender, and blood pressure: contributions to experimental pain report. Psychosom Med 2001;63(4):545–50.

[150] Sanford SD, Kersh BC, Thorn BE, et al. Psychosocial mediators of sex differences in pain responsivity. J Pain 2002;3(1):58–64.

[151] Dionne RA. Pharmacologic advances in orofacial pain: from molecules to medicine. J Dent Educ 2001;65(12):1393–403.

THE DENTAL
CLINICS
OF NORTH AMERICA

ELSEVIER
SAUNDERS

Dent Clin N Am 51 (2007) 19–44

Peripheral Mechanisms
of Odontogenic Pain

Michael A. Henry, DDS, PhD*,
Kenneth M. Hargreaves, DDS, PhD

*Department of Endodontics,
University of Texas Health Science Center at San Antonio School of Dentistry,
Mail Code 7892, 7703 Floyd Curl Drive, San Antonio, TX 78229, USA*

These are exciting times in the field of pain research. Every day brings advances in our understanding of pain mechanisms, and with each new advancement there is hope that these findings will lead to the development of novel and more effective analgesics not only for acute pain, but also for the more difficult and challenging to manage chronic pain conditions. The field of pain research represents an evolving field, where early studies identified basic pain pathways and the characterization of different fiber types and receptors that were activated by noxious stimuli. With this basic knowledge, the receptors and transmitters involved in the activation and inhibition of these different pathways were identified, and significant changes in their expressions were seen after inflammatory and nerve lesions. These changes in receptors and transmitters were also correlated with the increased activity of pain pathways in pathologic conditions. Advances in brain imaging techniques have led to the concept of pain as a widely distributed system involving many different nervous system structures that represent the affective and sensory aspects of the pain experience. Molecular approaches are being used to map the intricacies of the intracellular signaling pathways that are activated when molecules bind to a receptor or channels open in response to specific stimuli. Genetic analyses allow comparisons in the makeup and the identification of possible polymorphisms that might underlie differences in the way that individuals respond to painful stimuli and insults. Pain researchers have the challenging task to consider this wealth of

This work was supported by NIH Grants DE013942 and DE015576 (M. Henry) and DA016179 and DA19585 (K. Hargreaves).

* Corresponding author.
E-mail address: henrym2@uthscsa.edu (M.A. Henry).

doi:10.1016/j.cden.2006.09.007   *dental.theclinics.com*

knowledge regarding pain mechanisms when designing experiments, and clinicians who treat pain are anxiously waiting the time when these advances will make their treatments more effective. In one respect, the activation of the peripheral nociceptor and sensory neuron represents our first key step to our understanding of nociception. In this article, we review the key basic mechanisms associated with this phenomena and more recently identified mechanisms that are current areas of interest. Although many of these pain mechanisms apply throughout the body, we attempt to describe these mechanisms in the context of trigeminal pain.

Peripheral pain mechanisms associated with odontogenic or temporomandibular disorders and other orofacial pain conditions are generally similar to those seen elsewhere in the body. These similarities include the types of sensory neurons involved and the receptors, channels, and intracellular signaling pathways responsible for the transduction, modulation, and propagation of peripheral stimuli. Even though there are some structural features associated with the tooth pulp that make pulpal pain unique, the tooth pulp is considered as a model system to illustrate peripheral pain mechanisms associated with the trigeminal system. This also seems appropriate because toothache is a common presenting symptom for patients seeking dental care [1]. The use of the tooth as a model system for studying pain mechanisms is well established, and advantages include a rich representation of pain fibers [2] and that the stimulation of pulpal nerves produces mostly a pain sensation [3–5]. In this regard, the tooth as a sensory organ can be considered as a specialized receptor for nociception.

The tooth pulp is composed of connective tissue that is highly vascular and rich in fibroblasts. Within this connective tissue stroma are bundles of axons that provide innervation to the tooth pulp [6]. The distribution and overall pattern of nerve fibers within pulpal tissues have been studied extensively, including in humans and experimental animals. The majority of the axons enter the apex of the tooth, but others may enter accessory foramina when present and ascend the radicular pulp within fiber bundles composed of myelinated and unmyelinated nerve fibers (Fig. 1). Nerve fibers located in these fiber tracts ascend the pulp and terminate as free nerve endings within the pulp or after entering the sub-odontoblastic plexus sequentially along this path. The sub-odontoblastic plexus is located just inside the odontoblasts and represents a fine network of many small and mostly unmyelinated fibers, many of which originate from thinly myelinated fibers. The sub-odontoblastic plexus (plexus of Raschkow) is extensive and especially elaborate in the region of pulp horns. The odontoblasts outline the entire periphery of the dental pulp and are located at the pulpodentin junction. Many of the unmyelinated nerve fibers located in the subodontoblastic plexus pass toward and terminate in the odontoblastic layer as free nerve endings, whereas others terminate in the predentin or enter dentin by way of dentinal tubules where they extend about 100 μm [7]. Although more than 40% of dentinal tubules are innervated in the tip of pulp horns, far

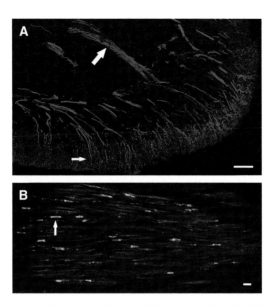

Fig. 1. Confocal micrographs of nerve fibers in the human tooth as identified with the indirect immunofluorescence technique. (*A*) The coronal aspect of the pulp contains nerve fibers as identified with the neuronal marker PGP9.5 (*red*) located within fiber bundles (*large arrow*) and small axons that traverse the odontoblastic layer (*small arrow*). Scale bar, 100 μm. (*B*) Nerve fibers located in the radicular pulp contain sodium channels (*red*) that are prominent at nodes of Ranvier (*arrow*) as identified by the paranodal staining of caspr (*green*). Scale bar, 10 μm.

fewer tubules are innervated in more apical locations, with less than 1% of tubules innervated in the midradicular region [8]. Stimulation of unmyelinated nerve fibers located in the pulp typically produces a dull throbbing and poorly localized pain sensation, whereas stimulation of the dentin produces a sharp, shooting pain that implicates the activation of more rapidly conducting myelinated fibers.

The nerve fiber density within human teeth is quite impressive. A number of ultrastructural studies have evaluated the type (as based on fiber diameter and presence or lack of myelin) and number of axons that innervate anterior and posterior teeth. Comprehensive studies of nerve fibers within posterior teeth are limited to single-rooted premolars (reviewed in [9]). Nair [9] concluded that human premolar teeth contain 2300 axons at the apex; 87% of these are unmyelinated, and the remainder are myelinated. The vast majority of the myelinated fibers are thinly myelinated and fall in the A-delta class, and the remaining 7% represent the more thickly myelinated A-beta nerve fibers. Even though the "average" premolar tooth has a significant nerve density, this can vary depending on the developmental stage and type of tooth [10–12] and can vary widely among individual samples. The innervation density is also dynamic because it can increase in human teeth with caries [12]. Other axons that enter the tooth pulp originate from postganglionic sympathetic neurons located in the superior cervical ganglion and whose role involves vasoconstriction [13], whereas parasympathetic fibers may be lacking that provide a vasodilatory role elsewhere [14]. Pulpal vasodilation can be achieved by the release of vasoactive neuropeptides from primary afferent terminals, a process that is integral to the production of neurogenic inflammation [15]. This process most likely involves arterioles because these vessels are most densely innervated in the tooth pulp [16].

Studies in experimental animals have also described the innervation of teeth, but, unlike in human studies, these studies allow a characterization of the sensory neurons within the trigeminal ganglion that supplies the innervation to pulpal tissues. Sensory neurons that supply the tooth pulp have been identified after the retrograde transport of fluorogold to exposed dentin. These studies have found that pulpal afferents typically originate from cell bodies with small, medium, and large diameters [17,18]. The cytochemistry of sensory neurons in the spinal system has been extensively evaluated, and in general these studies have identified two broad classes of neurons: (1) those that include peptidergic neurons that respond to nerve growth factor (NGF) and that express the trkA receptor and peptides such as calcitonin gene-related peptide (CGRP) and substance P (SP) and (2) nonpeptidergic neurons that respond to glial cell line–derived neurotrophic factor (GDNF) that express GDNF receptor alpha-1 and receptor tyrosine kinase (RET) and that bind the isolectin B4 (IB4). The IB4-binding neurons usually also express P2X3, an ATP-gated ion channel. In comparison, studies that have evaluated the cytochemical content of pulpal sensory neurons show some important differences when compared with the spinal system. Most notable is the lack of IB4 binding [19,20]. Even though these pulpal afferents do not express IB4 binding, they do express the P2X3 receptor, which is also a marker of the nonpeptidergic class and is usually coexpressed with IB4 binding in the spinal system. A recent study has found that many of the pulpal sensory neurons express the GDNF receptor alpha-1 and that many of these coexpressed the trkA receptor [18]. Therefore, pulpal afferent neurons express markers for peptidergic and nonpeptidergic neurons within the same neurons and do not follow patterns typically seen in the spinal system.

Many of the peptides and other molecules that have been identified as important in the activation of nociceptors in the spinal system have also been identified in the trigeminal system. Some of the peptides identified in tooth pulp include the tachykinins SP [21] and neurokinin A [22], vasoactive intestinal peptide [23], neuropeptide Y (NPY) [24], methionine- and leucine-enkephalin [25], CGRP [26], cholecystokinin and somatostatin [27], and galanin [28]. Peptides as a group are important in nociception because the expression of some change considerably with injury or after inflammatory insults. Sprouting of CGRP fibers is seen in the rat tooth pulp after inflammatory lesions [29], and similar results involving increased fibers with CGRP, NPY, SP, and vasoactive intestinal peptide have been described in human teeth with carious lesions [30,31]. These same neuropeptides are especially implicated in inflammatory processes because sensory nerve stimulation can lead to their local release by way of an axon-reflex [32], or they may be released from nerves that innervate blood vessels, leading to vasodilation and protein extravasation, which results in a neurogenic inflammation [33]. Neurogenic inflammation seems especially important in the trigeminal system because it represents a basic mechanism associated with the pathophysiology of migraine [34] and may be an important event associated with the inflammation of periodontal disease [35] and in the regulation of the immune response to infection [36]. Neurogenic inflammation and local tissue injury are associated with the release or activation of many different molecules that are involved in the sensitization of peripheral nociceptors, including their ability to further enhance the release of CGRP and SP. These substances include cytokines, NGF, prostaglandins, histamine, bradykinin, ATP, serotonin, lipids, nitric oxide, and hydrogen ions. The local release of CGRP and SP from peripheral terminals may bind to CGRP and SP receptors on immune cells, and this binding may be involved in the regulation of the immune response in a paracrine fashion. For example, SP released from nerve terminals can bind to mast cells, leading to degranulation and the release of histamine [37]. The degranulation of mast cells also releases tryptase, which is effective in the cleavage and activation of a new class of protease-activated receptors (PARs) and especially the PAR-2 receptor. PARs are colocalized with SP and CGRP receptors on nerve terminals and when activated can result in the additional release of SP and CGRP, thus perpetuating the inflammatory response. The effects of most neuropeptides are mediated by receptor binding, and many of these are G-protein–coupled receptors (GPCRs), which are discussed in greater detail in this article. The local release of neuropeptides that occurs in inflamed tissues represents an important event leading to the sensitization of peripheral nociceptors, and the specific mechanisms involved in this process will most likely remain a focus of pain research in the future.

Based upon these considerations, peripheral terminals of nociceptors can be envisioned as environmental detectors [38]. Although peripheral nociceptors have a relatively simple morphology of free nerve endings (Fig. 1A), they are biochemically specialized by the expression and localization of various receptors and ion channels, which confer to these cells the ability to detect noxious chemical, thermal, and mechanical stimuli. These nociceptive "polymodal detectors" can trigger this local release of neuropeptides (ie, the axon reflex), leading to coordinated inflammatory and healing responses in the injured tissue and evoking action potentials that provide sensory information back to the central nervous system (CNS).

From the perspectives of understanding peripheral pain mechanisms and management, the following section reviews the major classes of receptors and ion channels that confer the ability of nociceptors to "detect" noxious changes in their peripheral area. Fig. 2 summarizes these major classes of receptors and ion channels. Understanding their pharmacology (Table 1)

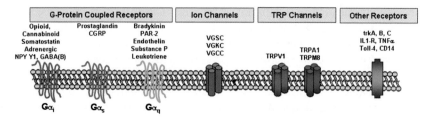

Fig. 2. Cartoon depicting major classes of receptor or ion channels proposed to be present on peripheral terminals of sensory neurons that serve to transduce external stimuli into altered neuronal function. Not all receptors or ion channels are present on all neurons, and several have been shown to be altered during inflammation or nerve injury. PAR-2, protease-activated receptor subtype 2; PG, prostaglandin; TRPA1, transient receptor potential A1; TRPM8, transient receptor potential M8; TRPV1, transient receptor potential V1 (aka the capsaicin receptor); VGCC, voltage-gated calcium channel; VGKC, voltage-gated potassium channel; VGSC, voltage-gated sodium channel.

provides insight into the pharmacologic strategies for peripheral pain control and permits appreciation of ongoing research designed to develop new peripherally acting analgesics. For example, the demonstration that dental pulp contains opioid receptors [39] and that peripherally administered opioids reduces pain in endodontic patients [40] suggests that locally active opioid analgesics might represent a novel class of drugs useful to treat endodontic pain patients. Because peripherally active opioid analgesics are under active development, it can be appreciated that a knowledge of peripheral pain mechanisms can improve our understanding of current and future pain control strategies [41].

Mechanisms for detecting stimuli and clinical implications

G-protein–coupled receptors

The G-protein–coupled receptors (GPCRs) comprise a large superfamily of receptors. The GPCRs share a common structure (seven transmembrane regions on the protein) and are called "G-protein–coupled" because they share a common signaling mechanism via activation of a certain class of GTP-binding proteins (aka G-proteins). Thus, the GPCR undergoes a conformational change when a drug or endogenous substance binds to the receptor, resulting in the GPCR binding to a G-protein and initiating a second messenger signaling pathway [42]. Although there are many subtypes of G-proteins and second messenger systems, and the actual signaling pathways are far more complicated than space permits, for our purposes we focus on the three major subtypes of G-proteins: $G\alpha_{i/o}$, $G\alpha_s$, and $G\alpha_q$ and their classic signaling pathways.

GPCRs that are coupled to the $G\alpha_{i/o}$ signaling pathway include opioid, cannabinoid, somatostatin, certain adrenergic subtypes, NPY, and GABA(B) receptors. In general, activating a $G\alpha_i$ signaling pathway leads to the inhibition of neuronal function by reducing cAMP levels, opening certain potassium channels (leading to a more negative membrane potential, called "hyperpolarization," and thus reducing the probability of triggering an action potential) and inhibiting certain calcium channels. As a first approximation, drugs that activate the $G\alpha_i$ GPCRs that are expressed on nociceptors would be predicted to be peripherally active analgesics. Drugs that activate peripheral opioid, cannabinoid, adrenergic, Y1, or GABA(B) receptors produce peripheral analgesia or inhibit peripheral neuronal function [40,43–45]. Clinicians use several drugs that activate $G\alpha_i$ GPCRs, and many additional drugs are in development as analgesics that act by these mechanisms.

In many respects, the $G\alpha_s$ GPCRs are complimentary to the $G\alpha_i$ family of GPCRs because these receptors typically increase cAMP levels, leading to cellular excitation. Examples of GPCRs that are coupled to the $G\alpha_s$ signaling pathway include prostaglandins and CGRP (Table 1). Recent molecular studies have demonstrated that of the four known subtypes of prostaglandin receptor, only the EP2 and EP3 subtypes are expressed in trigeminal sensory neurons [46]. Thus, local increases in prostaglandin E2 in dental pulp [47,48] or periradicular exudates [49,50] are likely to contribute to odontogenic pain mechanisms via activation of EP2 or EP3 receptors expressed on trigeminal sensory neurons. Although EP receptor antagonists have been developed, the current clinical strategy to control this receptor system is via the use of nonsteroidal anti-inflammatory drugs (NSAIDs) or via glucocorticoid steroids. Both classes of drugs block prostaglandin synthesis by interfering with the function of cyclooxygenase I/II (NSAIDs) or with phospholipase A2 (steroids).

Several GPCRs are coupled to the $G\alpha_q$ signaling pathway, including bradykinin, protease-activated receptors, endothelin, SP, and leukotriene receptors. In general, activation of a $G\alpha_q$–coupled GPCR leads to activation of the phospholipase C/protein kinase C signaling pathways. This can evoke a considerable stimulatory effect on nociceptors, leading to sensitization of the capsaicin receptor, transient receptor potential V1(TRPV1). Recent studies have demonstrated that activation of the phospholipase C signaling pathway can reduce the normally high threshold for activating TRPV1 from temperatures of $\sim 43°C$ to as low as $\sim 37°C$ [51]. This would lead to spontaneous activation of TRPV1 at body temperatures, possibly contributing to the spontaneous pain in patients who have irreversible pulpitis or acute apical periodontitis or other orofacial pain conditions. Prior studies have provided evidence for activation or functional activity of the bradykinin, endothelin, SP, and leukotriene systems in dental pulp [52–59].

Voltage-gated ion channels

Voltage-gated ion channels (VGICs) are transmembrane, pore-forming proteins that allow the selective passage of certain ions in a

Table 1
Examples of neuronal receptors, their ligands, and drugs that likely modulate odontogenic pain

Receptor class	Receptor subtype	Natural ligand or stimulus	Drug	In dental pulp	In trigeminal ganglia
Opioid	Mu (MOR)	β-endorphin	Opiates	[39,176]	
	Delta (DOR)	Met-enkephalin	None available		
	Kappa (KOR)	Dynorphin (?)	Pentazocine		
Cannabinoid	CB1	Anandamide	None available		[175]
	CB2	?	None available		[175]
Somatostatin	Sst1-5	Somatostatin	Octreotide	[176]	
Adrenergic	Alpha (family)	Norepinephrine	"Vasoconstrictors"	[44]	
	Beta (family)	Epinephrine	Albuterol, etc.	[177]	
GABA	GABA (B)	GABA	Baclofen	[178]	
NPY	Y1 (etc.)	Neuropeptide Y	None available		
Prostaglandin	EP2, EP3 (etc.)	PGE2	NSAIDs, steroids		[46]
CGRP	CGRP-R1, -R2	CGRP	CGRP28-37		
Bradykinin	B1	Kallidin	Des-Tyr HOE140		
	B2	Bradykinin	HOE140, steroids		[179]
Protease (PAR)	PAR2 (etc.)		?		

Endothelin	ETA, ETB	Endothelin	Atrasentan (antagonist)	?
Substance P	NK1, NK2	Substance P	L-703,606	
Leukotriene	BLT1, 2 and CysLT1, 2	LTB4, LTD4	Monteleukast, zafirlukast	[55]
VGSC	Na$_v$1.1 (etc.)		Local anesthetics	
VGCC			?	
VGKC			?	
TRP	TRPV1	Heat, acid, some lipid-like compounds	Capsaicin	
	TRPA1	Cold (?)	Mustard oil, garlic	
	TRPM8.	Cold	Menthol	
Trk	trkA (etc.)		?	[172]
Cytokine	IL1-RI, IL1-RII	IL1	Anakinra	
	TNF	TNFα	Adalimumab	
Innate PAMPS	Toll4	Endotoxin (LPS)		[180]
	CD14	Endotoxin (LPS)		[180]

Presence in dental pulp as evaluated by anatomical, biochemical, or pharmacologic methods.

Abbreviation: PAMPS, pathogen-associated molecular patterns.

voltage-dependent manner. There are more than 140 members of this superfamily representing one of the largest collections of proteins involved in signal
transduction [60]. They also represent key therapeutic targets given their importance in transduction. Within this superfamily are several important classes of ion channels that include the potassium (K^+), calcium (Ca^{2+}), and
sodium (Na^+) VGICs. The activation of these classic channels is a key process
involved in the initiation and propagation of action potentials and in the release of neurotransmitters involved in synaptic transmission. Their importance in pain pharmacology is recognized because analgesics exist that
function directly on the Na^+ and Ca^{2+} VGICs, and the actions of many different drugs produce analgesia indirectly through effects on K^+ channels.

There is a great deal of similarity in the structure of these different classic
VGICs, and this homology suggests a similar origin of not only these classic
channels but of the entire superfamily [61]. The K^+ channels represent the
ones with the simplest structure, whereas the Ca^{2+} and Na^+ channels represent modifications of this structural motif. The Na^+ channel was the first of
these to be described [62,63] and consists of an alpha subunit consisting of
four homologous domains (I–IV) that surround a central pore for ion passage [64,65]. In addition to the pore, the alpha subunit contains a selectivity
filter that allows only certain types of ions to pass and a voltage-sensor that
allows a conformational change and opening of the pore based on voltage.
Each domain consists of six transmembrane α-helices referred to as S1
through S6. The structure of the Ca^{2+} channel is similar to Na^+ channels
[66], whereas the K^+ channel consists of a tetramer of an identical protein
monomer that resembles one homologous domain of Na^+ and K^+ channels
[67]. Auxiliary subunits are typically associated with the α-subunit, and, in
the case of Na^+ channels, these beta subunits can modulate the expression,
localization, and gating properties of the α-subunits [68] and thus represent
possible therapeutic targets. Summary statements regarding the distributions, functional significance, and possible therapeutic roles of each of the
channels included in the superfamily of voltage-gated ion channels have recently been published. These statements include descriptions of the standardized nomenclature used to denote the different members of this class
[60].

Although it is difficult and most likely unfair to summarize the contribution of each of these classic VGICs in neuronal function, the following gen-
eralizations can be made. The activation of Na^+ channels is critical for
action potential (nerve impulse) initiation and propagation. The opening
of the voltage-gated Na^+ channels occurs when a transient generator potential is created by the activity of other ion channels (such as transient receptor
potential [TRP]), thus reaching the critical level needed to open the pore. If
enough Na^+ ions enter the axon, a depolarizing threshold is reached, resulting in the initiation of an action potential. Thus, drugs that block sodium
channels (eg, lidocaine) play a critical role in dental therapeutics. The activation of the K^+ channel is necessary to hyperpolarize (bringing the resting

potential within the nerve membrane back to a negative potential) and thus terminating the action potential. Therefore, the activation of the classic voltage-gated Na^+ channel initiates this activity, whereas the opening of K^+ channel results in the termination of nerve activity. The role of the voltage-gated Ca^{2+} channels in nerve activity is more complex because calcium entry into neurons can produce profound short- and long-lasting effects on many different cellular functions due to its role as a second messenger and involvement in intracellular signaling pathways. Important functions of voltage-gated Ca^{2+} channels include its influence on cell body excitability and the ability to gate the entry of calcium into nerve terminals, leading to vesicle fusion and release of neurotransmitter during synaptic transmission. Each of these channels, and especially the various subtypes, represents possible therapeutic targets to control the altered excitability of nociceptors. Evidence for the role of each of these classic VGICs and related members in pain conditions is discussed below.

Sodium channels: the Na_vs

Much recent interest has been focused on the contribution of altered voltage-gated sodium channel expression to pain states [69–71]. The importance of sodium channels on pain transmission is well known because the successful practice of "painless" dentistry largely depends on the sodium channel blocking effect of local anesthetics. Sodium channels are important in action potential initiation and propagation in response to normal stimuli [72], but they also seem to have a role in increased neuronal excitability and especially spontaneous and ectopic activity associated with inflammatory and neuropathic pain states. The association of altered sodium channel function with basic neuropathic pain mechanisms is strengthened by the relative effectiveness of medications with a sodium channel blocking effect, such as the anticonvulsant carbamazepine in the treatment of neuropathic pain conditions and especially trigeminal neuralgia [73,74]. The tricyclic antidepressants also represent a useful neuropathic pain medication, and some of their effectiveness may be due to a sodium channel–blocking effect [75].

Sodium channels are recognized as a diverse group consisting of at least nine different subtypes, or isoforms, localized to nervous system tissues and designated as $Na_v1.1$ through 1.9 [76]. Although all nine show similarities in structure and as a group show more similarity in function than the Ca^{2+} and K^+ families, some important differences exist. These include a differential nervous system distribution [76] and important differences in expression after inflammatory or axotomy insults [77]. The relative differences in expressions are important physiologically because each sodium channel has unique gating properties [66] that can influence action potential initiation. The isoforms that are normally expressed in sensory neurons include the $Na_v1.1$, -1.2, -1.6, -1.7, -1.8, and -1.9 isoforms. The $Na_v1.1$, -1.2, and -1.6 isoforms are also found in the CNS, whereas $Na_v1.3$ is seen in the developing nervous system [78]. The $Na_v1.6$ isoform is the predominant sodium channel located at nodes of Ranvier throughout the nervous system [79,80] and thus is critically linked to the saltatory conduction of action potentials in myelinated fibers. The $Na_v1.7$, -1.8, and -1.9 isoforms are preferentially expressed in the peripheral nervous system and seen in a subset of nociceptors [81–83]. Their peripheral nervous system location makes them attractive targets for the development of pharmacologic agents because such agents may lack the CNS side effects associated with many of the current medications that block sodium channels, such as anticonvulsants.

Nerve injury models have implicated the $Na_v1.3$, -1.7, -1.8, and -1.9 isoforms in the generation of neuropathic pain. Nerve injury models result in an upregulation of the previously non-expressed $Na_v1.3$ gene in DRG neurons [84], in dorsal horn neurons [85], and in dorsal horn and thalamic neurons after spinal cord injury [86]. Peripheral nerve injury is associated with a downregulation or loss of $Na_v1.8$ and $Na_v1.9$ in the DRG but with fewer changes of both isoforms at the site of injury [87–89]. The $Na_v1.8$ isoform has also been implicated in nerve injury hyperalgesia [90,91], including an upregulation in nearby uninjured c-fibers [92]. Axotomy of the inferior alveolar nerve also decreases $Na_v1.8$ mRNA in trigeminal ganglion neurons, like most studies done in the spinal system [93]. Recent human studies have also found increased $Na_v1.7$, -1.8, and -1.9 immunoreactivity and protein in injured nerves, an association of increased $Na_v1.8$ with hyperalgesia, and decreased expression in the injured DRG neurons [94–97]. Primary erythermalgia, a disease characterized by sporadic attacks of swollen, red, and warm extremities, has recently been defined as a neuropathic pain disorder due to mutations in the SCN9A gene that encodes for the $Na_v1.7$ protein [98]. Other recent findings show no change in neuropathic pain behavior in rats treated with $Na_v1.3$ antisense oligonucleotides [99] and in knockout mice lacking $Na_v1.7$ and -1.8 [100], whereas a specific blocker of $Na_v1.7$ and -1.8 [101] and $Na_v1.8$ [102] inhibited neuropathic behaviors. The role of altered sodium channel expression in neuropathic pain states remains an active area of research. The recent development of isoform-specific blockers is encouraging, and the development of other specific blockers should help to define the role of altered isoform expression to the development of neuropathic pain states.

Other studies have evaluated the effect of inflammation on specific isoform expression, and these results have suggested the involvement of $Na_v1.7$ and the tetrodotoxin-resistant isoforms $Na_v1.8$ and -1.9 in inflammatory pain mechanisms [103–109]. The expression of these isoforms may be mediated through prostaglandin signaling [110,111], and pretreatment with ibuprofen can prevent the augmentation of $Na_v1.7$ and -1.8 seen after injection of complete Freud's adjuvant [112]. Nerve growth factor is also involved in the expression of $Na_v1.7$ [113] and $Na_v1.8$ [114]. There is interest in studying sodium channel expression in human dental pulp [115], and recent studies have shown an increase in $Na_v1.8$ in painful tooth pulp when compared with normal tooth pulp [116,117]. One possible consequence of an increased expression is a higher incidence of local anesthesia failures encountered when treating painful teeth [118]. Although differences in the expression of the various isoforms are seen after nerve injury and inflammatory insults, the isoform that contributes most to the development of altered neuronal excitability is unknown.

Potassium channels: the voltage-gated potassium channels and others

The potassium-selective channels represent the largest class of ion channels and consist of diverse subtypes. The voltage-gated potassium (K_v) channels are one subtype and represent about 40 of the 70 known potassium-selective channels. Other K^+–selective channels include the inward rectifying, two-pore, and Ca^{2+}–activated K^+ channels. The Ca^{2+}–activated K^+ channels include the big, intermediate, and small conductance K^+ channels.

Each of the K_v genes encodes a single peptide subunit. The active K_v channel is composed of four subunits that can be homotetramers of the same subunit or heterotetramers composed of various subunits from within the family. The K_v family members, as designated with the IUPHAR [119] nomenclature and followed by the HUGO Gene Nomenclature Committee nomenclature in parentheses, include $K_v1.1$–1.8 (KCNA1–7, 10), $K_v2.1$–2.2 (KCNB1–2), $K_v3.1$–3.4 (KCNC1–4), $K_v4.1$–4.3 (KCND1–3), $K_v5.1$ (KCNF1), $K_v6.1$–6.4 (KCNG1–4), $K_v7.1$–7.5 (KCNQ1–5), $K_v8.1$–8.2 (KCNV1–2), $K_v9.1$–9.3 (KCNS1–3), $K_v10.1$–10.2 (KCNH1–2), $K_v11.1$–11.3 (KCNH2,6,7), and $K_v12.1$–12.3 (KCNH8,3,4). The K_v7 family represents the most interesting family from a pharmacologic aspect because mutations in four of the subunits have been associated with diseases such as long QT syndrome, deafness, and seizures. The $K_v7.2$ to 7.5 subtypes are considered possible targets for the development of anticonvulsants, and, due to the effectiveness of other anticonvulsants in neuropathic pain management, they may also represent pharmacologic targets for pain management. This association seems to hold true because the anticonvulsant retigabine (an opener of the $K_v7.2$–7.5 subtypes) seems effective in some models of neuropathic and chronic pain [120]. Other K_v subtypes that may be implicated in pain include $K_v1.4$, which is found in small-diameter dorsal root ganglion neurons [121], and the $K_v4.2$ subtype, which is localized to dorsal horn neurons and when inactivated by extracellular signal-related kinase after injury is inactivated and no longer able to inhibit neuronal firing [122].

Other K^+ channels that are implicated in pain mechanisms include two members of the inward rectifying family, the K_{ATP} subtype and the G-protein regulated inward rectifier K^+ channels (GIRK or $K_{ir}3$). The K_{ATP} subtype is implicated in peripheral analgesia because peripheral injections of the specific blockers pinacidil and diazoxide produced antinociception in a paw pressure test [123]. The opening of K_{ATP} and GIRK channels seems to be a critical step in the antinociceptive effects of many analgesic medications, including opioids. This occurs indirectly because opioid binding activates $G_{i/o}$ proteins, which open the K_{ATP}, GIRK1, and GIRK2 subtype K^+ channels, thus contributing to antinociception [124,125]. Opioid receptors located spinally primarily affect GIRK1 and GIRK2 [126], whereas peripheral opioid analgesia primarily affects the K_{ATP} K^+ channels [127]. The activation of GPCRs by non-opioid agonists and the subsequent opening of K^+ channels underlie the analgesic action of many different medications, including adrenoceptors, adenosine, 5-HT1A receptor agonists, muscarinic and dopamine receptors, cannabinoid receptors, $GABA_B$ receptors, some NSAIDs, tricyclic antidepressants, antihistamines, and gabapentin [120]. Evidence suggests the involvement of the big and small conductance K^+ channel subtypes of the Ca^{2+}–activated K^+ channel family in some of these effects. In summary, the activation and subsequent opening of a number of different K^+ channels seems to be a promising area of research that may lead to the development of new classes of analgesics through a direct opening effect on K^+ channels or indirectly through the activation of GPCRs.

Calcium channels: the voltage-gated Ca^{2+} channels and a few others

Activation of the voltage-gated Ca^{2+} (Ca_v) channels have broad-reaching effect on cellular function due to the role of calcium as an important intracellular second messenger system in addition to critical roles in the control of neuronal excitability and the release of neurotransmitters. The structure of the Ca_v is similar to that of the Na_v, consisting of four homologous domains with each domain consisting of a six-transmembrane α-helix segment [128,129]. The α1 subunit may also be associated with β and α2-δ and -γ subunits, which modify the gating characteristics of the α1 subunit. Currents due to calcium channel activation were initially characterized based on their physiologic properties (L, N P/Q, and R) and then by an alphabetical nomenclature based on that used to classify the K_v [129]. This classification includes $Ca_v1.1$ through $Ca_v1.4$ (L current), $Ca_v2.1$ (P/Q current), $Ca_v2.2$ (N current), $Ca_v2.3$ (R current), and $Ca_v3.1$ through $Ca_v3.3$ (T current).

The Ca_v2 (P/Q, N, and R currents) channels are of great interest with regard to pain mechanisms [130] because they are blocked by peptides isolated from the venom of spiders and snails [131]. Ziconotide represents a new intrathecally administered analgesic that is approved for chronic pain resistant to other therapies and that specifically blocks activity at the $Ca_v2.2$ channel and its N current [132]. It is a synthetic peptide based on the venom from the marine snail *Conus magus* and inhibits the release of excitatory amino acids from primary afferent terminals [133]. Inhibition of the N current is also achieved with the opioid receptor like receptor 1 agonist, nociceptin, which triggers a PKC-dependent internalization of N-type channels [134]. Mice lacking the $Ca_v2.2$ channel show decreased inflammatory and neuropathic pain behaviors [135], suggesting important influences of this channel on the neurotransmission of nociceptive stimuli. The analgesic action of various venoms may not be limited to the $Ca_v2.2$ channel because the venom from the spider *Phoneutria nigriventer* inhibits all three currents associated with the Ca_v2 channels [136]. The $Ca_v3.2$, T-type channel also represents a target because antisense knockdown of this gene inhibits pain behaviors in a neuropathic pain model [137]. Other potential targets related to the Ca_v include the β3 [138] and the α2-δ type 1 [139] subunits. Pregabalin is another new medication that is related to gabapentin. Pregabalin is approved to treat postherpetic neuralgia and diabetic neuropathy pain, and its analgesic action may include its ability to bind to the α2-δ type 1 subunit [140]. The modification of Ca^{2+} currents by drugs and venoms has led to the development of new analgesics, and hopefully more medications with specific action and fewer side-effects will be developed in this class.

The transient receptor potential channels

The TRP channels represent a family of six different members including some that that act broadly in the transduction of sensory stimuli related to pain, temperature, vision, hearing, taste, and pheromone detection [141]. Most are weakly gated by voltage and as a class act as nonselective cation channels that allow the passage of Na^+, sometimes Mg^{2+}, and especially Ca^{2+} into cells. Because Ca^{2+} plays an important role as an intracellular second messenger, they are implicated in the control of many cellular processes, including exocytosis, contraction, apoptosis, migration, cell development, and neuronal excitability. They often work in concert with other receptors, including GCPRs and tyrosine kinases. Tyrosine kinase activates phospholipase C, leading to Ca^{2+} release from the endoplasmic reticulum [142]. The TRP family is somewhat related in structure to the K^+ channels and consists of six transmembrane loops. They can form homomeric functional units or can form associations with other members, allowing the formation of heteromeric units. The six subfamilies of the TRPs include the vanilloid receptor TRPs (TRPVs), the melastatin or long TRPs (TRPMs), the ankyrin transmembrane protein 1 (ANKTM1 or TRPA1), the classic TRPs, the mucolipins, and the polycystins [143]. Four individual members within these subfamilies (TRPV1, TRPV2, TRPM8, and TRPA1) have been strongly implicated in pain signaling or some aspects of thermoreception, and all allow the passage of Ca^{2+} preferentially more than other cations.

The TRPV subfamily consists of six different members (TRPV1–6); TRPV1 is the most intensely studied and best understood member of this group [144,145]. The TRPV1 receptor was the first molecule to be found that is gated by temperature ($\geq 43°C$) and that represents the capsaicin receptor and was first described as the vanilloid receptor (VR1). It is primarily a Ca^{2+}–permeable channel that is also gated by hydrogen ions and polyunsaturated fatty acids and represents a possible receptor for the endogenous cannabinoid anandamide [146]. TRPV1 knockout mice have shown that the expression of this ligand-gated channel is critical for the development of inflammatory hyperalgesia [147,148] but is not necessary for the detection of heat in normal (uninflamed) tissues [149]. Capsaicin produces a neurogenic inflammation (by evoking peripheral neuropeptide release) and primary and secondary hyperalgesia [150] and highlights the importance of this receptor in this process. The receptor can be sensitized by inflammatory mediators such as bradykinin, prostaglandins, serotonin, ATP, and adenosine [151]. This sensitization can lead to a potentiation of currents through the channel and can result in lowering the temperatures needed to activate the channel [152]. The TRPV1 channel also shows the ability to become desensitized after prolonged stimulation. The TRPV1 channel represents an attractive pharmacologic target because it is widely expressed in the trigeminal and dorsal root ganglion in small-diameter cell bodies that typically give rise to unmyelinated axons, consistent with a nociceptive phenotype [153]. The TRPV1 receptor is seen in nociceptive tissues such as the human tooth pulp [116], is found in peptidergic and nonpeptidergic sensory neurons [154,155], and may play a role in neuropathic pain mechanisms [156]. Given the importance that TRPV1 plays in inflammatory pain mechanisms, it is widely regarded as a phenotypic marker for nociceptive neurons.

The TRPV2 receptor is another member of the TRPV subfamily and may play a role in the detection of noxious heat [157]. It is activated by higher temperatures, with a threshold of 52°C, and is not activated by protons or the vanilloids. The TRPV2 receptor is seen in larger cell bodies within sensory ganglia, A-delta and A-beta myelinated fibers, and in different cells than TRPV1 [158]. More recently, the heat receptor story has been complicated by the finding that TRPV1 and TRPV2 knockout mice respond normally to heat responses [149]. This surprising finding has led to their hypotheses that under normal conditions there is a population of IB4-negative neurons that respond to heat in ways that do not involve TRPV1 and TRPV2 and that TRPV1 is active only after injury or in disease states. Even though TRPV1 and TRPV2 have been implicated in the processing of noxious heat stimuli, additional studies are needed to more fully describe the role of each in this response.

The TRPM8 receptor was first called the cold menthol-receptor 1 because it binds menthol, thus producing its cooling effect [159,160]. Activity is increasingly activated by cool and noxious cold temperatures that range from 28 to 8°C and by other cooling compounds, such as icilin [161]. The activation by menthol is important because this compound can initiate a painful response when applied to human skin [162], leading to cold allodynia but without the development of an axon reflex [163]. Menthol can also produce a sensitization of the receptor, leading to an increase in the temperature, which is needed to activate the channel. TRPM8 has been identified in primary afferent neuronal cell bodies that give rise to myelinated A-fibers and unmyelinated C-fibers and has been seen in a different subset of neurons than TRPV1 [153]. This study also classified the different

TRP receptors based on their associations with trk receptors and found an important correlation of TRPM8 with the high-affinity nerve growth factor receptor trkA, which is seen as a marker of neurons that are critically involved in inflammatory pain mechanisms [164]. These studies have identified the TRPM8 receptor as a cold receptor.

The TRPA1 receptor (first called ANKTM1) was initially identified as a cold receptor [165]. It is activated by temperatures below 17°C, but conflicting evidence exists regarding its role in the signaling of noxious cold [166–168]. This receptor is activated by different naturally occurring compounds (eg, allyl isothiocyanates, such as mustard oil and wasabi; thiosulfinate allicin, which is found in garlic; and cinnamon) that, when applied to skin, can produce pain and neurogenic inflammation. Activation of TRPA1 also mediates the inflammatory response to environmental irritants, such as tear gas and car exhaust [166], bradykinin [167], and some of the effects of peripherally administered cannabinoids [169]. This receptor may also be involved in the detection of mechanical stimuli [167], an ability that may be related to the presence of multiple ankyrin repeats also seen in the TRPN1 receptor that mediates mechanotransduction in flies [170]. The TRPA1 receptor is found mainly in a subset of unmyelinated nociceptors and is colocalized in a subpopulation of TRPV1 neurons [153]. Due to its role in inflammation, activation by many different compounds that produce pain when applied topically, and its colocalization with TRPV1, it represents an important receptor involved in the transduction and modulation of painful stimuli.

In summary, the TRPs represent an important class of receptors involved in the pain associated with peripheral inflammation. The activation of some of these receptors by thermal stimuli in pathologic conditions represents an important finding. Given the ability of thermal stimuli and especially cold in the production of a painful response in inflamed teeth, the evaluation of these receptors in pulp from normal and painful human extracted teeth could provide additional insights into thermally mediated pain mechanisms.

Several other receptor systems are expressed on nociceptors and modulate the activity of this important class of sensory neurons (Table 1). The neurotrophin receptors trkA, trkB, and trkC are expressed on sensory neurons and detect tissue levels of NGF, BDNF, and GDNF, respectively. Of particular interest to dentists, NGF has been shown to increase during pulpal inflammation [171,172], to sensitize TRPV1 [173], and to evoke hyperalgesia after injection in human volunteers [174]. Inflammation likely increases more than one neurotrophin, and these potent mediators significantly alter sprouting of trigeminal neurons [175].

The future: toward a molecular model of pain diagnosis and management

The last few decades have seen a tremendous change in the pain field. Although the gate control theory of the 1960s emphasized the importance of differences in patterns of afferent input as pivotal in pain perception, contemporary research has focused extensive effort toward understanding the role of receptors and ion channels in the detection of noxious stimuli and in the transmission and processing of this information. Because this article focuses on peripheral mechanisms of odontogenic pain, we have discussed those receptors and ion channels located in terminals innervating dental pulp. This information has two major applications. First, a better understanding of peripheral pain mechanisms contributes to strategies for dental pain control using currently available drugs and the next generation of analgesics. Equally important, knowledge of peripheral pain mechanisms is likely to contribute to our understanding of many chronic pain conditions and supports the development of hypothesis-driven translational clinical research that is likely to increase our understanding of the pathophysiology of many forms of acute and chronic pain.

Although we have focused on the detection of peripheral noxious stimuli and its transmission, it would be overly simplistic to conclude that this is the only important component in pain perception. For example, knowledge of central pain mechanisms, including central sensitization, is equally important in understanding and managing clinical pain conditions. In addition, understanding the affective component of pain and its modulation by psychosocial issues plays an important role in pain control, particularly in chronic pain conditions. Today's skilled clinician must diagnose and treat pain conditions based not on anecdotal lore but on a firm understanding of the biology of pain conditions, the pharmacology of traditional and nontraditional analgesics, and the outcomes from evidence-based clinical trials. Our patients deserve no less.

References

[1] Lipton JA, Ship JA, Larach-Robinson D. Estimated prevalence and distribution of reported orofacial pain in the United States. J Am Dent Assoc 1993;124:115–21.

[2] Fearnhead R. Innervation of dental tissues. In: Miles A, editor. Structure and chemical organization of teeth. New York: Academic Press; 1967. p. 247–81.

[3] Anderson DJ, Hannam AG, Mathews B. Sensory mechanisms in mammalian teeth and their supporting structures. Physiol Rev 1970;50:171–95.

[4] McGrath PA, Gracely RH, Dubner R, et al. Non-pain and pain sensations evoked by tooth pulp stimulation. Pain 1983;15:377–88.

[5] Mumford JM, Bowsher D. Pain and protopathic sensibility: a review with particular reference to the teeth. Pain 1976;2:223–43.

[6] Pashley D, Liewehr F. Structure and functions of the dentin-pulp complex. In: Cohen S, Hargreaves K, editors. Pathways of the pulp. St. Louis (MO): Mosby Elsevier; 2006. p. 460–513.

[7] Byers MR, Narhi MV. Dental injury models: experimental tools for understanding neuroinflammatory interactions and polymodal nociceptor functions. Crit Rev Oral Biol Med 1999;10:4–39.

[8] Fearnhead RW. Histological evidence for the innervation of human dentine. J Anat 1957; 91:267–77.

[9] Nair PN. Neural elements in dental pulp and dentin. Oral Surg Oral Med Oral Pathol Oral Radiol Endod 1995;80:710–9.

[10] Johnsen D, Johns S. Quantitation of nerve fibres in the primary and permanent canine and incisor teeth in man. Arch Oral Biol 1978;23:825–9.

[11] Johnsen DC. Innervation of teeth: qualitative, quantitative, and developmental assessment. J Dent Res 1985;64:555–63.

[12] Rodd HD, Boissonade FM. Innervation of human tooth pulp in relation to caries and dentition type. J Dent Res 2001;80:389–93.

[13] Aars H, Brodin P, Andersen E. A study of cholinergic and beta-adrenergic components in the regulation of blood flow in the tooth pulp and gingiva in man. Acta Physiol Scand 1993; 148:441–7.

[14] Sasano T, Shoji N, Kuriwada S, et al. Absence of parasympathetic vasodilatation in cat dental pulp. J Dent Res 1995;74:1665–70.

[15] Olgart L, Gazelius B, Brodin E, et al. Release of substance P-like immunoreactivity from the dental pulp. Acta Physiol Scand 1977;101:510–2.

[16] Rodd HD, Boissonade FM. Immunocytochemical investigation of neurovascular relationships in human tooth pulp. J Anat 2003;202:195–203.

[17] Fristad I, Berggreen E, Haug SR. Delta (delta) opioid receptors in small and medium-sized trigeminal neurons supporting the dental pulp of rats. Arch Oral Biol 2006;51:273–81.

[18] Yang H, Bernanke JM, Naftel JP. Immunocytochemical evidence that most sensory neurons of the rat molar pulp express receptors for both glial cell line-derived neurotrophic factor and nerve growth factor. Arch Oral Biol 2006;51:69–78.

[19] Fried K, Arvidsson J, Robertson B, et al. Combined retrograde tracing and enzyme/immunohistochemistry of trigeminal ganglion cell bodies innervating tooth pulps in the rat. Neuroscience 1989;33:101–9.

[20] Kvinnsland IH, Luukko K, Fristad I, et al. Glial cell line-derived neurotrophic factor (GDNF) from adult rat tooth serves a distinct population of large-sized trigeminal neurons. Eur J Neurosci 2004;19:2089–98.

[21] Olgart L, Hokfelt T, Nilsson G, et al. Localization of substance P-like immunoreactivity in nerves in the tooth pulp. Pain 1977;4:153–9.

[22] Wakisaka S, Ichikawa H, Nishikawa S, et al. Neurokinin A-like immunoreactivity in feline dental pulp: its distribution, origin and coexistence with substance P-like immunoreactivity. Cell Tissue Res 1988;251:565–9.

[23] Uddman R, Bjorlin G, Moller B, et al. Occurrence of VIP nerves in mammalian dental pulps. Acta Odontol Scand 1980;38:325–8.

[24] Uddman R, Grunditz T, Sundler F. Neuropeptide Y: occurrence and distribution in dental pulps. Acta Odontol Scand 1984;42:361–5.

[25] Gronblad M, Liesi P, Munck AM. Peptidergic nerves in human tooth pulp. Scand J Dent Res 1984;92:319–24.

[26] Uddman R, Grunditz T, Sundler F. Calcitonin gene related peptide: a sensory transmitter in dental pulps? Scand J Dent Res 1986;94:219–24.

[27] Casasco A, Calligaro A, Casasco M, et al. Peptidergic nerves in human dental pulp: an immunocytochemical study. Histochemistry 1990;95:115–21.

[28] Wakisaka S, Itotagawa T, Youn SH, et al. Distribution and possible origin of galanin-like immunoreactive nerve fibers in the mammalian dental pulp. Regul Pept 1996;62: 137–43.

[29] Byers MR. Dynamic plasticity of dental sensory nerve structure and cytochemistry. Arch Oral Biol 1994;39(Suppl):13S–21S.

[30] Rodd HD, Boissonade FM. Substance P expression in human tooth pulp in relation to caries and pain experience. Eur J Oral Sci 2000;108:467–74.

[31] Rodd HD, Boissonade FM. Comparative immunohistochemical analysis of the peptidergic innervation of human primary and permanent tooth pulp. Arch Oral Biol 2002; 47:375–85.

[32] Lynn B. Neurogenic inflammation caused by cutaneous polymodal receptors. Prog Brain Res 1996;113:361–8.

[33] Jancso N, Jancso-Gabor A, Szolcsanyi J. Direct evidence for neurogenic inflammation and its prevention by denervation and by pretreatment with capsaicin. Br J Pharmacol Chemother 1967;31:138–51.

[34] Goadsby P. Migraine pathophysiology. Headache 2005;45:S14–24.

[35] Lundy FT, Linden GJ. Neuropeptides and neurogenic mechanisms in oral and periodontal inflammation. Crit Rev Oral Biol Med 2004;15:82–98.

[36] Byers MR, Taylor PE. Effect of sensory denervation on the response of rat molar pulp to exposure injury. J Dent Res 1993;72:613–8.

[37] Lorenz D, Wiesner B, Zipper J, et al. Mechanism of peptide-induced mast cell degranulation: translocation and patch-clamp studies. J Gen Physiol 1998;112:577–91.

[38] Jordt SE, Tominaga M, Julius D. Acid potentiation of the capsaicin receptor determined by a key extracellular site. Proc Natl Acad Sci USA 2000;97:8134–9.

[39] Jaber L, Swaim WD, Dionne RA. Immunohistochemical localization of mu-opioid receptors in human dental pulp. J Endod 2003;29:108–10.

[40] Dionne RA, Lepinski AM, Gordon SM, et al. Analgesic effects of peripherally administered opioids in clinical models of acute and chronic inflammation. Clin Pharmacol Ther 2001;70:66–73.

[41] Hargreaves KM. Peripheral opioid regulation of nociceptors: focus on "morphine directly inhibits nociceptors in inflamed skin". J Neurophysiol 2006;95:2031.

[42] Schoneberg T, Schultz G, Gudermann T. Structural basis of G protein-coupled receptor function. Mol Cell Endocrinol 1999;151:181–93.

[43] Gibbs JL, Flores CM, Hargreaves KM. Attenuation of capsaicin-evoked mechanical allodynia by peripheral neuropeptide Y Y(1) receptors. Pain 2006;124:167–74.

[44] Hargreaves KM, Jackson DL, Bowles WR. Adrenergic regulation of capsaicin-sensitive neurons in dental pulp. J Endod 2003;29:397–9.

[45] Richardson JD, Kilo S, Hargreaves KM. Cannabinoids reduce hyperalgesia and inflammation via interaction with peripheral CB1 receptors. Pain 1998;75:111–9.

[46] Cerka-Withers K, Patwardhan A, Hargreaves K. Characterization of prostaglandin receptors mediating sensitization of trigeminal nociceptors. J Dent Res 2006;1174.

[47] Cohen JS, Reader A, Fertel R, et al. A radioimmunoassay determination of the concentrations of prostaglandins E2 and F2alpha in painful and asymptomatic human dental pulps. J Endod 1985;11:330–5.

[48] Isett J, Reader A, Gallatin E, et al. Effect of an intraosseous injection of depo-medrol on pulpal concentrations of PGE2 and IL-8 in untreated irreversible pulpitis. J Endod 2003;29:268–71.

[49] Alptekin NO, Ari H, Haliloglu S, et al. The effect of endodontic therapy on periapical exudate neutrophil elastase and prostaglandin-E2 levels. J Endod 2005;31:791–5.

[50] Takayama S, Miki Y, Shimauchi H, et al. Relationship between prostaglandin E2 concentrations in periapical exudates from root canals and clinical findings of periapical periodontitis. J Endod 1996;22:677–80.

[51] Prescott ED, Julius D. A modular PIP2 binding site as a determinant of capsaicin receptor sensitivity. Science 2003;300:1284–8.

[52] Goodis HE, Bowles WR, Hargreaves KM. Prostaglandin E2 enhances bradykinin-evoked iCGRP release in bovine dental pulp. J Dent Res 2000;79:1604–7.

[53] Kim S, Dorscher-Kim J. Hemodynamic regulation of the dental pulp in a low compliance environment. J Endod 1989;15:404–8.

[54] Lepinski AM, Hargreaves KM, Goodis HE, et al. Bradykinin levels in dental pulp by microdialysis. J Endod 2000;26:744–7.

[55] Madison S, Whitsel EA, Suarez-Roca H, et al. Sensitizing effects of leukotriene B4 on intradental primary afferents. Pain 1992;49:99–104.

[56] Ohkubo T, Shibata M, Yamada Y, et al. Role of substance P in neurogenic inflammation in the rat incisor pulp and the lower lip. Arch Oral Biol 1993;38:151–8.

[57] Okiji T, Morita I, Suda H, et al. Pathophysiological roles of arachidonic acid metabolites in rat dental pulp. Proc Finn Dent Soc 1992;88(Suppl):433–8.

[58] Sunakawa M, Chiang CY, Sessle BJ, et al. Jaw electromyographic activity induced by the application of algesic chemicals to the rat tooth pulp. Pain 1999;80:493–501.

[59] Yu CY, Boyd NM, Cringle SJ, et al. An in vivo and in vitro comparison of the effects of vasoactive mediators on pulpal blood vessels in rat incisors. Arch Oral Biol 2002;47: 723–32.

[60] Yu FH, Yarov-Yarovoy V, Gutman GA, et al. Overview of molecular relationships in the voltage-gated ion channel superfamily. Pharmacol Rev 2005;57:387–95.

[61] Yu FH, Catterall WA. The VGL-chanome: a protein superfamily specialized for electrical signaling and ionic homeostasis. Sci STKE 2004;2004:re15.

[62] Agnew WS, Moore AC, Levinson SR, et al. Identification of a large molecular weight peptide associated with a tetrodotoxin binding protein from the electroplax of Electrophorus electricus. Biochem Biophys Res Commun 1980;92:860–6.

[63] Beneski DA, Catterall WA. Covalent labeling of protein components of the sodium channel with a photoactivable derivative of scorpion toxin. Proc Natl Acad Sci USA 1980;77: 639–43.

[64] Noda M, Shimizu S, Tanabe T, et al. Primary structure of Electrophorus electricus sodium channel deduced from cDNA sequence. Nature 1984;312:121–7.

[65] Noda M, Numa S. Structure and function of sodium channel. J Recept Res 1987;7:467–97.

[66] Catterall WA, Goldin AL, Waxman SG. International Union of Pharmacology. XLVII. Nomenclature and structure-function relationships of voltage-gated sodium channels. Pharmacol Rev 2005;57:397–409.

[67] Papazian DM, Schwarz TL, Tempel BL, et al. Cloning of genomic and complementary DNA from Shaker, a putative potassium channel gene from Drosophila. Science 1987; 237:749–53.

[68] Isom L. Sodium channel beta subunits: anything but auxiliary. Neuroscientist 2001;7: 42–54.

[69] Lai J, Hunter JC, Porreca F. The role of voltage-gated sodium channels in neuropathic pain. Curr Opin Neurobiol 2003;13:291–7.

[70] Lai J, Porreca F, Hunter J, et al. Voltage-gated sodium channels and hyperalgesia. Annu Rev Pharmacol Toxicol 2004;44:371–97.

[71] Wood JN. Recent advances in understanding molecular mechanisms of primary afferent activation. Gut 2004;53:9ii–12.

[72] Hille B. Ionic channels of excitable membranes. 3rd ed. Sunderland (MA): Sinauer; 2001.

[73] Jensen TS. Anticonvulsants in neuropathic pain: rationale and clinical evidence. Eur J Pain 2002;6(Suppl):61–8.

[74] McQuay HJ. Neuropathic pain: evidence matters. Eur J Pain 2002;6(Suppl A):11–8.

[75] Bielefeldt K, Ozaki N, Whiteis C, et al. Amitriptyline inhibits voltage-sensitive sodium currents in rat gastric sensory neurons. Dig Dis Sci 2002;47:959–66.

[76] Goldin AL, Barchi RL, Caldwell JH, et al. Nomenclature of voltage-gated sodium channels. Neuron 2000;28:365–8.

[77] Amir R, Argoff CE, Bennett GJ, et al. The role of sodium channels in chronic inflammatory and neuropathic pain. J Pain 2006;7(Suppl 3):S1–29.

[78] Waxman SG, Kocsis JD, Black JA. Type III sodium channel mRNA is expressed in embryonic but not adult spinal sensory neurons, and is reexpressed following axotomy. J Neurophysiol 1994;72:466–70.

[79] Caldwell JH, Schaller KL, Lasher RS, et al. Sodium channel Na(v)1.6 is localized at nodes of ranvier, dendrites, and synapses. Proc Natl Acad Sci USA 2000;97:5616–20.

[80] Krzemien DM, Schaller KL, Levinson SR, et al. Immunolocalization of sodium channel isoform NaCh6 in the nervous system. J Comp Neurol 2000;420:70–83.

[81] Akopian A, Sivilotti L, Wood J. A tetrodotoxin-resistant voltage-gated sodium channel expressed by sensory neurons. Nature 1996;379:257–62.

[82] Fang X, Djouhri L, Black JA, et al. The presence and role of the tetrodotoxin-resistant sodium channel Na(v)1.9 (NaN) in nociceptive primary afferent neurons. J Neurosci 2002;22:
7425–33.

[83] Toledo-Aral J, Moss B, He Z, et al. Identification of PN1, a predominant voltage-dependent sodium channel expressed principally in peripheral neurons. Proc Natl Acad Sci
USA 1997;94:1527–32.

[84] Black JA, Cummins TR, Plumpton C, et al. Upregulation of a silent sodium channel
after peripheral, but not central, nerve injury in DRG neurons. J Neurophysiol 1999;
82:2776–85.

[85] Hains BC, Saab CY, Klein JP, et al. Altered sodium channel expression in second-order spinal sensory neurons contributes to pain after peripheral nerve injury. J Neurosci 2004;24:
4832–9.

[86] Hains BC, Saab CY, Waxman SG. Changes in electrophysiological properties and sodium
channel Nav1.3 expression in thalamic neurons after spinal cord injury. Brain 2005;128:
2359–71.

[87] Decosterd I, Ji RR, Abdi S, et al. The pattern of expression of the voltage-gated sodium
channels Na(v)1.8 and Na(v)1.9 does not change in uninjured primary sensory neurons
in experimental neuropathic pain models. Pain 2002;96:269–77.

[88] Dib-Hajj S, Black JA, Felts P, et al. Down-regulation of transcripts for Na channel alpha-
SNS in spinal sensory neurons following axotomy. Proc Natl Acad Sci USA 1996;93:
14950–4.

[89] Dib-Hajj SD, Fjell J, Cummins TR, et al. Plasticity of sodium channel expression in DRG
neurons in the chronic constriction injury model of neuropathic pain. Pain 1999;83:
591–600.

[90] Lai J, Gold M, Kim C, et al. Inhibition of neuropathic pain by decreased expression of the
tetrodotoxin-resistant sodium channel, NaV1.8. Pain 2002;95:143–52.

[91] Porreca F, Lai J, Bian D, et al. A comparison of the potential role of the tetrodotoxin-
insensitive sodium channels, PN3/SNS and NaN/SNS2, in rat models of chronic pain.
Proc Natl Acad Sci USA 1999;96:7640–4.

[92] Gold MS, Weinreich D, Kim CS, et al. Redistribution of Na(V)1.8 in uninjured axons enables neuropathic pain. J Neurosci 2003;23:158–66.

[93] Bongenhielm U, Nosrat CA, Nosrat I, et al. Expression of sodium channel SNS/PN3 and
ankyrin(G) mRNAs in the trigeminal ganglion after inferior alveolar nerve injury in the rat.
Exp Neurol 2000;164:384–95.

[94] Coward K, Plumpton C, Facer P, et al. Immunolocalization of SNS/PN3 and NaN/SNS2
sodium channels in human pain states. Pain 2000;85:41–50.

[95] Kretschmer T, Happel LT, England JD, et al. Accumulation of PN1 and PN3 sodium channels in painful human neuroma-evidence from immunocytochemistry. Acta Neurochir
(Wien) 2002;144:803–10 [discussion: 10].

[96] Shembalkar PK, Till S, Boettger MK, et al. Increased sodium channel SNS/PN3 immunoreactivity in a causalgic finger. Eur J Pain 2001;5:319–23.

[97] Yiangou Y, Birch R, Sangameswaran L, et al. SNS/PN3 and SNS2/NaN sodium channel-
like immunoreactivity in human adult and neonate injured sensory nerves. FEBS Lett 2000;
467:249–52.

[98] Drenth JP, te Morsche RH, Guillet G, et al. SCN9A mutations define primary erythermalgia as a neuropathic disorder of voltage gated sodium channels. J Invest Dermatol 2005;
124:1333–8.

[99] Lindia JA, Kohler MG, Martin WJ, et al. Relationship between sodium channel NaV1.3
expression and neuropathic pain behavior in rats. Pain 2005;117:145–53.

[100] Nassar MA, Levato A, Stirling LC, et al. Neuropathic pain develops normally in mice lacking both Nav1.7 and Nav1.8. Mol Pain 2005;1:24.

[101] Brochu RM, Dick IE, Tarpley JW, et al. Block of peripheral nerve sodium channels selectively inhibits features of neuropathic pain in rats. Mol Pharmacol 2006;69:823–32.

[102] Gaida W, Klinder K, Arndt K, et al. Ambroxol, a Nav1.8-preferring Na(+) channel blocker, effectively suppresses pain symptoms in animal models of chronic, neuropathic and inflammatory pain. Neuropharmacology 2005;49:1220–7.

[103] Akopian AN, Souslova V, England S, et al. The tetrodotoxin-resistant sodium channel SNS has a specialized function in pain pathways. Nat Neurosci 1999;2:541–8.

[104] Coste B, Osorio N, Padilla F, et al. Gating and modulation of presumptive NaV1.9 channels in enteric and spinal sensory neurons. Mol Cell Neurosci 2004;26:123–34.

[105] Gold MS. Tetrodotoxin-resistant Na + currents and inflammatory hyperalgesia. Proc Natl Acad Sci USA 1999;96:7645–9.

[106] Nassar M, Stirling L, Forlani G, et al. Nociceptor-specific gene deletion reveals a major role for Nav1.7 (PN1) in acute and inflammatory pain. Proc Natl Acad Sci USA 2004;101: 12706–11.

[107] Priest B, Murphy BA, Lindia JA, et al. Contribution of the tetrodotoxin-resistant voltage-gated sodium channel NaV1.9 to sensory transmission and nociceptive behavior. Proc Natl Acad Sci USA 2005;102:9382–7.

[108] Tanaka M, Cummins TR, Ishikawa K, et al. SNS Na+ channel expression increases in dorsal root ganglion neurons in the carrageenan inflammatory pain model. Neuroreport 1998; 9:967–72.

[109] Tate S, Benn S, Hick C, et al. Two sodium channels contribute to the TTX-R sodium current in primary sensory neurons. Nat Neurosci 1998;1:653–5.

[110] Baker MD, Chandra SY, Ding Y, et al. GTP-induced tetrodotoxin-resistant Na + current regulates excitability in mouse and rat small diameter sensory neurones. J Physiol 2003;548: 373–82.

[111] Gold MS, Reichling DB, Shuster MJ, et al. Hyperalgesic agents increase a tetrodotoxin-resistant Na+ current in nociceptors. Proc Natl Acad Sci USA 1996;93:1108–12.

[112] Gould HJ 3rd, England JD, Soignier RD, et al. Ibuprofen blocks changes in Na v 1.7 and 1.8 sodium channels associated with complete Freund's adjuvant-induced inflammation in rat. J Pain 2004;5:270–80.

[113] Gould HJ 3rd, Gould TN, England JD, et al. A possible role for nerve growth factor in the augmentation of sodium channels in models of chronic pain. Brain Res 2000;854: 19–29.

[114] Fjell J, Cummins TR, Davis BM, et al. Sodium channel expression in NGF-overexpressing transgenic mice. J Neurosci Res 1999;57:39–47.

[115] Henry MA, Sorensen HJ, Johnson LR, et al. Localization of the Nav1.8 sodium channel isoform at nodes of Ranvier in normal human radicular tooth pulp. Neurosci Lett 2005; 380:32–6.

[116] Renton T, Yiangou Y, Baecker PA, et al. Capsaicin receptor VR1 and ATP purinoceptor P2X3 in painful and nonpainful human tooth pulp. J Orofac Pain 2003;17: 245–50.

[117] Renton T, Yiangou Y, Plumpton C, et al. Sodium channel Nav1.8 immunoreactivity in painful human dental pulp. BMC Oral Health 2005;5:5.

[118] Reisman D, Reader A, Nist R, et al. Anesthetic efficacy of the supplemental intraosseous injection of 3% mepivacaine in irreversible pulpitis. Oral Surg Oral Med Oral Pathol Oral Radiol Endod 1997;84:676–82.

[119] Gutman GA, Chandy KG, Grissmer S, et al. International Union of Pharmacology. LIII. Nomenclature and molecular relationships of voltage-gated potassium channels. Pharmacol Rev 2005;57:473–508.

[120] Ocana M, Cendan CM, Cobos EJ, et al. Potassium channels and pain: present realities and future opportunities. Eur J Pharmacol 2004;500:203–19.

[121] Rasband MN, Park EW, Vanderah TW, et al. Distinct potassium channels on pain-sensing neurons. Proc Natl Acad Sci USA 2001;98:13373–8.

[122] Hu HJ, Carrasquillo Y, Karim F, et al. The kv4.2 potassium channel subunit is required for pain plasticity. Neuron 2006;50:89–100.

[123] Picolo G, Cassola AC, Cury Y. Activation of peripheral ATP-sensitive K+ channels medi-
      ates the antinociceptive effect of Crotalus durissus terrificus snake venom. Eur J Pharmacol
      2003;469:57–64.
[124] Mark MD, Herlitze S. G-protein mediated gating of inward-rectifier K+ channels. Eur J
      Biochem 2000;267:5830–6.
[125] Wada Y, Yamashita T, Imai K, et al. A region of the sulfonylurea receptor critical for
      a modulation of ATP-sensitive K(+) channels by G-protein betagamma-subunits.
      EMBO J 2000;19:4915–25.
[126] Marker CL, Stoffel M, Wickman K. Spinal G-protein-gated K + channels formed by
      GIRK1 and GIRK2 subunits modulate thermal nociception and contribute to morphine
      analgesia. J Neurosci 2004;24:2806–12.
[127] Ortiz MI, Torres-Lopez JE, Castaneda-Hernandez G, et al. Pharmacological evidence for
      the activation of K(+) channels by diclofenac. Eur J Pharmacol 2002;438:85–91.
[128] Catterall WA, Perez-Reyes E, Snutch TP, et al. International Union of Pharmacology.
      XLVIII. Nomenclature and structure-function relationships of voltage-gated calcium
      channels. Pharmacol Rev 2005;57:411–25.
[129] Ertel EA, Campbell KP, Harpold MM, et al. Nomenclature of voltage-gated calcium chan-
      nels. Neuron 2000;25:533–5.
[130] Vanegas H, Schaible H. Effects of antagonists to high-threshold calcium channels upon spi-
      nal mechanisms of pain, hyperalgesia and allodynia. Pain 2000;85:9–18.
[131] Miljanich GP, Ramachandran J. Antagonists of neuronal calcium channels: struc-
      ture, function, and therapeutic implications. Annu Rev Pharmacol Toxicol 1995;
      35:707–34.
[132] Miljanich GP. Ziconotide: neuronal calcium channel blocker for treating severe chronic
      pain. Curr Med Chem 2004;11:3029–40.
[133] Santicioli P, Del Bianco E, Tramontana M, et al. Release of calcitonin gene-related peptide
      like-immunoreactivity induced by electrical field stimulation from rat spinal afferents is me-
      diated by conotoxin-sensitive calcium channels. Neurosci Lett 1992;136:161–4.
[134] Altier C, Khosravani H, Evans RM, et al. ORL1 receptor-mediated internalization of
      N-type calcium channels. Nat Neurosci 2006;9:31–40.
[135] Saegusa H, Kurihara T, Zong S, et al. Suppression of inflammatory and neuropathic pain
      symptoms in mice lacking the N-type Ca2+ channel. EMBO J 2001;20:2349–56.
[136] Vieira LB, Kushmerick C, Hildebrand ME, et al. Inhibition of high voltage-activated cal-
      cium channels by spider toxin PnTx3-6. J Pharmacol Exp Ther 2005;314:1370–7.
[137] Bourinet E, Alloui A, Monteil A, et al. Silencing of the Cav3.2 T-type calcium channel
      gene in sensory neurons demonstrates its major role in nociception. EMBO J 2005;24:
      315–24.
[138] Murakami M, Fleischmann B, De Felipe C, et al. Pain perception in mice lacking the beta3
      subunit of voltage-activated calcium channels. J Biol Chem 2002;277:40342–51.
[139] Li CY, Song YH, Higuera ES, et al. Spinal dorsal horn calcium channel alpha2delta-1 sub-
      unit upregulation contributes to peripheral nerve injury-induced tactile allodynia. J Neuro-
      sci 2004;24:8494–9.
[140] Bian F, Li Z, Offord J, et al. Calcium channel alpha2-delta type 1 subunit is the major bind-
      ing protein for pregabalin in neocortex, hippocampus, amygdala, and spinal cord: an ex
      vivo autoradiographic study in alpha2-delta type 1 genetically modified mice. Brain Res
      2006;1075:68–80.
[141] Montell C. The TRP superfamily of cation channels. Sci STKE 2005;2005:re3.
[142] Clapham DE. Calcium signaling. Cell 1995;80:259–68.
[143] Clapham DE, Julius D, Montell C, et al. International Union of Pharmacology. XLIX. No-
      menclature and structure-function relationships of transient receptor potential channels.
      Pharmacol Rev 2005;57:427–50.
[144] Caterina MJ, Julius D. The vanilloid receptor: a molecular gateway to the pain pathway.
      Annu Rev Neurosci 2001;24:487–517.

[145] Caterina MJ, Schumacher MA, Tominaga M, et al. The capsaicin receptor: a heat-activated ion channel in the pain pathway. Nature 1997;389:816–24.
[146] Zygmunt PM, Petersson J, Andersson DA, et al. Vanilloid receptors on sensory nerves mediate the vasodilator action of anandamide. Nature 1999;400:452–7.
[147] Caterina MJ, Leffler A, Malmberg AB, et al. Impaired nociception and pain sensation in mice lacking the capsaicin receptor. Science 2000;288:306–13.
[148] Davis JB, Gray J, Gunthorpe MJ, et al. Vanilloid receptor-1 is essential for inflammatory thermal hyperalgesia. Nature 2000;405:183–7.
[149] Woodbury CJ, Zwick M, Wang S, et al. Nociceptors lacking TRPV1 and TRPV2 have normal heat responses. J Neurosci 2004;24:6410–5.
[150] Szolcsanyi J. Forty years in capsaicin research for sensory pharmacology and physiology. Neuropeptides 2004;38:377–84.
[151] Julius D, Basbaum AI. Molecular mechanisms of nociception. Nature 2001;413:203–10.
[152] Tominaga M, Caterina MJ. Thermosensation and pain. J Neurobiol 2004;61:3–12.
[153] Kobayashi K, Fukuoka T, Obata K, et al. Distinct expression of TRPM8, TRPA1, and TRPV1 mRNAs in rat primary afferent neurons with adelta/c-fibers and colocalization with trk receptors. J Comp Neurol 2005;493:596–606.
[154] Amaya F, Shimosato G, Nagano M, et al. NGF and GDNF differentially regulate TRPV1 expression that contributes to development of inflammatory thermal hyperalgesia. Eur J Neurosci 2004;20:2303–10.
[155] Hwang SJ, Oh JM, Valtschanoff JG. Expression of the vanilloid receptor TRPV1 in rat dorsal root ganglion neurons supports different roles of the receptor in visceral and cutaneous afferents. Brain Res 2005;1047:261–6.
[156] Jordt SE, McKemy DD, Julius D. Lessons from peppers and peppermint: the molecular logic of thermosensation. Curr Opin Neurobiol 2003;13:487–92.
[157] Caterina MJ, Julius D. Sense and specificity: a molecular identity for nociceptors. Curr Opin Neurobiol 1999;9:525–30.
[158] Lewinter RD, Skinner K, Julius D, et al. Immunoreactive TRPV-2 (VRL-1), a capsaicin receptor homolog, in the spinal cord of the rat. J Comp Neurol 2004;470:400–8.
[159] McKemy DD, Neuhausser WM, Julius D. Identification of a cold receptor reveals a general role for TRP channels in thermosensation. Nature 2002;416:52–8.
[160] Peier AM, Moqrich A, Hergarden AC, et al. A TRP channel that senses cold stimuli and menthol. Cell 2002;108:705–15.
[161] Behrendt HJ, Germann T, Gillen C, et al. Characterization of the mouse cold-menthol receptor TRPM8 and vanilloid receptor type-1 VR1 using a fluorometric imaging plate reader (FLIPR) assay. Br J Pharmacol 2004;141:737–45.
[162] Wasner G, Schattschneider J, Binder A, et al. Topical menthol–a human model for cold pain by activation and sensitization of C nociceptors. Brain 2004;127:1159–71.
[163] Namer B, Seifert F, Handwerker HO, et al. TRPA1 and TRPM8 activation in humans: effects of cinnamaldehyde and menthol. Neuroreport 2005;16:955–9.
[164] Woolf CJ. Phenotypic modification of primary sensory neurons: the role of nerve growth factor in the production of persistent pain. Philos Trans R Soc Lond B Biol Sci 1996;351:441–8.
[165] Story GM, Peier AM, Reeve AJ, et al. ANKTM1, a TRP-like channel expressed in nociceptive neurons, is activated by cold temperatures. Cell 2003;112:819–29.
[166] Bautista DM, Jordt SE, Nikai T, et al. TRPA1 mediates the inflammatory actions of environmental irritants and proalgesic agents. Cell 2006;124:1269–82.
[167] Kwan KY, Allchorne AJ, Vollrath MA, et al. TRPA1 contributes to cold, mechanical, and chemical nociception but is not essential for hair-cell transduction. Neuron 2006;50:277–89.
[168] Obata K, Katsura H, Mizushima T, et al. TRPA1 induced in sensory neurons contributes to cold hyperalgesia after inflammation and nerve injury. J Clin Invest 2005;115:2393–401.
[169] Jordt SE, Bautista DM, Chuang HH, et al. Mustard oils and cannabinoids excite sensory nerve fibres through the TRP channel ANKTM1. Nature 2004;427:260–5.

[170] Walker RG, Willingham AT, Zuker CS. A Drosophila mechanosensory transduction channel. Science 2000;287:2229–34.

[171] Byers MR, Wheeler EF, Bothwell M. Altered expression of NGF and P75 NGF-receptor by fibroblasts of injured teeth precedes sensory nerve sprouting. Growth Factors 1992;6:41–52.

[172] Wheeler EF, Naftel JP, Pan M, et al. Neurotrophin receptor expression is induced in a sub-population of trigeminal neurons that label by retrograde transport of NGF or fluoro-gold following tooth injury. Brain Res Mol Brain Res 1998;61:23–38.

[173] Bonnington JK, McNaughton PA. Signalling pathways involved in the sensitisation of mouse nociceptive neurones by nerve growth factor. J Physiol 2003;551:433–46.

[174] Dyck PJ, Peroutka S, Rask C, et al. Intradermal recombinant human nerve growth factor induces pressure allodynia and lowered heat-pain threshold in humans. Neurology 1997;48:501–5.

[175] Price TJ, Helesic G, Parghi D, et al. The neuronal distribution of cannabinoid receptor type 1 in the trigeminal ganglion of the rat. Neuroscience 2003;120:155–62.

[176] Mudie AS, Holland GR. Local opioids in the inflamed dental pulp. J Endod 2006;32:319–23.

[177] Bowles WR, Flores CM, Jackson DL, et al. beta 2-Adrenoceptor regulation of CGRP release from capsaicin-sensitive neurons. J Dent Res 2003;82:308–11.

[178] Wurm C, Richardson JD, Bowles W, et al. Evaluation of functional GABA(B) receptors in dental pulp. J Endod 2001;27:620–3.

[179] Patwardhan AM, Berg KA, Akopain AN, et al. Bradykinin-induced functional competence and trafficking of the delta-opioid receptor in trigeminal nociceptors. J Neurosci 2005;25:8825–32.

[180] Wadachi R, Hargreaves KM. Trigeminal nociceptors express TLR-4 and CD14: a mechanism for pain due to infection. J Dent Res 2006;85:49–53.

ELSEVIER
SAUNDERS

THE DENTAL
CLINICS
OF NORTH AMERICA

Dent Clin N Am 51 (2007) 45–59

Central Mechanisms of Orofacial Pain

Robert L. Merrill, DDS, MS

*Graduate Orofacial Pain Program, UCLA School of Dentistry,
13-089C CHS, 10833 Le Conte Avenue, Los Angeles, CA 90095-1668, USA*

A review of the literature for temporomandibular disorders (TMD) has shown little appreciation for basic pain science, but with the expansion of the perspective into the broader context of orofacial pain, there is a developing interest in understanding the pathophysiology of pain as it relates to TMD and orofacial pain. The possibility of TMD being associated with neuropathic pain has received little attention.

The International Association for the Study of Pain has defined pain as "an unpleasant, sensory and emotional experience associated with actual or potential tissue damage, or described in terms of such damage." This definition includes not only the sensory aspect of pain but also the emotional and interpretive or cognitive aspects of pain. The emotional factors are more significant in chronic than in acute pain and assert a significant influence that usually has to be recognized and addressed to effectively treat the patient who has chronic pain. Often, chronic pain treatment failures can be traced to ignoring the psychologic issues that are affecting the patient's pain condition.

The understanding of chronic pain has advanced significantly in the last 10 years. This understanding has led to improved diagnosis and treatment strategies for pain. Until recently, patients who had facial pain that did not fit the existing understanding and taxonomy were given the diagnosis of "atypical facial pain." The recent IHS Classification of Headache provides a comprehensive classification system for head and neck pain and has removed the "atypical facial pain" diagnosis in favor of "persistent idiopathic facial pain." This is an important step in disengaging the less understood facial pain condition from a co-psychosomatic diagnosis that was implied in atypical facial pain [23].

To be able to diagnose and treat orofacial pain, one must understand basic neurophysiology of pain from the periphery to the central nervous

---

E-mail address: rmerrill@ucla.edu

0011-8532/07/$ - see front matter © 2007 Elsevier Inc. All rights reserved.
doi:10.1016/j.cden.2006.09.010
dental.theclinics.com

system (CNS). This article describes the basis of central sensitization as it relates to orofacial pain.

Pain transmission from periphery to central nervous system

Afferent sensory system: C-polymodal nociceptors and A-δ and A-β fibers

A basic understanding of the peripheral and CNS is necessary to understand pain mechanisms and to understand how central sensitization develops. Most text books on pain discuss dorsal horn mechanisms when referring to the CNS. For orofacial pain, the trigeminal correlate of the dorsal horn is the trigeminal nucleus within the pontine brain stem. Peripherally, the trigeminal nerve provides sensory input from the anterior part of the head, including the intraoral structures. Because the nociceptive endings of pain fibers lack specialized receptors, they are named from their afferent fiber and the stimulus that activates them. The sensory fibers are divided into A-β mechanoreceptors and three types of nociceptors: A-δ fibers, C–polymodal nociceptors (C-PMNs), and silent or sleeping nociceptors, which are unmyelinated or thinly myelinated. The A-β fibers that respond to light-touch mechanostimulation are large diameter, fast conducting, and myelinated. No matter what the frequency or intensity of the stimulus, these fibers normally encode only low-frequency, non-noxious stimuli that are interpreted as light touch [36]. After trauma, the A-β fibers may begin to signal pain. The A-δ fibers respond to painful mechanical stimuli with an output in the high-frequency range. This is perceived as sharp or stabbing pain. Because the A-δ fibers are myelinated, the convey impulses more rapidly than the C-PMNs (Fig. 1) [7–9]. The silent nociceptors are normally mechanically insensitive. They become active when tissue is injured. These fibers add to the nociceptive input to the CNS [18,26,27]. The afferent impulses from all the sensory fibers travel from the periphery through the trigeminal ganglion and trigeminal root, enter the pons, and descend in the trigeminal tract to enter the trigeminal nucleus. Once the fibers have entered the pons, they are in the CNS.

The trigeminal nerve innervates the anterior of the head. These fibers travel to the trigeminal ganglion and to the trigeminal nucleus in the pons. The trigeminal nucleus is subdivided into three parts: the uppermost subnucleus oralis, the middle subnucleus interpolaris, and the subnucleus caudalis (Fig. 2) [24]. Most of the pain fibers synapse in the subnucleus caudalis. For pain, the wide dynamic range neurons (WDRs) are the most important second-order neurons in the subnucleus caudalis. They receive convergent sensory input from primary afferent nociceptors and low-threshold mechanoreceptors.

Certain features of pain have long puzzled clinicians and researchers. The stimulation of pain from a normally nonpainful stimulus has defied explanation. Conversely, Beecher [1] puzzled over a battlefield phenomenon he

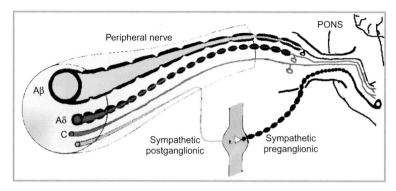

Fig. 1. Afferent and efferent fibers. This figure shows diagrammatically the make up of a typical bundle of afferent sensory nerves going from periphery to the central nervous system. The efferent sympathetic nerves follow a separate route from the central nervous system but eventually innervate the peripheral area in close proximity to the afferent sensory fibers. The large-diameter Aβ fibers are mechanoreceptors that respond only to non-noxious mechano-stimulation. The Aδ and C fibers carry noxious stimulation. Figure suggested by Fields [7] and altered for the trigeminal system. (*Adapted from* Fields HL. Pain. New York: McGraw-Hill Book Company; 1987. p. 14.)

noted during the Second World War on Enzio Beach in Italy. Beecher attracted attention to the role of cognitive appraisal with his observations that soldiers wounded during battle complain far less than civilians comparably injured during accidents, presumably because the soldiers were

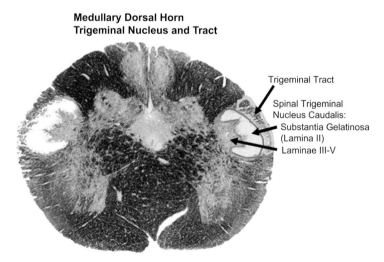

Fig. 2. The trigeminal nucleus caudalis has been outlined in the medullary dorsal horn. Note the lateral position of the nucleus and the somatotopic arrangement, which is similar to the spinal cord dorsal horn Rexed laminar arrangement. Nociceptor axons descend in the trigeminal tract and cross into lamina I/II or substantia gelatinosa at the level of the subnucleus caudalis. The A-β fibers synapse in lamina IV and V.

relieved that they had escaped from the battlefield and expected to return home, whereas the civilians evaluated the injury as a threat to comfortable, established lives. Contrasting findings have shown that people who "catastrophize" or self-alarm by focusing negatively upon their distress suffer higher levels of anxiety and are the most disabled and benefit the least from conventional medical care [14,21]. Patients who have chronic low back pain and are depressed have also been found to misinterpret or distort the nature and significance of their pain. These observations highlight the presence of pain-modulating systems in the body that can turn down or turn up the volume control for pain. This had been implied by Melzack and Wall [20] but was poorly understood when they proposed the Gate Control Theory in 1965.

Second-order neurons

The first interface between the peripheral nociceptors and the CNS occurs in the spinal cord or trigeminal nucleus, the brainstem extension of the spinal cord dorsal horn (see Fig. 2). There are many types of receptors and ion channels associated with the cell membrane of the WDR that modulate cell activity. Modulatory circuits can suppress WDR activity and decrease pain or facilitate pain transmission.

The Gate Control Theory and pain modulation

Fig. 3 shows the Gate Control of Pain that was proposed by Melzack and Wall in 1962 [20] and republished in 1965. Although there have been some modifications to the original theory, most of the system features have been confirmed by research.

The Melzack and Wall model describes modulation of pain transmission through the interneuron connections in the substantia gelatinosa. Past research had identified a pain-modulating effect of afferent activity from large-diameter A-β fibers. The gate control model identified the spinal cord substantia gelatinosa as one of the areas where pain is modulated. Fig. 3 illustrates the modulating effect of the L (light touch fibers) in reducing the effect of afferent activity from the S (c-nociceptors) fibers. Melzack and Wall [20] also theorized that there were descending inhibitory and facilitatory influences, but little was known of these mechanisms in 1965, and it has only been within the last few years that descending inhibitory and facilitatory systems have been identified.

Central pain processing and central sensitization

The phenomenon of peripheral sensitization develops from an injury-induced inflammatory response. Allodynia and hyperalgesia in this model are due to the inflammatory mediators being released at the site of injury.

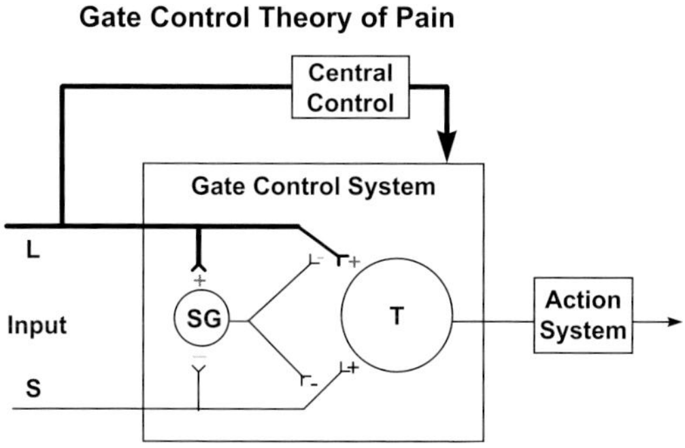

Gate Control Theory of Pain

Fig. 3. Melzack and Walls Gate Control of pain proposed that light-touch myelinated mecha-noreceptors (L) modulated or decreased the gain of the small-diameter unmyelinated pain fibers (S) in the substantia gelatinosa or dorsal horn lamina II through the intermediary effect of seg-mental interneurons in that lamina (SG). The action potential synapsed with the second-order wide dynamic range neurons (T) to bring about the response to the signals (Action System). Further modulation was suggested by other poorly understood mechanisms, including descend-ing facilitatory and inhibitory mechanisms (Central Control).

In a tooth extraction site, the inflamed area is marked by increased sensitiv-ity to pressure (static hyperalgesia) that is mediated by sensitized nocicep-tors. It is expected that this reaction will resolve within a reasonable period of time due to the decreasing activity of the nociceptors and conse-quent decrease in afferent activity to the dorsal horn. If the inflammatory process and consequent afferent activity is of sufficient intensity and if there has been neuronal damage, a central process is established that increases sensitization, lowers the threshold of response, and causes ectopic discharges (physiologic changes). Additionally, A-β fibers begin signaling pain (dy-namic mechanical allodynia), and their inhibitory effect is lost (anatomic changes and disinhibition). There is now an increased central release of ex-citatory mediators, such as glutamate and nitric oxide production (neuro-chemical changes). These changes stimulate the MAP kinase cascades, resulting in messenger RNA–mediated changes that alter the phenotype of nociceptors and mechanoreceptors such that normal cell response becomes genetically changed to a pathologic state (Fig. 4).

Central sensitization is a form of neuroplasticity in which nociceptor ac-tivity triggers a prolonged increase in the excitability of dorsal horn neurons. It is initiated by a brief burst of C-fiber activity. The peripheral manifesta-tion of this central process is dynamic hyperalgesia. Torebjork [36] has pro-vided evidence showing that once central sensitization has occurred, Aβ fiber afferents begin to evoke painful response (allodynia) [36]. C-nociceptors have been identified as the primary nociceptor involved in the initiation of central sensitization due to the slow synaptic currents they generate and the low-stimuli repetition rates that cause an increased rate of depolarization in the dorsal horn [35]. This occurs as a result of the activation of ligand-gated ion channels, initially the alpha-amino-3-hydroxy-5-methyl-4-isoxazole

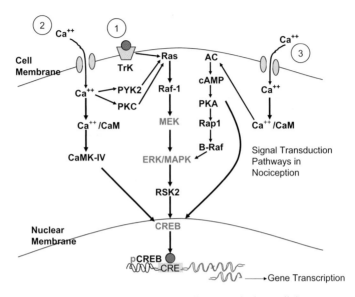

Fig. 4. The MAP kinase cascades. This diagram illustrates the intracellular responses to noci-ceptor depolarization. There are three main pathways of the MAP kinase cascades that result in the stimulation of cAMP response element binding protein and in the transcription of genes that produce target proteins altering the phenotypic expression of the nociceptors and postsynaptic neurons in the nociceptive chain. The gene transcription causes long-term potentiation and cell memory for pain. *Abbreviations:* CamK, calmodulin kinase; CRE, cAMP response element; CREB, cAMP response element binding protein; ERK, extracellular signal-regulated protein kinase; MAPK, mitogen-activated protein kinase; MEK, MAPK/ERK kinase; Ras/Raf-1, pro-teins that are molecular switches in the MAPK pathway; TRK, tyrosine kinase

proprionate (AMPA) receptor allowing calcium to enter the cell through the calcium channels. In addition, activation of the metabotropic glutamate and neurokinin receptors by glutamate and substance P causes a G-protein–coupled transduction signal that releases calcium from intracellular stores, further increasing the intracellular calcium levels. This calcium activates a calcium-dependent enzyme system, including protein kinases that phosphor-ylate the N-methyl-D-aspartate (NMDA) receptor. The NMDA receptor at normal resting membrane potentials has a magnesium ion block in the channel, but when the receptor is phosphorylated, the ion is released. Before phosphorylation, the NMDA receptor generates little inward current when glutamate is bound, but after phosphorylation and release of the ion channel block, the NMDA receptor generates inward synaptic currents at normal rest-ing membrane potentials [39]. This process causes increased glutamate sensi-tivity and is the underlying mechanism that is represented by the expansion of receptive fields and a decrease in the threshold of the dorsal horn neurons.

Aβ fiber–mediated dynamic hyperalgesia may also be the result of central reorganization of neuronal connections in the dorsal horn. Woolf and others [4,39] have found that A-β fibers sprout into dorsal horn lamina I and II after peripheral injury, forming new connections in areas normally occupied only by c-fiber nociceptors. These new connections can apparently signal pain. Additionally, it has been reported that with the neuronal organization and transcriptional changes induced by the sensitization, Aβ fibers begin expressing substance P, previously thought to be associated only with c-fibers [22]. μ−Opioid receptors are found presynaptically on c-fibers but not on A-β fibers. Part of the descending inhibitory system uses endogenous opioid action on presynaptic μ-opioid receptor. Because these receptors are not found on A-β fibers, this may account for the relative lack of response to opioid agonists in neuropathic pain.

The influx of calcium through voltage-gated ion channels also occurs on the inhibitory interneurons in lamina II. Calcium may induce excitotoxic cell death, resulting in a loss of inhibitory connections [33,38]. Mao and colleagues [17] showed that pretreatment with NMDA receptor antagonists seemed to protect the dorsal horn from changes that produced prolonged sensory hypersensitivity. Nitric oxide, arachidonic acid, superoxide, and intracellular calcium overload are the ultimate mediators of neuronal death.

Pain-modulating circuits

Pain is strongly affected by emotions. In the presence of anger, fear, or elation, major injury may be essentially painless. Conversely, in situations associated with dysphoria or when pain is anticipated, subjects often report the occurrence or worsening of pain without additional noxious stimulation. Psychologic factors influence the firing of dorsal horn pain transmission neurons.

It has been observed that stimulation of the periaquaductal gray area in the midbrain increased tail-flick latency in rats that were given a painful stimulus. The periaquaductal gray area was demonstrated to be heavily innervated with serotonergic neurons. Subsequently it has been demonstrated that there are connections to the nucleus raphe magnus of the rostral ventral medulla and thence to the nucleus caudalis of the trigeminal nucleus or the dorsal horn of the spinal cord. This system is part of the descending inhibitory system mediated by serotonin. Additionally, a descending system modulated by norepinephrine travels from cortical stimulatory centers to the periaquaductal gray and on to the dorsolateral pontine tegmentum area of the medulla, also connecting to the relay neurons (wide dynamic range) in the nucleus caudalis or dorsal horn. The dorsolateral pontine tegmentum is directly linked to the periaquaductal gray and rostral ventral medulla and projects directly to the spinal cord dorsal horn and the nucleus caudalis. Pain modulation requires action from both circuits acting in tandem (Fig. 5).

Many of the centrally acting medications used to modulate pain act within these two systems to bring about a reduction of pain that does not involve the opioid system and consequently does not build tolerance to

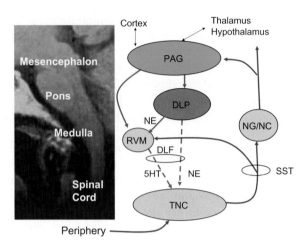

Fig. 5. Pain-modulating circuitry in the dorsal horn. Action potentials from trigeminal nociceptors enter the trigeminal nucleus caudalis (TNC), where they synapse with second-order neurons. In the TNC, the relayed signals "ascend" in the spinothalamic tract (SST), going to the
rostroventromedial medulla (RVM) and through the nucleus gracilis (NG) from the lower
body or the nucleus cuneatus (NC) from the upper body to the periaquaductal gray (PAG),
the hypothalamus and thalamus where tertiary synapses occur. One of the major descending
inhibitory systems in the pathways is the linkage with the serotonergic cells of the PAG and
RVM. An additional inhibitory pathway involves a descending connection from the PAG to
the dorsolateral pontine tegmentum (DLP), which is modulated by norepinephrine. The inhibitory signals from the RVM and the DLP descend in the dorsolateral faniculus (DLF) to the
TNC, mediating TNC nociceptive activity. The information is transmitted to the cortex and
can be modulated (inhibited or disinhibited) through cortical influence.

the effects of the medications. One of the most widely used classes of medications for chronic pain is the tricyclic antidepressants. Medications such as
amitriptyline and nortriptyline are commonly used for central pain conditions such as postherpetic neuralgia and diabetic neuropathy and work
within the serotonin system. Another tricyclic antidepressant, desipramine,
works primarily through the norepinephrine system. Their pain inhibitory
effects are not linked to the antidepressant effects.

Glial influences on pain

Glial cells (microglia and astrocytes) have been viewed classically as support cells in the CNS and were not seen to have an active role in pain transmission because they did not possess axons. This view has changed with
recent research, and there is evidence that glia have an important role in
the development of central sensitization. This role is being defined as research explores the interactions from dorsal horn neurons to the glia and
the glia to the dorsal horn neurons. Consequently, glia are no longer viewed
as only passive support cells but as active participants in modulating pain
transmission and other types of neuronal activity in the CNS.

Synapses in the CNS are surrounded by glial cells, and neurotransmitter receptors have been identified on these glia. The implication is that the glia can respond to central neurotransmitter release from presynaptic nociceptor endings [13,25]. Furthermore, transport mechanisms have been identified in glia that oversee the uptake and release of neurotransmitters from the glia [28,15]. More recently, glial cells have been shown to be involved in the development of hyperalgesia due to nerve trauma and other conditions that can lead to central sensitization [5,34].

Because glia possess receptors and transport mechanisms for neurotransmitters, one might assume that they release neurotransmitters in the synaptic cleft that would have a presynaptic and postsynaptic effect on pain modulation. Watkins [37] demonstrated that glia were involved in central sensitization from nerve injury when hyperalgesia was reduce by disrupting glial activation [37]. It has also been observed that glia are normally involved only in pathologic pain processes [19].

The classical model of central sensitization did not include glial influence, but current evidence has shown that glial activation is intimately involved in the central sensitization process.

Part of the mechanism responsible for enhancing glial-mediated central sensitization is the release of the neurotransmitter nitric oxide, prostaglandins, and excitatory amino acids such as glutamate that have been linked to the development of central sensitization in the classic model [37]. A central synaptic feedback loop has been described that involves the second-order neurons and the central terminals of the nociceptors. Now, a similar feedback loop is described between the glia and the central synaptic neurons that would further affect central sensitization.

Impact of central sensitization on orofacial pain and temporomandibular disorders

Myofascial pain

Myofascial pain probably represents a neurosensory disorder involving peripheral and centrally sensitized muscle nociceptors. There are many characteristics of the disorder that are best accounted for by equating the pain phenomena with a neurosensory pathophysiology. For example, the primary indication of myofascial pain is the characteristic radiation of the pain from the primary site of palpation to unrelated sites that can be in different dermatomes. This most likely occurs secondarily to central phenomena, including convergence and activation of adjacent second-order neurons, which would explain the expansion of the receptive field, the lowering of the threshold to stimulation, and the allodynia associated with active trigger points.

Simons proposed a central mechanism for the development of the disorder [12,29–31]. He postulated that the muscle nociceptors, when activated by peripheral injury, released substance P, which would diffuse and spread between segments of the spinal cord to activate other adjacent nociceptors and second-order neurons. As we now understand central sensitization, there are many neurotransmitters and ion channels that become involved in the central sensitization process in addition to glial activation (Fig. 6). The ultimate result is activation of the NMDA receptors on the second-order neurons. When the NMDA receptor is activated, the pain becomes modulated primarily in the CNS and is only partially affected by peripheral mechanisms. In neuropathic pain conditions, NMDA activation connotes a more protracted change in pain. In neuropathic pain, these changes seem to be permanently persistent or at least of long duration. Central sensitization has also been associated with migraine. This situation does not typically have an enduring impact on migraine because the headache tends to resolve within hours. Timely treatment of the migraine can stop the sensitization, and the headache will resolve, or if left untreated, will resolve by itself. Therefore, the sensitization that occurs is of shorter duration. This may be the case with myofascial pain.

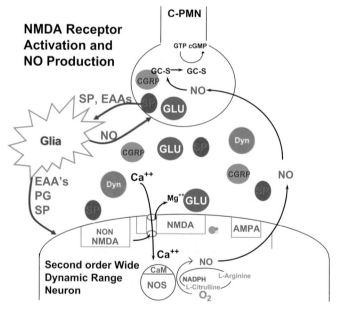

Fig. 6. Glial activation and central sensitization. Classic description of central sensitization involved central release neurotransmitters from nociceptors (C-PMN) that caused a cascade of events in the second-order neuron, including activation of the NMDA receptor and opening of its ion channel, allowing calcium to flow into the wide dynamic range neurons. The calcium interacts with the calmodulin protein complex, nitric oxide synthetase, and L-arginine to form nitric oxide (NO). NO diffuses out of the postsynaptic neuron and stimulates further release of excitatory amino acids (EAAs) and neurokinins from the presynaptic buton to continue the process. This process is understood to be enhanced by a similar response in the glial cells (glial activation).

Although the focus of this article is on central sensitization, peripheral sensitization needs to be considered as a component leading to central changes. If myofascial pain is a disorder with characteristics of peripheral and central sensitization, the other phenomena of myofascial pain become more understandable. For example, the trigger point may represent peripheral sensitization of muscle nociceptors. A component of peripheral sensitization is the activation of nociceptors that release neurotransmitters such as substance P, calcitonin gene related peptide (CGRP), and prostaglandins. These neurotransmitters cause a localized inflammatory reaction by acting on neurokinin and prostaglandin receptors on the nociceptors and on the blood vessels resulting in the expansion of the blood vessels and plasma extravasation (swelling = taut bands), increased pain with palpation (local allodynia and twitch response) at the site neurotransmitter release, and expansion of the pain into the area immediately around the site (static mechanical allodynia = decreased threshold to palpation resulting in twitch response). The dorsal horn reflex causes muscle tightening when the nociceptors relay pain to the dorsal horn. These mechanisms are consistent with mechanism of peripheral sensitization in neuropathic pain. The action of trigger point injections also would be consistent with peripheral neurosensory mechanisms when myofascial pain is viewed as a neurosensory disorder. Injecting a local anesthetic would block sodium channels in the pain fibers, stopping the release of neurotransmitters peripherally and centrally. The net effect of this would be to decrease the local neurogenic inflammatory response. Heating the area, stretching the muscle fibers, and the irritation by dry needling would increase the blood flow to the area, diluting or washing out the neurotransmitters and eventually decreasing the neurogenic inflammation. Centrally, these effects decrease the release of neurotransmitters that are responsible for the central sensitization that is characterized by expansion of the peripheral receptive field and autonomic activation through parasympathetic fiber release of norepinephrine.

Temporomandibular joint pain

Pain of the temporomandibular joint (TMJ) joint is commonly associated with redness and swelling and allodynia of the skin over the joint. These reactions are modulated by release of peripheral neurotransmitters in the joint space, causing peripheral sensitization. Occasionally, an inflamed joint continues to be painful despite appropriate treatment aimed at decreasing joint inflammation and pain. In some patients, attempting to quell the joint inflammation with intracapsular injections can be met with a significant increase rather than a decrease in pain. This reaction may be seen in patients who have had long-standing TMJ inflammation subsequent to trauma or surgery. This reaction is difficult to manage with traditional conservative TMJ therapy. The clinician may begin to suspect that a centralized neuropathy has developed in the joint. These joints may not respond to local anesthetic injections, and, if epinephrine is injected with the local anesthetic, the pain can become significantly worse, suggesting that sympathetically mediated pain has developed. Often, these patients are recommended to have another surgery to try to correct what is thought to be a musculoskeletal problem but which is a peripheral or central neuropathy. Temporomandibular joints can develop peripheral and centralized neuropathy, and once this occurs, the treatment needs to focus on the types of treatment used in neuropathic pain, such as antiseizure medications, tricyclic antidepressants, narcotics, and sympathetic ganglion blocks to evaluate for sympathetically mediated pain.

Neurovascular disorders

Neurovascular disorders relate primarily to headaches. Until recently, the "science" of headache disorders did not try to equate them with known mechanisms of central neurophysiology. Burstein [2,3,16,32] published several articles in the late 1990s that showed that migraine and other headache disorders were affected by the same central pathophysiology as neuropathic pain. The mechanisms of central sensitization made some of the characteristics of migraine more understandable, such as the lack of response to analgesics and triptans, if they are taken too late in the development of the headache attack. Additionally, the development of central sensitization causes static and dynamic mechanical allodynia of the head and neck, including the masticatory and cervical muscles. It is not uncommon for a patient to report to an OFP clinician that they get moderate to severe jaw and neck pain with a headache. When a patient is seen during one of these attacks, administration of a triptan or DHE-45 can stop the attack and relieve the jaw and neck pain within minutes. The clinician needs to differentiate between jaw and neck pain due to secondary or central sensitization associated with headache and headache due to painful TMJ and muscle inputs into the CNS that result in headache. In the first case, treating the headache relieves the muscle pain; in the last case, treating the muscle pain can relieve the headache.

Neuropathic pain

Neuropathic pain is commonly seen in the orofacial region. It may develop as a consequence of trauma, simple dental treatment, extractions, endodontic treatment, oral surgery, implants, or orthognathic surgery. The development of a neuropathy does not imply improper or poor treatment. It is not understood why some dental patients develop neuropathies when most do not, even in the face of fairly severe neurotrauma that can occur in everyday general dentistry. Researchers are beginning to suspect that there is a genetic diathesis due to variables such as receptor polymorphism that may predispose someone to develop a neuropathy [6].

Neuropathic pain in the oral environment due to central sensitization is characterized by chronic aching and burning pain that is persistent over a 24-hour period but which may fluctuate in intensity during this time. The distinguishing characteristic of centralized neuropathic pain is the lack of response to a topical, local, or regional anesthetic. Neurosensory testing may find that the painful area has pin-prick hyperalgesia and dynamic mechanical allodynia. These neurosensory responses are mediated by central sensitization and A-β fiber stimulation. The classical dental term for this oral neuropathy is "atypical odontalgia" [10,11]. Marbach, in the 1990s, suggested that they were phantom tooth pains [40]. Neither of these terms indicates a mechanism behind the pain. In reviewing the characteristics of these two conditions, it becomes apparent that both are describing peripheral and central neuropathies. A more useful title should reference the likely mechanism underpinning the condition. If the tooth pain is blockable and is characterized by static mechanical allodynia, it is a chronic peripheral neuropathy. If the tooth pain is not blockable and is characterized by dynamic mechanical allodynia or pinprick hyperalgesia, it is a chronic centralized neuropathy [9]. Treatment of these conditions differs, and it is important to distinguish whether the pain is due to peripheral sensitization or central sensitization.

Summary

The orofacial pain clinician must understand the difference between peripheral and central mechanisms of pain. Particularly, one has to understand the process of central sensitization as it relates to the various orofacial pain conditions to understand orofacial pain. Understanding leads to more effective treatment.

References

[1] Beecher HK. Relationship of significance of wound to pain experienced. JAMA 1956;161: 1609–13.
[2] Burstein R. Deconstructing migraine headache into peripheral and central sensitization. Pain 2001;89:107–10.
[3] Burstein R, Cutrer MF, Yarnitsky D. The development of cutaneous allodynia during a migraine attack clinical evidence for the sequential recruitment of spinal and supraspinal nociceptive neurons in migraine. Brain 2000;123:1703–9.
[4] Chong MS, Woolf Clifford J, Haque NS, et al. Axonal regeneration from injured dorsal roots into the spinal cord of adult rats. J Comp Neurol 1999;410:42–54.
[5] Colburn RW, DeLeo JA. The effect of perineural colchicine on nerve injury-induced spinal glial activation and neuropathic pain behavior. Brain Res Bull 1999;49:419–27.
[6] Diatchenko L, Slade GD, Nackley AG, et al. Genetic basis for individual variations in pain perception and the development of a chronic pain condition. Hum Mol Genet 2005;14: 135–43.
[7] Fields HL. Pain. New York: McGraw-Hill Book Company; 1987.

[8] Fields HL, Basbaum A. Central nervous system mechanisms of pain modulation. In: Wall P, Melzack R, editors. Textbook of pain. London: Churchill Livingstone; 1999. p. 309–29.

[9] Fields HL, Rowbotham M, Baron R. Postherpetic neuralgia: irritable nociceptors and deafferentation. Neurobiol Dis 1998;5:209–27.

[10] Graff-Radford SB, Solberg WK. Atypical odontalgia. CDA J 1986;14:27–32.

[11] Graff-Radford SB, Solberg WK. Atypical odontalgia. J Craniomandib Disord Facial Oral Pain 1992;6:260–5.

[12] Hong CZ, Simons DG. Pathophysiologic and electrophysiologic mechanisms of myofascial trigger points. Arch Phys Med Rehabil 1998;79:863–72.

[13] Inagaki N, Fukui H, Ito S, et al. Single type-2 astrocytes show multiple independent sites of Ca2+ signaling in response to histamine. Proc Natl Acad Sci USA 1991;88:4215–9.

[14] Jacobsen PB, Butler RW. Relation of cognitive coping and catastrophizing to acute pain and analgesic use following breast cancer surgery. J Behav Med 1996;19:17–29.

[15] Koller H, Thiem K, Siebler M. Tumour necrosis factor-alpha increases intracellular Ca2+ and induces a depolarization in cultured astroglial cells. Brain 1996;119:2021–7.

[16] Malick A, Burstein R. Peripheral and central sensitization during migraine. Funct Neurol 2000;15(Suppl 3):28–35.

[17] Mao J, Price D, Hayes R, Lu J, et al. Intrathecal treatment with dextrorphan or ketamine potently reduces pain-related behaviors in rad model of peripheral monoeneuropathy. Brain Res 1993;605:164–8.

[18] McMahon SB, Koltzenburg M. Silent afferents and visceral pain. In: Fields HL, Liebeskind JC, editors. Pharmacological approaches to the treatment of chronic pain: new concepts and critical issues. Seattle (WA): IASP Press; 1994. p. 11–30.

[19] Meller ST, Dykstra C, Grzybycki D, et al. The possible role of glia in nociceptive processing and hyperalgesia in the spinal cord of the rat. Neuropharmacology 1994;33:1471–8.

[20] Melzack R, Wall PD. Pain mechanisms: a new theory. Science 1965;150:971–9.

[21] Meredith PJ, Strong J, Feeney JA. The relationship of adult attachment to emotion, catastrophizing, control, threshold and tolerance, in experimentally-induced pain. Pain 2006; 120:44–52.

[22] Noguchi K, Kawai Y, Fukuoka T, et al. Substance P induced by peripheral nerve injury in primary afferent sensory neurons and its effect on dorsal column nucleus neurons. J Neurosci 1995;15:7633–43.

[23] Olesen J. The international classification of headache disorders. Cephalalgia 2004; 24(Suppl 1):133.

[24] Olszewski J. On the anatomical and functional organization of the trigeminal nucleus. J Comp Neurol 1950;92:401–13.

[25] Palma C, Minghetti L, Astolfi M, et al. Functional characterization of substance P receptors on cultured human spinal cord astrocytes: synergism of substance P with cytokines in inducing interleukin-6 and prostaglandin E2 production. Glia 1997;21:183–93.

[26] Schmidt R, Schmelz M, Forster C, et al. Novel classes of responsive and unresponsive C nociceptors in human skin. J Neurosci 1995;15:333–41.

[27] Schmidt RF, Schaible HG, MeBlinger K, et al. Silent and active nociceptors: structure, functions, and clinical implication. In: Gebhart GF, Hammond DL, Jensen TS, editors. Proceedings of the 7th World Congress on Pain. Seattle (WA): IASP Press; 1994. p. 213–50.

[28] Shao Y, McCarthy KD. Plasticity of astrocytes. Glia 1994;11:147–55.

[29] Simons DG. The nature of myofascial trigger points. Clin J Pain 1995;11:83–4.

[30] Simons DG. Neurophysiological basis of pain caused by trigger points. J Am Pain Soc 1994; 3:17–9.

[31] Simons DG. Travell & Simons' myofascial pain and dysfunction: the trigger point manual. Baltimore (MD): Williams & Wilkins; 1999.

[32] Strassman AM, Raymond SA, Burstein R. Sensitization of meningeal sensory neurons and the origin of headaches. Nature 1996;384:560–4.

[33] Sugimoto T, Bennett GJ, Kajander K. Transsynaptic degeneration in the superficial dorsal horn after sciatic nerve injury: effects of a chronic constriction injury, transection, and strychnine. Pain 1990;42:201–13.

[34] Sweitzer SM, Colburn RW, Rutkowski M, et al. Acute peripheral inflammation induces moderate glial activation and spinal IL-1beta expression that correlates with pain behavior in the rat. Brain Res 1999;829:209–21.

[35] Thompson S, Woolf CJ, Sivilotti L. Small caliber afferents produce a heterosynaptic facilitation of the synaptic responses evoked by primary afferent A fibres in the neonatal rat spinal cord in vitro. J Neurophysiol 1993;69:2116–28.

[36] Torebjork HI, Lundberg LE, LaMotte RH. Central changes in processing of mechanoreceptive input in capsaicin-induced secondary hyperalgesia in humans. J Physiol 1992;448: 765–80.

[37] Watkins LR, Maier SF. The pain of being sick: implications of immune-to-brain communication for understanding pain. Annu Rev Psychol 2000;51:29–57.

[38] Wilcox GL. Spinal mediators of nociceptive neurotransmission and hyperalgesia. J Am Pain Soc 1993;2:265–75.

[39] Woolf CJ. Molecular signals responsible for the reorganization of the synaptic circuitry of the dorsal horn after peripheral nerve injury: the mechanisms of tactile allodynia. In: Barsook D, editor. Molecular neurobiology of pain. Seattle (WA): IASP Press; 1997. p. 171–200.

[40] Marbach JJ. Is phantom tooth pain a deafferentation (neuropathic) syndrome? Part 1: evidence derived from pathophysiology and treatment. Oral Surg Oral Med Oral Pathol 1993;75(1):95–105.

ELSEVIER
SAUNDERS

THE DENTAL
CLINICS
OF NORTH AMERICA

Dent Clin N Am 51 (2007) 61–83

Myogenous Temporomandibular Disorders: Diagnostic and Management Considerations

James Fricton, DDS, MS

*Diagnostic and Biological Sciences, University of Minnesota School of Dentistry,
6-320 Moos, Minneapolis, MN 55455, USA*

Myogenous temporomandibular disorders (or masticatory myalgia) are characterized by pain and dysfunction that arise from pathologic and functional processes in the masticatory muscles. There are several distinct muscle disorder subtypes in the masticatory system, including myofascial pain, myositis, muscle spasm, and muscle contracture (Box 1) [1].

Myofascial pain is the most common muscle pain disorder [2]. It is an acute to chronic condition that includes the presence of regional pain associated with tender areas, called trigger points (TrPs), which are expressed in taut bands of skeletal muscles, tendons, or ligaments. Although the pain occurs most often in the region over the TrP, pain can be referred to areas distant from the TrPs (eg, temporalis referring to the frontal area and masseter referring into the ear or the posterior teeth). Often, reproducible duplication of pain complaints with specific palpation of the tender area is diagnostic.

Myositis is an acute condition with localized or generalized inflammation of the muscle and connective tissue, and associated pain and swelling overlying the muscle. Most areas in the muscle are tender, with pain in active range of motion. Usually, the inflammation is due to local causes, such as overuse, excessive stretch, drug use (ie, Ecstasy), local infection from pericoronitis, trauma, or cellulitis. It also is termed delayed-onset muscle soreness in cases of acute overuse.

Muscle spasm also is an acute disorder that is characterized by a brief involuntary tonic contraction of a muscle. It can occur as a result of overstretching of a previously weakened muscle; protective splinting of an injury; as a centrally mediated phenomenon, such as Compazine-induced

E-mail address: frict001@umn.edu

0011-8532/07/$ - see front matter © 2007 Elsevier Inc. All rights reserved.
doi:10.1016/j.cden.2006.10.002   *dental.theclinics.com*

Box 1. Diagnostic criteria for masticatory myalgia disorders

Myofascial pain: repetitive strain
Dull aching pain in the jaw, face, ear, temples, or forehead
Localized tenderness (TrPs) in specific taut muscle bands with
    tenderness on the same side as the pain. See Fig. 1 for sites
    and referral patterns.
Duplicate the pain with palpation of the tender TrPs

Muscle spasm: acute overuse
Acute onset of pain in the jaw, face, ear, or temples at rest and
    in function
Moderate to severe acute limited range of motion due to
    continuous muscle contraction. In lateral pterygoid spasm, the
    jaw has a shift to one side with subsequent acute malocclusion
    that is reversible.
Generalized tenderness of the muscle

Myositis: injury or infection
Pain, usually continuous, in a localized muscle area following
    injury or infection that is increased with mandibular
    movement.
Diffuse tenderness over the entire muscle area involved
Moderate to severe limited range of motion
Swelling over muscle area involved

Muscle contracture: muscle fibrosis
Gross limited range of mandibular motion
Unyielding firmness on passive stretch (hard end feel)
Little or no pain unless the involved muscle is forced to
    lengthen
Long-term history of trauma, infection, or long period of disuse
    and limited range of motion

---

spasm of the lateral pterygoid muscle; or overuse of a muscle. A muscle in spasm is acutely shortened, and painful, with limited range of motion. Lateral pterygoid spasm on one side also can cause a shift of the occlusion to the contralateral side.

Muscle contracture is a chronic condition that is characterized by continuous gross shortening of the muscle with significant limited range of motion. It can begin because of factors such as trauma, infection, or prolonged hypomobility. If the muscle is maintained in a shortened state, muscular fibrosis and contracture may develop over several months. Often, pain can be minimal in the process from protection of the muscle.

Clinical presentation

The major characteristics of masticatory myalgia include pain, muscle tenderness, limited range of motion, and other symptoms, such as fatigability, stiffness, and subjective weakness. Comorbid conditions and complicating factors also are common and are discussed. Each is discussed for the different subtypes.

Pain

The common sites of pain in the masticatory system include jaw pain; facial pain; temple, frontal, or occipital headaches; preauricular pain; earache; and neck pain. Often, the pain is a constant steady dull ache that fluctuates in intensity and can be acute to chronic. The duration may vary from hours to days.

Muscle tenderness

In myofascial pain (MFP), the tenderness, termed trigger points (TrPs), is deep, localized, and about 2–5 mm in diameter. It is located in a taut band of skeletal muscle and is associated with consistent patterns of pain referral, whereas in myositis and muscle spasm, the tenderness can be generalized over the whole muscle. Myofascial TrPs are common and may be active or latent. Active TrPs are hypersensitive and display continuous pain in the zone of reference that can be altered with specific palpation. Latent TrPs display only hypersensitivity with no continuous pain. This localized tenderness is a reliable indicator of the presence and severity of MFP with manual palpation and pressure algometers [3–5]; however, the presence of taut bands seems to be a characteristic of skeletal muscles in all subjects, regardless of the presence of MFP. Palpating the active TrP with sustained deep, single-finger pressure on the taut band elicits an alteration of the pain (intensification or reduction) in the zone of reference (area of pain complaint) or causes radiation of the pain toward the zone of reference. This can occur immediately or be delayed a few seconds. The pattern of referral is reproducible and consistent with patterns of other patients who have similar TrPs (Fig. 1). This enables a clinician to use the zone of reference as a guide to locate the TrP for purposes of treatment.

Limited range of motion

In myofascial pain, limitation in range of motion may be slight (10%–20%) and unrelated to joint restriction, whereas in muscle spasm, myositis, and contracture, it may be gross limitation ($\geq 50\%$). A study of jaw range of motion in patients who had MFP and no joint abnormalities demonstrated a slightly diminished range of 35 to 45 mm ($\sim 10\%$ compared with normals) and pain in full range of motion. This is considerably less limitation than was found with joint locking that is due to a temporomandibular joint

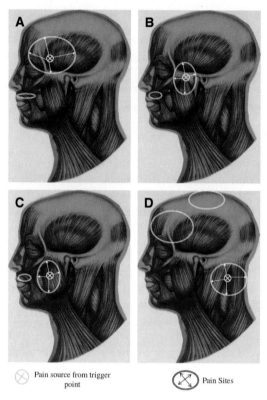

Fig. 1. Trigger points in myofascial pain associated with local or distant patterns of pain referral in the jaw, head, and neck, as indicated by the white circles. (*A*) The pain source is the anterior temporalis trigger point. The pain sites include temple, frontal, and retro-orbital headaches and pain in the maxillary anterior teeth. These muscles are activated by clenching, bruxism, and other oral parafunctional habits. (*B*) The pain source is the deep masseter trigger point. The pain sites include preauricular pain, earaches, and pain in the maxillary posterior teeth. These muscles also are activated by clenching, bruxism, and other oral parafunctional habits. (*C*) The pain source is the middle masseter trigger point. The pain sites include temple, frontal, and retro-orbital headaches and pain in the maxillary anterior teeth. These muscles also are activated by clenching, bruxism, and other oral parafunctional habits. (*D*) The pain source is the splenius capitus trigger point in the posterior cervical area. The pain sites include posterior cervical region, vertex headache, and frontal headaches. These muscles also are activated by clenching and forward head posture.

(TMJ) internal derangement (20–35 mm) [6]. This restriction may perpetuate the TrP and develop other TrPs in the same muscle and agonist muscles. This can cause multiple TrPs with overlapping areas of pain referral and changes in pain patterns as TrPs are inactivated. Other causes of diminished mandibular opening, which include structural disorders of the TMJ (eg, ankylosis, internal derangements, coronoid hypertrophy, gross osteoarthritis), must be ruled out with radiographs and clinical examination.

Other symptoms

Other associated signs and symptoms may occur, including increased fatigability, stiffness, subjective weakness, and pain in movement; otologic symptoms, including dizziness, tinnitus, and plugged ears; paresthesias, including numb feelings, decreased sensation, and tingling; and dermatographia, including increased redness of the skin upon palpation or rolling. The affected muscles also may display an increased fatigability, stiffness, subjective weakness, pain in movement, and slight restricted range of motion that is unrelated to joint restriction [1,7–10]. The muscles are painful when stretched, which causes the patient to protect the muscle through poor posture and sustained contraction [11]. No neurologic deficits are associated with muscle pain disorders unless a nerve entrapment syndrome with weakness and diminished sensation coincides with the muscle tightness. Although routine clinical electromyographic (EMG) studies show no significant abnormalities associated with TrPs, some specialized EMG studies reveal differences [12–15]. The consistency or firmness of soft tissues over the TrPs has been found to be more than adjacent muscles [16,17]. Skin overlying the TrPs in the masseter muscle seems to be warmer as measured by infrared emission [18,19].

Comorbid conditions and complicating factors

There are many comorbid conditions to myogenous temporomandibular disorder (TMD) pain that reflect common etiologic factors and mechanisms of pain. In most recent classifications, the regional pain that is found with MFP is distinguished from the widespread muscular pain that is associated with fibromyalgia (FM). These two disorders have similar characteristics and may represent two ends of a continuous spectrum. For example, as Simons [20] pointed out, 16 of the 18 tender point sites in FM lie at well-known TrP sites. Many of the clinical characteristics of FM, such as fatigue, morning stiffness, and sleep disorders, also can accompany MFP. Bennett [21] compared these two disorders and concluded that they are two distinct disorders that may have a similar underlying pathophysiology. The clinical significance of distinguishing between them lies in the more common centrally generated contributing factors in FM (sleep disorders, depression, stress) versus the more common regional contributing factors in MFP (trauma, posture and muscle tension habits) as well as the better prognosis in treatment of MFP as compared with FM.

Other comorbid conditions that often have been cited to accompany myogenous disorders include joint disk displacement and osteoarthritis, malocclusion and functional occlusal dysfunction, connective tissue diseases, neuropathic pain disorders, migraine and tension-type headaches, gastrointestinal disorders, and hypothyroidism. The underlying mechanism for the coexistence of these comorbid conditions is not clear. Common underlying central and peripheral mechanisms and etiologies may play a role.

Furthermore, many associated behavioral and psychosocial factors can accompany the chronic pain that is associated with myogenous disorders. Behavioral factors include muscle tension, oral parafunctional, and maladaptive postural habits; psychological factors include frustration, anxiety, and depression; secondary gain from pain behaviors include pain verbalization and avoidance of activities, medication dependencies, and sleep disturbance.

Etiology and epidemiology

Prevalence

Muscle pain disorders are the most common cause of persistent pain in the head and neck; they affect about 50% of a population that has chronic head and neck pain population [22]. They also are a common cause of pain in the general population, with 20% to 50% having the disorder; about 6% have symptoms that are severe enough to warrant treatment [23,24].

Etiologic factors

Onset factors for myogenous TMDs include direct or indirect macrotrauma to the muscle and repetitive strain activities [9]. Macrotraumatic events include a direct blow to the jaw, and opening the mouth too wide or for too long a period during activities, such as dental visits, eating, yawning, and sexual activity. In some cases, indirect trauma that is due to a whiplash-type of injury may initiate muscle pain. Local infection and trauma may cause myositis and lead to muscle contracture if not resolved. Occupational and repetitive strain injury may cause myofascial pain and muscle spasm if acute. Sleep disturbance and nocturnal habits can contribute to myofascial pain.

Oral parafunctional muscle tension–producing habits, such as teeth clenching, jaw thrusting, gum chewing, and jaw tensing can add repetitive strain to the masticatory muscles and cause tenderness and pain. Postural strain that is caused by a forward head posture, increased cervical or lumbar lordosis, some occlusal abnormalities, and poor positioning of the head or tongue also have been implicated in myofascial pain. Psychosocial stressors, such as relationship conflicts, monetary problems, feeling hurried or overscheduled, or poor pacing skills can play an indirect role.

Pathophysiology and mechanisms

Because there are no specific anatomic changes with myogenous pain, no conclusive mechanisms are identified in cases of non-traumatic etiology.

Thus, several processes may explain the development and persistence of masticatory myogenous pain [9].

Repetitive strain hypotheses

Repetitive strain from oral parafunctional habits contribute to localized progressive increases in oxidative metabolism and depleted energy supply (decrease in the levels of ATP, ADP, and phosphoryl creatine; abnormal tissue oxygenation). These changes result in the muscle nociception, particularly with type I muscle fiber types associated with static muscle tone and posture. Tenderness and pain in the muscle involve types III and IV muscle nociceptors that are activated by noxious substances, such as potassium, histamine, kinins, or prostaglandins, which are released locally and cause tenderness.

Neurophysiologic hypothesis

Tonic muscular hyperactivity may be a normal protective adaptation to pain instead of its cause. Phasic modulation of excitatory and inhibitory interneurons that are supplied by high-threshold sensory afferents may be involved.

Central hypotheses

Convergence of multiple afferent inputs from the muscle and other visceral and somatic structures in the lamina I or V of the dorsal horn on the way to the cortex can result in perception of local and referred pain [10].

Central biasing mechanism

Multiple peripheral and central factors may inhibit or facilitate central input through modulatory influence of the brain stem. This may explain the diverse factors that can exacerbate or alleviate the pain, such as stress, repetitive strain, poor posture, relaxation, medications, temperature change, massage, local anesthetic injections, and electrical stimulation.

Diagnostic tests

Typically, the diagnoses of masticatory myalgia are determined through clinical diagnostic criteria (see Box 1); however, some diagnostic strategies can be helpful. In myofascial pain, injections of local anesthetic into the active TrP reduce or eliminate the referred pain and the tenderness. Generally, blood and urine studies are normal unless caused by a concomitant disorder. Imaging studies, including radiographs and MRI, are normal. Routine clinical EMG studies are abnormal in muscle spasm only. Some specialized EMG studies (twitch response) reveal differences in myofascial pain. Pain questionnaires, such as the Chronic Pain Battery and TMJ Scale, may identify contributing factors, including emotional issues, somatization, secondary gain, and disability.

Treatment

Simple to complex

Myogenous pain can range from simple cases with transient single muscle syndromes, to complex cases that involve multiple muscles and many interrelating contributing factors. Many investigators have found success in treating myogenous pain using a wide variety of techniques, such as exercise, TrP injections, vapocoolant spray and stretch, transcutaneous electrical nerve stimulation, biofeedback, posture correction, tricyclic antidepressants, muscle relaxants and other medications, and addressing perpetuating factors [12,23–25]. The difficulty in management lies in the critical need to match the level of complexity of the management program with the complexity of the patient. Failure to address the entire problem, including all involved muscles, concomitant diagnoses, and contributing factors, may lead to failure to resolve the pain and perpetuation of the pain.

Although no controlled studies have examined the progression of chronic pain syndromes, results from clinical studies reveal that many patients who have muscle pain have seen many clinicians, or received numerous medications and multiple other singular treatments for years without more than temporary improvement. In one study of 164 patients who had muscle pain, the mean duration of pain was 5.8 years for men and 6.9 years for women, with a mean of 4.5 clinicians seen [23]. In another study of 102 consecutive patients who had TMJ and craniofacial pain (59.8% had muscle pain), the mean duration of pain was 6.0 years, with 28.8 previous treatment sessions, 5.1 previous doctors, and 6.4 previous medications [26].

These and other studies of chronic pain suggest that regardless of the pathogenesis of muscular pain, a major characteristic of some of these patients is the failure of traditional approaches to resolve the problem. Each clinician who is confronted with a patient who has muscle pain needs to recognize and address the whole problem to maximize the potential for a successful outcome. Treating only those patients whose complexity matches the treatment strategy that is available to the clinician can improve success. Typically, simple cases with minimal behavioral and psychosocial involvement can be managed by a single clinician with self care as the initial focus of care (Box 2). Complex patients should be managed within an interdisciplinary pain clinic setting that uses a team of clinicians to address different aspects of the problem in a concerted fashion (Box 3). Fig. 2 presents a hierarchy of treatment strategies, depending on whether the condition is acute, simple, or complex.

The short-term goal is to restore the muscle to normal length, posture, and full joint range of motion with exercises and TrP therapy (Box 4). This is followed long term with a regular muscle stretching, postural, and strengthening exercise program as well as control of contributing factors. Long-term control of pain depends on patient education, self-responsibility,

---

Box 2. Palliative self-care program for acute episodes of masticatory myalgia

Eat a soft diet and avoid caffeine.
Keep your tongue up and resting gently on the palate. Keep teeth apart as the rest position of the jaw.
Chew on both sides at the same time or alternate sides to minimize strain to muscles.
Avoid oral parafunctional habits, such as clenching and grinding the teeth, jaw tensing, or gum chewing.
Avoid excessive or prolonged opening of mouth.
Avoid stomaching sleeping to minimize strain to the jaw during sleep.
Use over-the-counter analgesics or nonsteroidal anti-inflammatory drugs as needed for pain.
Use heat or ice over the tender muscles.

---

and development of long-term doctor–patient relationships. This often requires shifting the paradigms that are implicit in patient care (Table 1). Often, the difficulty in long-term management lies not in treating the TrPs, but rather in the complex task of changing the identified contributing factors, because they can be integrally related to the patient's attitudes, lifestyles, and social and physical environment. Interdisciplinary teams integrate various health professionals in a supportive environment to accomplish long-term treatment of illness and modification of these contributing factors

---

Box 3. Fulfilling any one of these criteria may suggest that this patient is complex and may require the use of the team to address the contributing factors and increase the prognosis

Persistent pain (daily or regular) that is longer than 6 months in duration
Significant lifestyle disturbances, such as loss of work, social activities, or home activities
High use of past health care, including medications for problem or related problems
Emotional difficulties related to problem, including depression, anxiety, or anger
Daily oral habits, such as clenching or grinding of the teeth
Significant stressful life events, such as pacing problems, divorce, or recent death in family

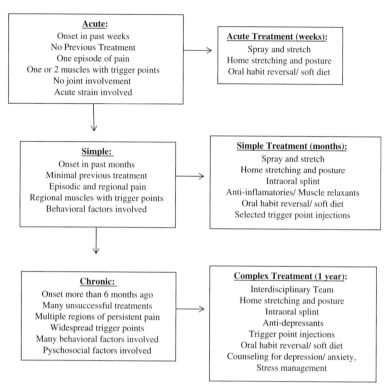

Fig. 2. Treatment strategies differ depending on whether the condition is acute, simple, and complex.

(Box 4). Many approaches, such as habit reversal techniques, biofeedback, and stress management have been used to achieve this result within a team approach (Box 5).

Management follows these goals and includes self-care, muscle exercises, muscle therapy, and reducing all contributing factors; it is directed at rehabilitating the muscle to improving range of motion, reducing tenderness, and reducing or eliminating contributing factors. Muscle rehabilitation is focused on exercise to improve range of motion, relaxation, and strength of the muscle. Reduction of contributing factors includes reducing biomechanical strain to the muscles from oral parafunctional habits, such as clenching, gum chewing, and other repetitive strain activities. In addition, improved posture of the head, neck, and tongue reduces sustained muscle activity and encourages healing. Reducing tenderness can be accomplished by inhibiting peripheral neural input through various treatment modalities, such as cold, heat, analgesic medications, massage, muscle injections, and transcutaneous electrical nerve stimulation. Reducing central modulating factors, include management of contributing factors (eg, improving stress, sleep, anxiety, and depression).

Box 4. Short- and long-term goals in treatment of myofascial pain

Short-term goals
Reduce pain
Restore muscle to normal length with full joint range of motion
Restore muscle to normal posture
Reduce sustained muscle activity

Long-term goals
Restore normal lifestyle activities
Reduce contributing factors
Regular stretching, postural, and conditioning exercises
Proper use of muscles

Self-care

Most acute recent symptoms are self-limited and resolve with minimal intervention. Initial treatment should be a self-care program to reduce repetitive strain of the masticatory system and encourage relaxation and healing of the muscles (see Box 2).

This strategy includes jaw range of motion and posture exercises (Fig. 3), oral habit change, and protective gentle use of the jaw. Most patients respond well to self-care in 4 to 6 weeks; if not, further assessment and treatment are indicated.

Orthopedic intraoral splints

These can encourage relaxation of the muscles, alter muscular recruitment patterns, and reduce oral habits. Stabilization splints allow passive protection of the jaw and reduction of oral habits as the result of the flat passive occlusal surface on mandibular or maxillary teeth. Mandibular splints can be smaller and result in higher patient satisfaction in some cases. They should be

Table 1
Shifting the doctor-patient paradigms involves each member of the team following the same concepts by conveying the same messages implicit in their dialogue with the patient

Concept	Statement
Self-responsibility	You have more influence on your problem than we do
Self-care	You will need to make daily changes to improve your condition
Education	We can teach you how to make the changes
Long-term change	It will take at least 6 months for the changes to have an effect
Doctor-patient relationship	We will support you as you make the changes
Patient motivation	Do you want to make the changes?

Box 5. Protocol checklist for managing masticatory and cervical myalgia pain

Evaluation
Identify masticatory and cervical muscles involved
Identify each area of pain
    Frequency
    Duration
    Intensity
Identify contributing factors
    Direct macrotrauma (eg, blow to jaw)
    Indirect macrotrauma (eg, whiplash injuries)
    Postural habits in the neck and shoulders (eg, phone bracing,
        shoulder shrugging, neck tensing)
    Oral parafunctional habits (eg, clenching and grinding
        of teeth)
    Dietary factors (eg, caffeine)
    Sleep disturbance
    Psychosocial stressors
    Anxiety and depression
Determine simple versus complex
    Simple: single clinician evaluation and treatment
    Complex: team evaluation including dentist, physical therapist
        or chiropractor, psychologist

Management
Acute care with palliative self-care
Simple case management with single clinician
    Self-care
    Splint
    Jaw exercises
    Vapocoolant spray or other modality with stretching
    Oral habit and muscle relaxation and posture instruction
Complex case management with the team
    Self care
    Splint
    Trigger point or muscle injections
    Medications (muscle relaxants and anti-inflammatory drugs
        as needed)
    Exercises with physical therapist
    Cognitive-behavioral therapy
    Counseling as needed

A   **B**

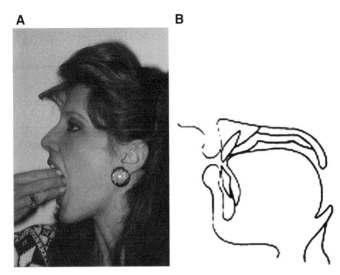

Fig. 3. (*A, B*) Jaw exercises. These jaw stretching exercises can be used for initial postural correction and range of motion restoration for masticatory myalgia. 1) Active stretching of the muscles increases the opening to the normal range and decreases the pain. The jaw should be stretched progressively slightly beyond the point of tightness and pain. Precautions should be made to avoid overstretching with acutely strained jaws or severe pain of the TMJ. Place one finger between your teeth for one minute. Rest and repeat. Then place two fingers between your teeth for one minute. Stretching can continue over weeks to months to achieve a three finger stretch. 2) Jaw relaxed with tongue up and teeth apart. Place the flat tip of the tongue gently on the palate (roof of the mouth) wherever it is most comfortable, while allowing the teeth to come apart and the jaw to be relaxed. The position of the tongue when you say "n" is often a comfortable position. Do not touch the teeth together at all during the day except occasionally; they touch lightly with swallowing.

adjusted to achieve mutually protected occlusion with bilateral balanced contact on all posterior teeth with the condyles in their most seated positions, with anterior guidance (lateral and protrusive) provided by the cuspids or incisors.

Anterior repositioning splints can be efficacious for concomitant joint problems with intermittent jaw locking with limited range of motion, especially upon awakening. They are recommended for short-term, part-time use, primarily during sleep, because they can cause occlusal changes if worn continuously or chronically.

Partial coverage splints may cause occlusal changes in some patients. Splints should cover all of the mandibular or maxillary teeth to prevent movement of uncovered teeth, with malocclusion.

Cognitive-behavioral therapy

Cognitive-behavioral therapy approaches can help to change maladaptive habits and behaviors that contribute to myalgia, such as jaw tensing, teeth clenching, neck and shoulder tensing, and teeth grinding. Although many simple habits are abandoned easily when the patient becomes aware of them, changing persistent habits requires a structured program that is facilitated by a clinician who is trained in behavioral strategies. Habits do not change themselves. Patients are responsible for initiating and maintaining behavior changes.

Habit reversal can be accomplished by becoming more aware of the habit, knowing how to correct it (ie, what to do with the teeth and tongue or neck and shoulders), and knowing why to correct it. Combining the patient's commitment to conscientious self-monitoring and the patient's focus upon the goal, habits will gradually change over several weeks time. Furthermore, correcting the habits such as clenching during the day will help to reduce them at night. This can be supplemented with additional behavioral strategies, such as biofeedback, meditation, stress management, or relaxation techniques as needed. It also is important to address poor pacing or hurrying that is related to a day that is overloaded with commitments. In addition, addressing other contributing factors such as depression, anxiety, sleep disorders, and emotional problems through behavioral and psychologic therapy or medications may be critical to success.

Muscle exercises

The most useful exercise techniques for muscle rehabilitation include muscle stretching, posture, strengthening, and relaxation exercises [12,24,25,27,28]. In patients who have muscle pain, a home program of active and passive muscle stretching exercises reduces the activity of muscle pain, whereas postural exercises reduce its susceptibility to reactivation of pain by physical strain (see Fig. 3). Strengthening and cardiovascular fitness exercises improve circulation, strength, and durability of the muscles. Relaxation exercise can help reduce repetitive tensing and strain of the muscles.

Evaluating the present range of motion of muscles is the first step in prescribing a set of exercises to follow. For example, in the head and neck, range of motion should be determined for the jaw and neck at the initial evaluation. A limited mandibular opening in the jaw indicates if there is any pain within the elevator muscles: temporalis, masseter, and medial pterygoid. If mandibular opening is measured as the interincisal distance, the maximum range of opening is generally between 42 mm and 60 mm or approximately three knuckles' width (nondominant hand). A mandibular opening in the masseter is approximately 30 mm to 40 mm or two knuckles' width. If contracture of masticatory muscles is present, the mandibular opening can be as limited as 10 mm to 20 mm. Other causes of diminished mandibular opening include structural disorders of the TMJ, such as ankylosis, internal derangements, and gross osteoarthritis.

Passive and active stretching of the muscles increases the opening to the normal range and decreases the pain. Passive stretching of the masticatory muscles during counterstimulation of the tender muscle can be accomplished through placing tongue blades between the incisors or placing gentle pressure between the incisors with the thumb and middle finger while the spray-and-stretch technique is accomplished. It must be emphasized to avoid rapid, jerky stretching or overstretching of the muscle to reduce potential injury to the muscle.

Postural exercises are designed to teach the patient mental reminders to hold the body in a balanced relaxed position and to use the body with positions that afford the best mechanical advantage. This includes static postural problems, such as unilateral short leg, small hemipelvis, occlusal discrepancies, and scoliosis, or functional postural habits (eg, forward head, jaw thrust, shoulder phone bracing, lumbar lifting). In a study of postural problems in 164 patients who had head and neck muscle pain, poor sitting/standing posture in 96%, forward head in 84.7%, rounded shoulders in 82.3%, lower tongue position in 67.7%, abnormal lordosis in 46.3%, scoliosis in 15.9%, and leg length discrepancy in 14.0% contributed to muscle pain [23]. In improving posture, specific skeletal conditions, such as structural asymmetry or degenerative joint changes need to be considered. In the masticatory system, the patient should be instructed to place the tongue gently on the roof of the mouth and keep the teeth slightly apart. In the cervical spine, a forward or lateral head posture must be corrected by guiding the chin in and the head vertex up. The shoulders fall back naturally if the thorax is positioned up and back with proper lumbar support. Patients need to be instructed in proper posture for each position— sitting, standing, and lying down—as well as in movements that are done repetitively throughout the day, such as lifting or turning the head to the side. Sleeping posture on the side or back is particularly important for patients who wake up with soreness.

Improved posture also is facilitated by regular physical exercise and conditioning. Patients need to be placed on a conditioning program to facilitate increased flexibility, aerobic capacity and strength. Exercise programs, such as yoga, an exercise class, regular running, walking, biking, or swimming improve the comfort, flexibility, endurance, and functional status of patients who have muscle pain [6].

Muscle therapy

Many methods have been suggested for providing repetitive stimulation to tender muscles. Massage, acupressure, and ultrasound provide noninvasive mechanical disruption to reduce tenderness. Moist heat applications, ice pack, vapocoolant spray, and diathermy provide skin and muscle temperature change as a form of counterstimulation. Transcutaneous electrical nerve stimulation, electroacupuncture, and direct current stimulation provide electric currents to stimulate the muscles and TrPs. Acupuncture or TrP injections of local anesthetic, corticosteroids, or saline cause direct mechanical or chemical alteration of TrPs; however, the two most common techniques for treating a muscle pain include the spray-and-stretch technique and TrP injections.

With the spray-and-stretch technique, an application of a vapocoolant spray, such as Fluori-Methane, over the muscle with simultaneous passive stretching can provide immediate reduction of pain, although lasting relief requires a full management program [3]. The technique involves directing a fine stream of vapocoolant spray from the finely calibrated nozzle toward the skin directly overlying the muscle with the TrP. A few sweeps of the spray is passed over the TrP and zone of reference before adding sufficient manual stretch to the muscle to elicit pain and discomfort. The muscle is put on a progressively increasing passive stretch while the jet stream of spray is directed at an acute angle 30 to 50 cm (1–1.5 feet) away. It is applied in one direction from the TrP toward its reference zone in slow even sweeps over adjacent parallel areas, at a rate of about 10 cm per second. This sequence can be repeated up to four times if the clinician warms the muscle with his or her hand or warm moist packs to prevent overcooling after each sequence. Frosting the skin and excessive sweeps should be avoided, because they may reduce the underlying skeletal muscle temperature, which tends to aggravate TrPs. The range of passive and active motion can be tested before and after spraying as an indication of responsiveness to therapy. Failure to reduce TrPs with spray and stretch may be due to (1) inability to secure full muscle length because of bone or joint abnormalities, muscle contracture, or the patient avoiding voluntary relaxation; (2) incorrect spray technique; or (3) failure to reduce perpetuating factors. If spray and stretch fails with repeated trials, direct needling with TrP injections may be effective.

TrP muscle injections also have been shown to reduce pain, increase range of motion, increase exercise tolerance, and increase circulation of muscles [4,5,13]. The pain relief may last from the duration of the anesthetic to many months, depending on the chronicity and severity of TrPs, and the degree of reducing perpetuating factors. Because the critical factor in relief is the mechanical disruption of the TrP by the needle, precision in needling the exact TrP and the intensity of pain during needling seem to be the major factors in TrP inactivation [14]. Generally, TrP injections with local anesthetic are more effective and comfortable than are dry needling or injecting other substances (eg, saline), although acupuncture may be helpful for patients who have chronic TrPs in multiple muscles. The effect of needling can be complemented with local anesthetics in concentrations that are less than those required for a nerve conduction block. This can markedly lengthen the relative refractory period of peripheral nerves and limit the maximum frequency of impulse conduction. Local anesthetics can be chosen for their duration, safety, and versatility; local anesthetics without vasoconstrictors are suggested.

Pharmacotherapy

Pharmacotherapy is a useful adjunct to initial treatment of muscle pain. The most commonly used medications for pain are classified as nonnarcotic analgesics (nonsteroidal anti-inflammatory drugs [NSAIDs]), narcotic analgesics, muscle relaxants, tranquilizers, sedatives, and antidepressants. Analgesics are used to allay pain, muscle relaxants and tranquilizers for anxiety, fear, and muscle tension; sedatives for enhancing sleep; and antidepressants for pain, depression, and enhancing sleep [15].

Randomized clinical trials on NSAIDs, such as ibuprofen or piroxicam, suggest that for myalgia, their short-term use for analgesic or anti-inflammatory effects can be effective as a supplement to overall management. Chronic, long-term use is cautioned against because of the long-term systemic and gastrointestinal effects; however, cyclooxygenase-2 inhibitors may prove to be safer NSAIDs for long-term use with less gastrointestinal toxicity. If some therapeutic result is not apparent after 7 to 10 days or if the patient develops any side effects, especially gastrointestinal symptoms, the medication should be discontinued.

For muscle pain, especially with stress and sleep disturbance, benzodiazepines, including diazepam and clonazepam, are effective [1]. Experience suggests that these are best used before bedtime to minimize sedation while awake. Cyclobenzaprine also was shown, in clinical trials of myalgia, to be efficacious in reducing pain and improving sleep [29,30]; it can be considered when a benzodiazepine has side effects. These medications, with or without NSAIDs, also can be considered for a 2- to 4-week trial with minimal habitual potential; however, long-term use has not been tested adequately.

Research on medications for masticatory myalgia, especially in patients with sleep disturbances, indicates that tricyclic antidepressants, such as amitriptyline/Elavil, have a significant impact on sleep disturbances, anxiety, and pain. As such, these medications can be used on a long-term basis in the appropriate case [31]. The side effects with amitriptyline can be significant, however, nortriptyline can be considered an analogous medication with fewer side effects. Typically, the dosage for either of these medications in patients who do not have depression is in the range of 25 to 75 mg at bedtime. The use of selective serotonin reuptake inhibitors has been suggested for depression and pain, but they may have the common side effect of increasing oral habits, muscle tension and potentially aggravating the pain.

For chronic pain conditions that are resistant to interventions, opioids can be considered. Tramadol has been shown to be effective in fibromyalgia; however, no randomized, controlled trial has evaluated the appropriateness of opioids in the long-term treatment of chronic orofacial pain. Because of their side effects, including constipation, sedation, potential for dose escalation, and the unknown effects with long-term use, chronic opioid use is indicated mainly for patients who have chronic intractable severe pain conditions that are refractory to rehabilitation treatments.

Despite the advantages of medications for pain disorders, there is an opportunity for problems to occur as a result of their misuse. These problems include chemical dependency, behavioral reinforcement of continuing pain, inhibition of endogenous pain relief mechanisms, rebound pain, side effects, and adverse effects from the use of polypharmaceuticals. For this reason, medication should be used with proper caution.

Control of contributing factors

One of the common causes of a lack of success in managing masticatory myalgia is failure to recognize and control contributing factors that may perpetuate muscle restriction and tension. Postural contributing factors, whether behavioral or biologic, perpetuate muscle pain if not corrected. In general, a muscle is more predisposed to developing problems if it is held in sustained contraction in the normal position, and, especially, if it is in an abnormally shortened position. Such a situation exists with structural skeletal problems, such as loss of posterior teeth, an excessive lordosis of the cervical spine, a unilateral short leg, or a small hemipelvis [6]. An occlusal imbalance can be corrected short term with an occlusal stabilization splint, also termed a flat plane or full coverage splint. Other postural factors that can be corrected include a foot lift for a unilateral leg length discrepancy, a pelvic lift for a small hemipelvis, and proper height of arm rests in chairs for short upper arms.

Behavioral factors that cause sustained muscle tension also can occur with habits such as cradling a phone between the head and shoulder; a laborer lifting at the waist with lumbar strain; a student studying with the head forward for hours at a time; or bruxism, clenching, gum-chewing, or other oral parafunctional habits. Correcting poor habits through education and long-term reinforcement is essential in preventing pain from returning. Biofeedback, meditation, hypnosis, stress management counseling, psychotherapy, antianxiety medications, antidepressants, and even placebos have been reported to be effective in reducing contributing factors to masticatory myalgia [11,26,32–34]. Many of these treatments are directed toward reducing muscle tension–producing habits, such as bruxism or bracing of muscles. Teaching control of habits is a difficult process because of the relationship that muscle tension may have with psychosocial factors. Simply telling a patient to stop the habits may be helpful with some, whereas with others it may result in noncompliance, failure, and frustration. An integrated approach that involves education, increased awareness, and other treatments, such as behavior modification, biofeedback, hypnosis, or drug therapy, may prove to be more successful.

Pain clinic team management

Although each clinician may have limited success in managing the "whole" patient alone, the assumption behind a team approach is that it is vital to address different aspects of the problem with different specialists to enhance the overall potential for success [16–18]. Although these programs provide a broader framework for treating the complex patient, they have added another dimension to the skills that are needed by the clinician: working as part of a coordinated team. Failure to integrate care adequately may result in poor communication, fragmented care, distrustful relationships, and, eventually confusion and failure in management. Team coordination can be facilitated by a well-defined evaluation and management system that clearly integrates team members. Fig. 4 describes a defined patient flow from evaluation to assessment to treatment and follow-up.

A prerequisite to a team approach is an inclusive medical model and conceptual framework that places the physical, behavioral, and psychosocial aspects of illness on an equal and integrated basis [19,35]. With an inclusive theory of human systems and their relationship to illness, a patient can be assessed as a whole person by different clinicians from diverse backgrounds. Although each clinician understands a different part of the patient's problem, s/he can integrate them with other clinicians' perspectives and see how each part is interrelated in the whole patient. Each contributing identified factor becomes part of the problem list to be addressed in the treatment plan by all clinicians. In the process, the synergism of each factor in the etiology of the disorder can become apparent to clinicians. For example, social stressors can lead to anxiety, anxiety can lead to poor posture and muscle tension, the poor posture and muscle tension can lead to myofascial pain

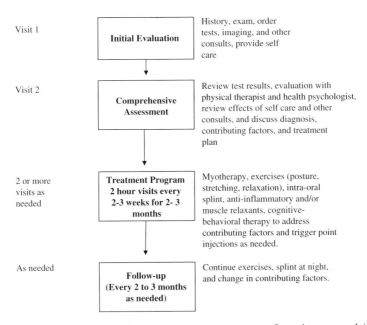

Fig. 4. Patient flow from evaluation to assessment to treatment of masticatory myalgia using a team approach includes many components. The key to successful management lies in matching the patient's needs with the unique combination of active treatment, education on contributing factors, and self-care that is appropriate for that patient.

syndrome, the pain contributes to more anxiety, and a cycle continues. Likewise, a reduction of each factor works synergistically to improve the whole problem. Treatment of only one factor may improve the problem, but relief may be partial or temporary. Treatment of all factors simultaneously can have a cumulative effect that is greater than the effects of treating each factor individually.

The problem list for a patient who has a specific chronic illness includes a physical diagnosis and a list of contributing factors. In establishing the problem list, the clinician needs to determine if the patient is complex and requires a team approach. Recommended criteria for determining complexity include any one of the following: multiple diagnoses, persistent pain longer than 6 months in duration, significant emotional problems (depression, anxiety), frequent use of health care services or medication, daily oral parafunctional habits, and significant lifestyle disturbances. The use of a screening instrument, such as research diagnostic criteria for temporomandibular disorders, the McGill Pain Questionnaire, or the Multidimensional Inventory, can readily elicit the degree of complexity of a case at initial evaluation [1,36–38]. The more complex the case, the greater is the need for a team approach. The decision to use a team must be made at the time of evaluation and not part way through a failing singular treatment plan. If a team is needed, the broad understanding of the patient is used to design a long-term management program that treats the physical diagnosis and helps to reduce these contributing factors.

The primary goals of the program include reducing the symptoms and their negative effects while helping the patient return to normal function without the need for future health care. The patient first participates in an educational session with each clinician to learn about the diagnoses and contributing factors, why it is necessary to change these factors, and how to do it. The dentist or physician is responsible for establishing the physical diagnosis, providing short-term medical or dental care, and monitoring medication and patient progress. The health psychologist is responsible for providing instruction about contributing factors; diagnosing, managing, or referring for primary psychologic disturbances; and establishing a program to support the patient and family in making changes. The physical therapist is responsible for evaluating musculoskeletal problems, providing support, instruction, and a management program on specifically assigned and common contributing factors, such as an exercise and posture program. Depending on the therapist's background and the patient's needs, this person also may provide special care, such as physical therapy modalities or occupational therapy. Each clinician also is responsible for establishing a trusting, supportive relationship with the patient while reaffirming the self-care philosophy of the program, reinforcing change, and assuring compliance. The patient is viewed as responsible for making the changes (see Table 1). The team meets weekly to review current patient progress and discuss new patients.

Summary

Goals of treatment of masticatory myalgia include reducing or eliminating pain, restoring normal jaw function, reducing the need for future health care, and restoring normal lifestyle functioning. The short-term strategy is to restore the muscle to normal length, posture, and full joint range of motion with exercises. The long-term strategy includes reducing the symptoms through muscle rehabilitation while helping the patient to reduce contributing factors, muscle tension and strain, and return to normal function without the need for future health care.

Recent-onset cases often can be managed with palliative self-care strategies that are designed to protect the muscles and encourage healing. Simple cases with minimal behavioral and psychosocial involvement can be managed by a single clinician with self-care, exercises, and a stabilization splint. Complex patients can be managed most effectively within an interdisciplinary pain clinic setting that uses a team of clinicians to address different aspects of the problem in a concerted fashion. Behavioral and psychosocial evaluations should be conducted on all patients who have persistent pain to determine complexity and contributing factors.

To improve outcomes, it is important to match the level of complexity of the management program with the complexity of the patients, and to use a pain clinic team approach to facilitate success in complex patients. Using clinical paradigms of self-care, education, and self-responsibility in care enhances long-term outcomes and maintains positive relationships between the patient and clinician.

References

[1] Okeson JP. Bell's orofacial pains. 5th edition. Chicago: Quintessence Publishing Co. Inc.; 1995. p. 239–49.

[2] Fricton J, Kroening R, Haley D, et al. Myofascial pain syndrome of the head and neck: a review of clinical characteristics of 164 patients. Oral Surg Oral Med Oral Pathol 1985;60(6): 615–23.

[3] Travell J. Myofascial trigger points: clinical view. In: Bonica JJ, et al, editors. Advances in pain research and therapy. New York: Raven Press; 1976. p. 919–26.

[4] Cifala J. Myofascial (trigger point pain) injection: theory and treatment. Osteopath Med 1979;31–6.

[5] Cooper AL. Trigger point injection: its place in physical medicine and rehabilitation. Arch Phys Med 1961;42:704–9.

[6] Travell J, Simons DG. Myofascial pain and dysfunction: the trigger point manual. Baltimore (MD): Williams & Wilkins Co.; 1998.

[7] Skootsky S, Jaeger B, Oye RK. Prevalence of myofascial pain in general internal medicine practice. West J Med 1989;151(2):157–60.

[8] Fricton JR. Recent advances in temporomandibular disorders and orofacial pain. J Am Dent Assoc 1991;122(11):24–32.

[9] Okeson JP, editor. Orofacial pain: guidelines for assessment, diagnosis, and management. Chicago: Quintessence Publishing Co., Inc.; 1996.

[10] Lund JP, Donga R, Widmer CG, et al. The pain-adaptation model: a discussion of the relationship between chronic musculoskeletal pain and motor activity. Can J Physiol Pharmacol 1991;69(5):683–94.

[11] Fricton JR. Myofascial pain. In: Masi AT, editor. Fibromyalgia and myofascial pain syndromes. London: BailliÈre Tindall; 1994. p. 857–80.

[12] Dall Arancio D, Fricton J. Randomized controlled study of exercises for masticatory myofascial pain. J Orofac Pain 1993;7(1):117.

[13] Jaeger B, Skootsky SA. Double blind, controlled study of different myofascial trigger point injection techniques [abstract]. Pain 1987;4(Suppl 1):S292.

[14] Lewit K. The needle effect in the relief of myofascial pain. Pain 1979;6(1):83–90.

[15] Fields HL, Liebeskind JC, editors. Pharmacological approaches to the treatment of chronic pain: new concepts and critical issues. Seattle: IASP Press; 1994.

[16] Ng LK, editor. New approaches to treatment of chronic pain: a review of multidisciplinary pain clinics and pain centers. Washington, DC: US Government Printing Office; 1981.

[17] Fricton J, Dall' AD. Interdisciplinary management of myofascial pain of the masticatory muscles. In: Fricton JR, Dubner R, editors. Orofacial pain and temporomandibular disorders. New York: Raven Press; 1995. p. 485–500.

[18] Aronoff GM, Evans WO, Enders PL. A review of follow-up studies of multidisciplinary pain units. Pain 1983;16(1):1–11.

[19] Rodin J. Biopsychosocial aspects of self management. In: Karoly P, Kanfer FH, editors. Self management and behavioral change: from theory to practice. New York: Pergamon Press; 1982.

[20] Simons D. Muscular pain syndromes. In: Fricton J, Awad EA, editors. Myofascial pain and fibromyalgia. New York: Raven Press; 1990. p. 1–43.

[21] Bennett R. Myofascial pain syndromes and the fibromyalgia syndrome: a comparative analysis. In: Fricton J, Awad EA, editors. Myofascial pain and fibromyalgia. New York: Raven Press; 1990. p. 43–66.

[22] Fricton JR. Myofascial pain syndrome: characteristics and epidemiology. In: Fricton JR, Awad EA, editors. Myofascial pain and fibromyalgia. New York: Raven Press; 1990. p. 107–28.

[23] Fricton JR, Kroening R. Practical differential diagnosis of chronic craniofacial pain. Oral Surg Oral Med Oral Pathol 1982;54(6):628–34.

[24] Shata R, Mehta NR, Forgione AG. Active resistance exercise for TMD related tension pain [abstract]. J Dent Res 2000;79:354.

[25] Au AR, Klineberg IJ. Isokinetic exercise management of temporomandibular joint clicking in young adults. J Prosthet Dent 1993;70(1):33–9.

[26] Fricton JR, Hathaway KM, Bromaghim C. Interdisciplinary management of patients with TMJ and craniofacial pain: characteristics and outcome. J Craniomandib Disord 1987;1(2):115–22.

[27] Magnusson T, Syren M. Therapeutic jaw exercises and interocclusal appliance therapy. A comparison between two common treatments of temporomandibular disorders. Swed Dent J 1999;23(1):27–37.

[28] Michellotti A, Steenks MH, Farella M, et al. The additional value of a home physical therapy regimen versus patient education only for the treatment of myofascial pain of the jaw muscles: short-term results of a randomized clinical trial. J Orofac Pain 2004;18(2):114–25.

[29] Dionne RA. Pharmacologic treatments for temporomandibular disorders. Oral Surg Oral Med Oral Pathol Oral Radiol Endod 1997;83(1):134–42.

[30] Singer E, Dionne R. A controlled evaluation of ibuprofen and diazepam for chronic orofacial muscle pain. J Orofac Pain 1997;11(2):139–46.

[31] Wedel A, Carlsson GE. Sick-leave in patients with functional disturbances of the masticatory system. Swed Dent J 1987;11(1–2):53–9.

[32] Clarke NG, Kardachi BJ. The treatment of myofascial pain-dysfunction syndrome using the biofeedback principle. J Periodontol 1977;48(10):643–5.

[33] Fricton J. Psychosocial characteristics of patients with low back pain compared to patients with head and neck pain [abstract]. Am Congress Rehab Med 1987:34.

[34] Graff-Radford SB, Reeves JL, Jaeger B. Management of chronic head and neck pain: effectiveness of altering factors perpetuating myofascial pain. Headache 1987;27(4):186–90.

[35] Schneider F, Kraly P. Conceptions of pain experience: the emergence of multidimensional models and their implications for contemporary clinical practice. Clin Psych Rev 1983;3:61–86.

[36] Fricton JR, Nelson A, Monsein M. IMPATH: microcomputer assessment of behavioral and psychosocial factors in craniomandibular disorders. Cranio 1987;5(4):372–81.

[37] Kerns RD, Turk DC, Rudy TE. The West Haven-Yale Multidimensional Pain Inventory (WHYMPI). Pain 1985;23(4):345–56.

[38] Turk DC, Rudy TE, Salovey P. The McGill Pain Questionnaire reconsidered: confirming the factor structure and examining appropriate uses. Pain 1985;21(4):385–97.

ELSEVIER
SAUNDERS

Dent Clin N Am 51 (2007) 85–103

THE DENTAL
CLINICS
OF NORTH AMERICA

Joint Intracapsular Disorders: Diagnostic and Nonsurgical Management Considerations

Jeffrey P. Okeson, DMD

Department of Oral Health Science, Orofacial Pain Program, D-530 University of Kentucky
College of Dentistry, Lexington, KY 40536-0297, USA

Temporomandibular disorders (TMD) refer to a large group of musculo-skeletal disorders that originate from the masticatory structures [1]. There are two broad types of TMD: those primarily involving the muscles and those primarily involving the temporomandibular joints. Muscle disorders are far more common than intracapsular disorders. This article focuses on the intracapsular disorders and is limited to the most common types encountered in the dental practice. The article begins with a brief review of normal temporomandibular joint (TMJ) anatomy and function followed by a description of the common types of disorders known as "internal derangements." Nonsurgical management is suggested based on the long-term scientific documentation. This article represents a brief review of these conditions. Other references are suggested for more in depth information [1–3].

Normal function of the temporomandibular joint

For clinicians to effectively manage dysfunction of the temporomandibular joint, they must have a sound understanding of normal joint function because the treatment goal for a patient with dysfunction is to re-establish normal function. A clinician cannot manage a disorder without a sound understanding of order.

The temporomandibular joint represents the articulation of the mandible to the temporal bone of the cranium (Fig. 1). The bony components of the joint are separated by a structure composed of dense fibrous connective tissue called the articular disc. Like any mobile joint, the integrity and

E-mail address: okeson@uky.edu

doi:10.1016/j.cden.2006.09.009   *dental.theclinics.com*

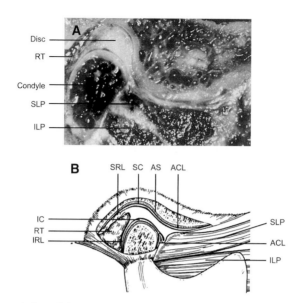

Fig. 1. (*A*) Lateral view of the temporomandibular joint. (*B*) Diagram revealing the following anatomic components: ACL, anterior capsular ligament; AS, articular surface; IC, inferior joint cavity; ILP, inferior lateral pterygoid muscle; IRL, inferior retrodiscal lamina; RT, retrodiscal tissues; SC superior joint cavity; SLP, superior and lateral pterygoid muscle; SRL, superior retrodiscal lamina. The lateral collateral discal ligament has not been drawn. (*From* Okeson JP. Management of temporomandibular disorders and occlusion. 5th edition. St. Louis (MO): C.V. Mosby Publishing; 2003. p. 10; with permission.)

limitations of the joint are maintained by ligaments. Ligaments are composed of collagenous fibers that have specific lengths. Ligaments do not actively participate in normal function of the joint; rather, they act as guide wires to restrict certain movements (border movements) while allowing other movements (functional movements). If joint movements consistently function against ligaments, the length of the ligaments can become altered. Ligaments have a poor ability to stretch, and therefore, when this occurs, they often elongate. This elongation creates a change in joint biomechanics and can lead to certain clinical changes discussed in this article.

Careful examination of the condyle and disc reveals that the disc is attached to the condyle medially and laterally by the discal collateral ligaments (Fig. 2). These ligaments allow rotation of the disc across the articular surface of the condyle in an anterior and posterior direction while restricting medial and lateral movements. The range of anterior and posterior rotation of the disc is also restricted by ligaments. The inferior retrodiscal lamina limits anterior rotation of the disc on the condyle, whereas the anterior capsular ligament limits posterior rotation of the disc (Fig. 1).

The morphology of the disc is extremely important. It is thinnest in the intermediate zone, thicker in the anterior border, and thickest in the posterior border. The condyle articulates on the intermediate zone of the disc and

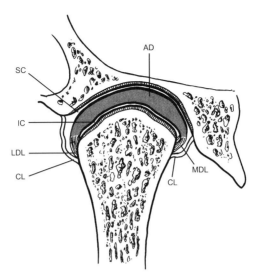

Fig. 2. Anterior view of the temporomandibular joint revealing the following anatomic components: AD, articular disc; CL, capsular ligament; IC, inferior joint cavity; LDL, lateral discal
ligament; MDL, medial discal ligament; SC, superior joint cavity. (*From* Okeson JP. Management of temporomandibular disorders and occlusion. 5th edition. St. Louis (MO): C.V. Mosby
Publishing; 2003. p. 14; with permission.)

is maintained in this position by constant interarticular pressure provided by
the elevator muscles (masseter, temporalis, and medial pterygoid). Although
the pressure between the condyle, disc, and fossa can vary according to the
activity of the elevator muscles, some pressure is maintained to prevent separation of the articular surfaces. If contact between the articular surfaces is
lost, a condition of dislocation exists (dislocation means separation of the
articular surfaces).

Posterior to the disc are the retrodiscal tissues. These tissues are highly
vascularized and well innervated. Anterior to the condyle-disc complex
are the superior and inferior lateral pterygoid muscles. The inferior pterygoid muscle inserts on the neck of the condyle, whereas the superior lateral
pterygoid muscle inserts on the neck of the condyle and the articular disc
(Fig. 1). The inferior lateral pterygoid is active with the depressing muscles
(mouth opening), and the superior lateral pterygoid muscle has been shown
to be active in conjunction with the elevator muscles (mouth closing) [4,5].
The superior lateral pterygoid muscle seems to be a stabilizing muscle for
the condyle–disc complex, especially during unilateral chewing.

When the condyle–disc complex translates down the articular eminence
(ie, the mouth opening), the disc rotates posteriorly on the condyle
(Fig. 3). The superior surface of the retrodiscal tissues is unlike any other
structure in the joint. The superior retrodiscal lamina is composed of loose
connective tissue and elastin fibers that allow the condyle–disc complex to
translate forward without damage to the retrodiscal tissues. In the closed

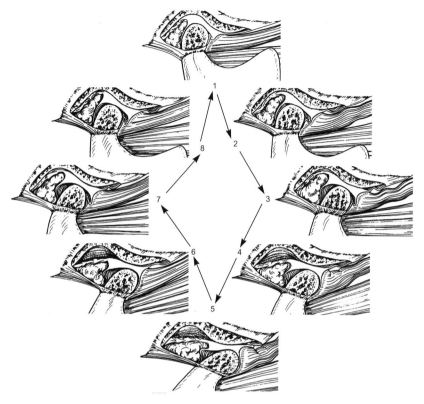

Fig. 3. Normal functional movement of the condyle and disc during the full range of opening and closing. The disc is rotated posteriorly on the condyle as the condyle is translated out of the fossa. The closing movement is the opposite of opening. (*From* Okeson JP. Management of temporomandibular disorders and occlusion. 5th edition. St. Louis (MO): C.V. Mosby Publishing; 2003. p. 29; with permission.)

mouth position, the superior retrodiscal tissues are passive and have little influence on disc position. During full mouth opening, the superior retrodiscal lamina is fully stretched and produces a posterior, retractive force on the disc (Fig. 3). This is the only structure in the temporomandibular joint capable of providing a retractive force on the articular disc.

During opening and closing, the disc and condyle move together, not because of ligamentous attachments, but because of two fundamental features: the morphology of the disc and interarticular pressure (pressure between the articular surfaces). Because some degree of interarticular pressure is always present, the condyle maintains itself on the thinnest intermediate zone of the disc. The thicker anterior and posterior borders of the disc force it to translate with the condyle during mouth opening and closing. It is the disc's morphology, therefore, that requires it to move with the condyle. If there is an alteration in interarticular pressure or a change in the morphology of the disc, condyle–disc movement can be altered. This begins the biomechanical changes associated with internal derangements.

Intracapsular disorders of the temporomandibular joint

Once change occurs in the structure of the condyle–disc complex, normal biomechanics can be altered. This alteration results in specific clinical signs and symptoms. It is by these signs and symptoms that a classification of disorders can be developed. Intracapsular disorders fall into one of two broad types: derangements of the condyle–disc complex and structural incompatibility of the articular surfaces [2]. Because of the brevity of this article, only derangements of the condyle–disc complex are discussed. These conditions include disc displacements with reduction and disc dislocations without reduction. In this section each category is described according to etiology, anamnestic, or history findings and clinical characteristics.

Disc displacement with reduction

Derangements of the condyle–disc complex arise from breakdown of the normal rotational movement of the disc on the condyle. This loss of normal disc movement can occur when there is elongation of the discal collateral ligaments and the inferior retrodiscal lamina. If the inferior retrodiscal lamina and the discal collateral ligament are elongated, the disc can be positioned more anteriorly by pull of the superior lateral pterygoid muscle. If this anterior pull is constant, a thinning of the posterior border of the disc may allow the disc to be displaced in a more anterior position (Fig. 4, position 1). With the condyle resting on a more posterior portion of the disc or retrodiscal tissues, an abnormal translatory shift of the condyle over the posterior border of the disc can occur during opening. Associated with the abnormal condyle–disc movement is a click that may be initially felt just during opening (single click) (Fig. 4, position 3) but later may be felt during opening and closing of the mouth (reciprocal clicking) (Fig. 4, position 8).

Etiology

The most common etiologic factor associated with breakdown of the condyle–disc complex is trauma. This may result from macrotrauma or microtrauma. Macrotrauma represents a single, often sudden, episode of trauma, such as a blow to the jaw [6–17]. Open mouth macrotrauma commonly produces elongation of the ligaments, whereas closed mouth trauma is more often associated with impact loading of the articular surfaces. Microtrauma is a produced by mild, frequent forces over a long period. Chronic muscle hyperactivity, such as bruxism, is an example of microtrauma. Although not well documented, chronic muscle hyperactivity may contribute to internal derangement disorders when significant orthopedic instability is present [2].

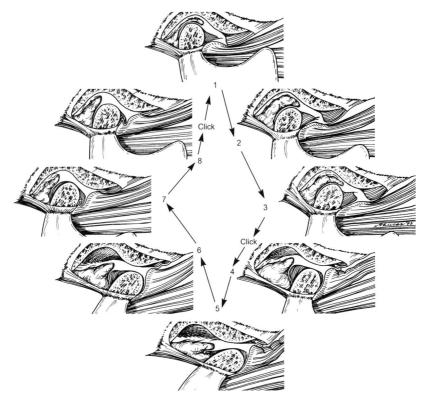

Fig. 4. Disc displacement (dislocation) with reduction. In position 1, the posterior border of the disc has been thinned, allowing activity of the superior lateral pterygoid to dislocate the disc anteriorly (and medially). Between positions 3 and 4, a click is felt as the condyle moves across the posterior border of the disc. Normal condyle–disc function occurs during the remaining opening and closing movement until the closed joint position is approached. A second click is heard as the condyle moves from the intermediate zone over the posterior border of the disc (between positions 8 and 1). (*From* Okeson JP. Management of temporomandibular disorders and occlusion. 5th edition. St. Louis (MO): C.V. Mosby Publishing; 2003. p. 213; with permission.)

History

It is common for a history of trauma to be associated with the onset of joint sounds. There may or may not be pain accompanying the disc displacement with reduction. If pain is present, it is intracapsular and associated with the dysfunction (the click).

Clinical characteristics

Examination reveals joint sounds during mouth opening and often during mouth closure. Disc displacement is characterized by a normal range of jaw movement during opening and eccentric movements. Any limitation is due to pain and not to a true structural dysfunction. When reciprocal clicking is present, the two clicks normally occur at different degrees of mouth opening, with the closing click usually occurring near the intercuspal position. Pain, if present, is directly related to joint function.

If the inferior retrodiscal lamina and discal collateral ligaments become further elongated and the posterior border of the disc sufficiently thinned, the disc can slip or be forced completely through the discal space. Because the disc and condyle no longer articulate, this condition is referred to as a "disc dislocation" (Fig. 4). If the patient can manipulate the jaw to reposition the condyle over the posterior border of the disc, the disc is said to be reduced. This represents a progression of the disc movement and may be accompanied by the patient report of joint catches and getting stuck. The patients may describe having to move the jaw around a little to get it back to functioning normally. The catching may or may not be painful, but if pain is present it is directly associated with the dysfunctional symptoms.

Disc dislocation without reduction

As the elasticity of the superior retrodiscal lamina is lost or the disc undergoes morphologic change, recapturing of the disc becomes more difficult. When the disc is not reduced, the forward translation of the condyle forces the disc further anteriorly (Fig. 5). This is clinically called a "closed lock" because the disc dislocation does not allow full mouth opening.

History

Most patients who have a history of disc dislocation without reduction know precisely when the dislocation occurred. They can readily relate it to an event such as biting into an apple or waking up with the condition. They report that the jaw is locked closed so that normal mouth opening cannot be achieved. Pain is commonly associated with dislocation without reduction. When pain is present, it usually accompanies trying to open beyond the point of joint restriction. The history also reveals that clicking occurred before the onset of locking but not since the disc dislocation has occurred.

Clinical characteristics

The range of mouth opening is commonly between 25 and 30 mm, and the mandible often deflects toward the involved joint during maximum opening. At the maximum point of opening, there is a hard end feel. In other words, if mild, steady, downward forward pressure is applied to the lower incisors, there is no increase in mouth opening. Eccentric movement is relatively normal to the ipsilateral side but restricted to the contralateral side. Loading the joint with bilateral manual manipulation is often painful because the condyle is seated on the retrodiscal tissues.

Nonsurgical management of intracapsular disorders

The correct management of TMJ intracapsular disorders is predicated on two factors: making a correct diagnosis and understanding the natural

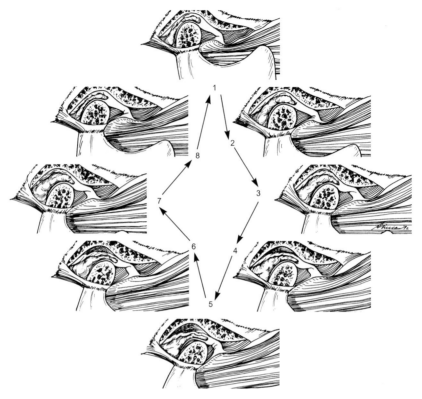

Fig. 5. Disc dislocation without reduction (closed lock). The disc is dislocated anterior to the condyle and never assumes a normal relationship during opening. This condition limits the distance the condyle can translate forward, resulting in limited mouth opening. (*From* Okeson JP. Management of temporomandibular disorders and occlusion. 5th edition. St. Louis (MO): C.V. Mosby Publishing; 2003. p. 214; with permission.)

course of the disorder. Each of the categories of internal derangements represents a clinical condition that is treated in a particular manner. An incorrect diagnosis leads to mismanagement and treatment failure.

Successful management of intracapsular disorders is also based on the clinician's understanding of the natural course of the disorder. Although the sequence of internal derangements is often clinically evident, it does not account for the outcome of all intracapsular disorders. The presence of chronic, unchanging, asymptomatic joint sounds suggests that intracapsular disorders are not always progressive. Epidemiologic studies reveal that asymptomatic joint sounds are common [18–22]. This poses an interesting question: If all joint sounds are not progressive, which sounds should be treated? It is my opinion that only joint sounds associated with pain should be considered for treatment provided that the pain is intracapsular in origin. In other words, patients who present with extracapsular muscle pain and a painless clicking joint should not be managed for the intracapsular disorder. Doing so leads to treatment failure because it does not address the source of the pain. Most painless joint sounds do not seem to lead to any major progressive disorders [22–29].

The management of disc displacement with reduction and disc dislocation without reduction is discussed separately because data suggest they should be managed differently.

Disc displacement with reduction

Definitive treatment for disc displacement with reduction (and disc dislocation with reduction) is to re-establish a normal condyle–disc relationship. Although this may sound relatively easy, it has not proven to be so. During the past 30 years, the dental profession's attitude toward management of intracapsular disc derangements has changed greatly. In the early 1970s, Farrar [30] introduced the anterior positioning appliance. This appliance provides an occlusal relationship that requires the mandible to be maintained in a forward position (Fig. 6). The position selected is one that places the mandible in the least protruded position that re-establishes a more normal condyle–disc relationship. This is usually achieved clinically by monitoring the clicking joint. Although eliminating the click does not always

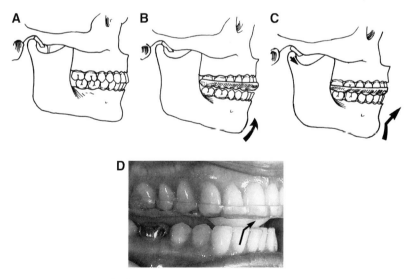

Fig. 6. The anterior positioning appliance. (*A*) The anterior positioning appliance causes the mandible to assume a forward position, creating a more favorable condyle–disc relationship. (*B*) During normal closure, the mandibular anterior teeth contact in the retrusive guiding ramp provided by the maxillary appliance. (*C*) As the mandible rises into occlusion, the ramp causes it to shift forward into the desired position that eliminates the disc derangement disorder. At the desired forward position, all teeth contact to maintain arch stability. (*From* Okeson JP. Management of temporomandibular disorders and occlusion. 5th edition. St. Louis (MO): C.V. Mosby Publishing; 2003. p. 441; with permission.)

denote successful reduction of the disc [31,32], it is a good clinical reference point for beginning therapy.

The idea behind the anterior positioning appliance was to position the condyle back on the disc (ie, to "recapture the disc"). It was originally suggested that this appliance be worn 24 h/d for as long as 3 to 6 months. Although this appliance is helpful in managing certain disc derangement disorders, its use has changed considerably due to results of recent studies.

It was quickly discovered that the anterior positioning appliance was useful in reducing painful joint symptoms [33,34]. When this appliance successfully reduced symptoms, a major treatment question was asked: What's next? Some clinicians believed that the mandible needed to be permanently maintained in this forward position [35,36]. Dental procedures were suggested to create an occlusal condition that maintained the mandible in this therapeutic relationship. Accomplishing this task was never a simple dental procedure [37]. Others felt that once the discal ligaments repaired, the mandible should be returned to its normal position in the fossa (the musculoskeletally stable position), and the disc would remain in proper position (recaptured). Although one approach is more conservative than the other, neither is supported by long-term data.

In early short-term studies [7,33,34,38–43], the anterior positioning appliance proved to be much more effective in reducing intracapsular symptoms than the more traditional stabilization appliance. This led to the belief that returning the disc to its proper relationship with the condyle was an essential part of treatment. The greatest insight regarding the appropriateness of a treatment modality is gained from long-term studies. Forty patients with various derangements of the condyle–disc complex were evaluated 2.5 years after anterior positioning therapy and a step-back procedure [38]. None received occlusal alterations. It was reported that 66% of the patients still had joint sounds, but only 25% were still experiencing pain problems. If the criteria for success in this study were the elimination of pain and joint sounds, then success was achieved in only 28%. Other long-term studies [7,44] have reported similar findings. If the presence of asymptomatic joint sounds is not a criterion for failure, then the success rate for anterior positioning appliances rises to 75%. The issue that must be addressed, therefore, is the clinical significance of asymptomatic joint sounds.

Joint sounds are common in the general population. In many cases [22–29], it seems that they are not related to pain or decreased joint mobility. If all clicking joints progressed to more serious disorders, then this would be a good indication to treat every joint that clicked. The presence of unchanging joint sounds over time indicates that the structures involved can adapt to less than optimum functional relationships.

Long-term studies reveal that anterior positioning appliances are not as effective as once thought. They seem to be helpful in reducing pain in 75% of the patients, but joint sounds seem to be much more resistant to therapy, and their persistence does not always indicate a progressive disorder. These studies provide insight into how the joint responds to anterior positioning therapy. In many patients, advancing the mandible forward temporarily prevents the condyle from articulating with the highly vascularized, well innervated, retrodiscal tissues. This is the likely explanation for an almost immediate reduction of intracapsular pain. During the forward positioning, the retrodiscal tissues undergo adaptive and reparative changes [45–56]. These changes result in dense fibrosis connective tissues that can be loaded by the condyle in the absence of pain.

Discs generally are not recaptured by anterior positioning appliances [57–59]. Instead, as the condyle returns to the fossa, it moves posteriorly to articulate on the adapted retrodiscal tissues. If these tissues have adequately adapted, loading occurs without pain. The condyle functions on the newly adapted retrodiscal tissues, although the disc is still anteriorly displaced. The result is a painless joint that may continue to click with condylar movement (Fig. 7). At one time the dental profession believed that the presence of joint sounds indicated treatment failure. Long-term follow-up studies have given the profession new insight regarding success and failure. We, like our orthopedic colleagues, have learned to accept that some dysfunction is likely to persist once joint structures have been altered. Controlling pain while allowing joint structures to adapt seems to be the most important role of the therapist.

A few long-term studies [36,60,61] support the concept that permanent alteration of the occlusal condition can be successful in controlling most major symptoms. This treatment requires extensive dental therapy, and one must question the need when natural adaptation seems to work well for most patients. Reconstruction of the dentition or orthodontic therapy should be reserved for patients who present with a significant orthopedic instability.

The continuous use of anterior positioning appliance therapy is not without consequence. A certain percentage of patients who wear these appliances may develop a posterior open-bite. A posterior open-bite is likely

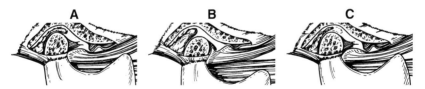

Fig. 7. Adaptive changes in the retrodiscal tissues. (*A*) An anteriorly displaced disc with the condyle articulating on the retrodiscal tissues producing pain. (*B*) An anterior positioning appliance is placed in the mouth to bring the condyle forward off of the retrodiscal tissues onto the disc. This relationship lessens the loading of the retrodiscal tissues, which decreases the pain. (*C*) Once the tissues have adapted, the condyle can assume the original musculoskeletally stable position and painless function on this new fibrotic tissues. A click may remain because the disc is still displaced. (*From* Okeson JP. Management of temporomandibular disorders and occlusion. 5th edition. St. Louis (MO): C.V. Mosby Publishing; 2003. p. 445; with permission.)

the result of a reversible, myostatic contracture of the inferior lateral ptery-goid muscle. When this condition occurs, a gradual relengthening of the muscle can be accomplished by converting the anterior positioning appliance to a stabilization appliance, which allows the condyles to assume the musculoskeletally stable position. This can also be accomplished by slowly decreasing use of the appliance.

The degree of myostatic contracture that develops is likely to be proportional to the length of time the appliance has been worn. When these appliances were first introduced, it was suggested that they be worn 24 h/d for 3 to 6 months. With 24-hour use, the development of a posterior open bite was common. The present philosophy is to reduce the time the appliance is being worn to limit the adverse effects on the occlusal condition. For most patients, full-time use is not necessary to reduce symptoms. The patient should be encouraged to wear the appliance only at night to protect the retrodiscal tissues from heavy loading (bruxism). During the day, the patient should not wear the appliance so that the mandible can return to its normal position. In most instances, this allows a mild loading of the retrodiscal tissue during the day, which enhances the fibrotic response of the retrodiscal tissues. If the symptoms can be adequately controlled without daytime use, myostatic contracture is avoided. This technique is appropriate for most patients, but if significant orthopedic instability exists, symptoms may not be controlled.

If the symptoms persist with only night-time use, the patient may need to wear the appliance more often. Daytime use may be necessary for a few weeks. As soon as the patient becomes symptom free, the use of the appliance should be gradually reduced. If reduction of use creates a return of symptoms, then the time allowed for tissue repair has not been adequate or orthopedic instability is present. It is best to assume that inadequate time for tissue repair is the reason for the return of symptoms. The anterior positioning appliance should therefore be reinstituted and more time given for tissue adaptation.

When repeated attempts to eliminate the appliance fail to control symptoms, orthopedic instability should be suspected. When this occurs, the anterior positioning appliance should be converted to a stabilization appliance that allows the condyle to return to the musculoskeletally stable position. Once the condyles are in the musculoskeletally stable position the occlusal condition should be assessed for orthopedic stability. If obvious orthopedic instability exists, dental procedures may need to be considered. In this author's experience, the need for dental procedures is rare.

Supportive therapies

In addition to appliance therapy, the patient should be educated about the mechanics of the disorder and the adaptive process that is essential for treatment. When pain is present, the patient needs to be encouraged to decrease loading of the joint when ever possible. Softer foods, slower chewing, and smaller bites should be promoted. The patient should be told not to allow the joint to click whenever possible. If inflammation is suspected, a nonsteroidal anti-inflammatory drug, such as ibuprofen (600–800 mg, three times a day), may be prescribed. Moist heat or ice can be used if the patient finds either helpful. Active exercises are not usually helpful because they cause joint movements that often increase pain. Passive jaw movements may be helpful, and distractive manipulation by a physical therapist may assist in healing. These general principles are appropriate for most intracapsular disorders.

Disc dislocation without reduction

In the case of disc displacement with reduction, the anterior positioning appliance re-establishes the normal condyle–disc relationship. Fabricating an anterior positioning appliance for a patient who has a disc dislocation without reduction aggravates the condition by forcing the disc further forward. Patients who present with disc dislocation without reduction (Fig. 5) need to be managed differently.

When the condition of disc dislocation without reduction is acute, the initial therapy should include an attempt to reduce or recapture the disc by manual manipulation. This manipulation is most successful with patients who are experiencing their first episode of locking. In these patients, there is a great likelihood that tissues are healthy and with minimal morphologic changes. Patients who have a long history of locking are likely to present with discs and ligaments that have undergone changes that will not allow reduction of the disc. As a general rule, when patients report a history of being locked for a week or less, manipulation is often successful. In patients who have a longer history, success begins to decrease rapidly.

The success of manual manipulation for the reduction of a dislocated disc depends on three factors. The first factor is the level of activity in the superior lateral pterygoid muscle. This muscle must be relaxed to permit successful reduction. If it remains active because of pain, it may need to be injected with local anesthetic before any attempt to reduce the disc. Second, the disc space must be increased so the disc can be repositioned on the condyle. When increased activity of the elevator muscles is present, the interarticular pressure is increased, making it more difficult to reduce the disc. The patient needs to be encouraged to relax and avoid forcefully closing the mouth. Third, the condyle must be in the maximum forward translatory position. The only structure that can produce a posterior or retractive force on the disc is the superior retrodiscal lamina, and if this tissue is to be effective, the condyle must be in the most forward protrusive position.

The first attempt to reduce the disc should begin by having the patient attempt to self-reduce the dislocation. With the teeth slightly separated, the patient is asked to move the mandible to the contralateral side of the dislocation as far as possible. From this position the mouth is opened maximally. If this is not successful at first, the patient should attempt this several times. If the patient is unable to reduce the disc, assistance with manual manipulation is indicated. The thumb is placed intraorally over the mandibular second molar on the affected side. The fingers are placed on the inferior border of the mandible anterior to the thumb position. Firm but controlled downward force is exerted on the molar at the same time that upward force is placed by the fingers on the outer inferior boarder of the mandible in the anterior region. The opposite hand helps stabilize the cranium above the joint that is being distracted. While the joint is being distracted, the patient is asked to assist by slowly protruding the mandible, which translates the condyle downward and forward out of the fossa. It may be helpful to bring the mandible to the contralateral side during the distraction procedure because the disc is likely to be dislocated anteriorly and medially, and a contralateral movement moves the condyle into it better.

Once the full range of laterotrusive excursion has been reached, the patient is asked to relax for 20 to 30 seconds while constant distractive force is applied to the joint. The clinician needs to be sure that unusual heavy forces are not placed on the uninvolved joint. Always ask the patient if he or she is feeling any discomfort in the uninvolved joint. If there is discomfort, the procedure should be immediately stopped and begun again with the proper directional force placed. A correctly performed manual manipulation to distract a TMJ should not jeopardize the healthy joint.

Once the distractive force has been applied for 20 to 30 seconds, the force is discontinued, and the fingers are removed from the mouth. The patient is asked to lightly close the mouth to the incisal end-to-end position on the anterior teeth. The patient is asked to relax for a few seconds and then to open wide and immediately return to this anterior position (not maximum intercuspation). If the disc has been successfully reduced, the patient should be able to open to the full range (no restrictions). When this occurs, the disc has likely been recaptured, and an anterior positioning appliance is immediately placed to prevent clenching on the posterior teeth, which would likely redislocate the disc. At this point, the patient has a normal condyle–disc relationship and should be managed in the same manner as discussed for the patient who has a disc dislocation with reduction, with one exception.

When an acute disc dislocation has been reduced, it is advisable to have the patient wear the anterior positioning appliance continuously for the first 2 to 4 days before beginning only night-time use. The rationale for this is that the dislocated disc may have become distorted during the dislocation, which may allow it to be redislocated more easily. Maintaining the anterior positioning appliance in place for a few days may help the disc reassume its more normal shape (thinnest in the intermediate band and thicker anterior and posterior). If the normal morphology is present, the disc is more likely to be maintained its normal position. If this disc has permanently lost its normal morphology, it is difficult to maintain its position. This is why manual manipulations for disc dislocations are attempted only in acute conditions when the likelihood of normal disc morphology exists.

If the disc is not successfully reduced, a second and possibly a third attempt can be attempted. Failure to reduce the disc may indicate a dysfunctional superior retrodiscal lamina or a general loss of disc morphology. Once these tissues have changed, the disc dislocation is most often permanent.

If the disc is permanently dislocated, what types of treatments are indicated? This question has been asked for many years. At one time it was felt that the disc needed to be in its proper position for health to exist. Therefore, when the disc could not be restored to proper position, a surgical repair of the joint seemed to be necessary. Over years of studying this condition, we have learned that surgery may not be needed for most patients. Studies [62–73] have revealed that over time many patients achieve relatively normal joint function even with the disc permanently dislocated. With these studies in mind, it would seem appropriate to follow a more conservative approach that would encourage adaptation of the retrodiscal tissues. Patients who have permanent disc dislocation should be given a stabilization appliance that reduces forces to the retrodiscal tissues (ie, decrease bruxism) [74].

Supportive therapy

Supportive therapy for a permanent disc dislocation should begin with educating the patient about the condition. Because of the restricted range of mouth opening, many patients try to force their mouth to open wider. If this is attempted too strongly, it aggravates the intracapsular tissues, producing more pain. Patients should be encouraged not to open too wide especially immediately after the dislocation. With time and tissue adaptation, they will be able to return to a more normal range of movement (usually > 40 mm) [63–69,71]. Gentle, controlled jaw exercise may be helpful in regaining mouth opening [75,76], but care should be taken to not be too aggressive, which may lead to more tissue injury. The patient must be told that this may take a year or more for full range to be attained.

The patient should be told to decrease hard biting, to avoid chewing gum, and to avoid anything that aggravates the condition. If pain is present, heat or ice may be used. Nonsteroidal anti-inflammatory drugs are indicated for pain and inflammation. Joint distraction and phonophoresis over the joint area may be helpful.

When a joint is not able to adapt to a dislocated disc, pain may become a significant symptom. This pain forces the clinician into more aggressive approaches. Therapies that may need to be considered are arthrocentesis, arthroscopy, and arthrotomy.

Summary

The treatment goals for managing intracapsular disorders of the temporomandibular joint have changed over the past 20 years. There is no longer an attitude that all discs must be properly positioned to maintain a healthy joint. Therapies for re-establishing disc position, for the most part, have failed. On the other hand, patients seem to adapt to abnormal disc positions and function relatively normally. Intracapsular disorders seem to follow a natural course that is influenced by many factors. Therapy does not seem to radically change this course. However, therapy can reduce the suffering that accompanies some of the stages of these disorders. It is the therapist's role to intervene when possible to decrease suffering. Reversible therapies are often adequate and should be attempted first. Only when reversible therapies fail to adequately reduce suffering should more aggressive therapies be considered. When suffering continues, re-evaluation of the clinical condition is necessary to assure that more aggressive therapy effectively alters the symptoms.

References

[1] Okeson J. Orofacial pain: guidelines for classification, assessment, and management. 3rd edition. Chicago: Quintessence; 1996.
[2] Okeson JP. Management of temporomandibular disorders and occlusion. 5th edition. St. Louis (MO): Mosby Year Book; 2003.
[3] Okeson JP. Bell's orofacial pains. 6th edition. Chicago, IL: Quintessence Publishing Co., Inc.; 2005.
[4] McNamara JA. The independent functions of the two heads of the lateral pterygoid muscle in the human temporomandibular joint. Am J Anat 1973;138:197–205.
[5] Mahan PE, Wilkinson TM, Gibbs CH, et al. Superior and inferior bellies of the lateral pterygoid muscle EMG activity at basic jaw positions. J Prosthet Dent 1983;50:710–8.
[6] Harkins SJ, Marteney JL. Extrinsic trauma: a significant precipitating factor in temporomandibular dysfunction. J Prosthet Dent 1985;54:271–2.
[7] Moloney F, Howard JA. Internal derangements of the temporomandibular joint: III. Anterior repositioning splint therapy. Aust Dent J 1986;31:30–9.
[8] Weinberg S, Lapointe H. Cervical extension-flexion injury (whiplash) and internal derangement of the temporomandibular joint. J Oral Maxillofac Surg 1987;45:653–6.
[9] Pullinger AG, Seligman DA. Trauma history in diagnostic groups of temporomandibular disorders. Oral Surg Oral Med Oral Pathol 1991;71:529–34.
[10] Westling L, Carlsson GE, Helkimo M. Background factors in craniomandibular disorders with special reference to general joint hypermobility, parafunction, and trauma. J Craniomandib Disord 1990;4:89–98.
[11] Pullinger AG, Seligman DA. Association of TMJ subgroups with general trauma and MVA. J Dent Res 1988;67:403.
[12] Pullinger AG, Monteriro AA. History factors associated with symptoms of temporomandibular disorders. J Oral Rehabil 1988;15:117.
[13] Skolnick J, Iranpour B, Westesson PL, et al. Prepubertal trauma and mandibular asymmetry in orthognathic surgery and orthodontic paients. Am J Orthod Dentofacial Orthop 1994; 105:73–7.
[14] Braun BL, DiGiovanna A, Schiffman E, et al. A cross-sectional study of temporomandibular joint dysfunction in post-cervical trauma patients. Journal of Craniomandibular Disorders Facial Oral Pain 1992;6:24–31.
[15] Burgess J. Symptom characteristics in TMD patients reporting blunt trauma and/or whiplash injury. J Craniomandib Disord 1991;5:251–7.
[16] De Boever JA, Keersmaekers K. Trauma in patients with temporomandibular disorders: frequency and treatment outcome. J Oral Rehabil 1996;23:91–6.

[17] Yun PY, Kim YK. The role of facial trauma as a possible etiologic factor in temporomandibular joint disorder. J Oral Maxillofac Surg 2005;63:1576–83.

[18] Gazit E, Lieberman M, Eini R, et al. Prevalence of mandibular dysfunction in 10–18 year old Israeli schoolchildren. J Oral Rehabil 1984;11:307–17.

[19] Osterberg T, Carlsson GE. Symptoms and signs of mandibular dysfunction in 70-year-old men and women in Gothenburg, Sweden. Community Dent Oral Epidemiol 1979; 7:315–21.

[20] Solberg WK, Woo MW, Houston JB. Prevalence of mandibular dysfunction in young adults. J Am Dent Assoc 1979;98:25–34.

[21] Swanljung O, Rantanen T. Functional disorders of the masticatory system in southwest Finland. Community Dent Oral Epidemiol 1979;7:177–82.

[22] Vincent SD, Lilly GE. Incidence and characterization of temporomandibular joint sounds in adults. J Am Dent Assoc 1988;116:203–6.

[23] Heikinheimo K, Salmi K, Myllarniemi S, et al. Symptoms of craniomandibular disorder in a sample of Finnish adolescents at the ages of 12 and 15 years. Eur J Orthod 1989;11: 325–31.

[24] Tallents RH, Katzberg RW, Murphy W, et al. Magnetic resonance imaging findings in asymptomatic volunteers and symptomatic patients with temporomandibular disorders. J Prosthet Dent 1996;75:529–33.

[25] Dibbets JM, van der Weele LT. Signs and symptoms of temporomandibular disorder (TMD) and craniofacial form. Am J Orthod Dentofacial Orthop 1996;110:73–8.

[26] Spruijt RJ, Wabeke KB. An extended replication study of dental factors associated with temporomandibular joint sounds. J Prosthet Dent 1996;75:388–92.

[27] Sato S, Goto S, Nasu F, et al. Natural course of disc displacement with reduction of the temporomandibular joint: changes in clinical signs and symptoms. J Oral Maxillofac Surg 2003; 61:32–4.

[28] Magnusson T, Egermark I, Carlsson GE. A longitudinal epidemiologic study of signs and symptoms of temporomandibular disorders from 15 to 35 years of age. J Orofac Pain 2000;14:310–9.

[29] Magnusson T, Egermarki I, Carlsson GE. A prospective investigation over two decades on signs and symptoms of temporomandibular disorders and associated variables: a final summary. Acta Odontol Scand 2005;63:99–109.

[30] Farrar WB. Differentiation of temporomandibular joint dysfunction to simplify treatment. J Prosthet Dent 1972;28:629–36.

[31] Tallents RH, Katzberg RW, Miller TL, et al. Arthrographically assisted splint therapy; painful clicking with a nonreducing meniscus. Oral Surg Oral Med Oral Pathol 1986;61:2–4.

[32] Raustia AM, Pyhtinen J. Direct sagittal computed tomography as a diagnostic aid in the treatment of an anteriorly displaced temporomandibular joint disk by splint therapy. Cranio 1987;5:240–5.

[33] Anderson GC, Schulte JK, Goodkind RJ. Comparative study of two treatment methods for internal derangement of the temporomandibular joint. J Prosthet Dent 1985;53:392–7.

[34] Lundh H, Westesson PL, Kopp S, Tillstrom B. Anterior repositioning splint in the treatment of temporomandibular joints with reciprocal clicking: comparison with a flat occlusal splint and an untreated control group. Oral Surg Oral Med Oral Pathol 1985;60:131–6.

[35] Summer JD, Westesson PL. Mandibular repositioning can be effective in treatment of reducing TMJ disk displacement: a long-term clinical and MR imaging follow-up. Cranio 1997;15: 107–20.

[36] Simmons HC 3rd, Gibbs SJ. Anterior repositioning appliance therapy for TMJ disorders: specific symptoms relieved and relationship to disk status on MRI. Cranio 2005;23:89–99.

[37] Joondeph DR. Long-term stability of mandibular orthopedic repositioning. Angle Orthod 1999;69:201–9.

[38] Okeson JP. Long-term treatment of disk-interference disorders of the temporomandibular joint with anterior repositioning occlusal splints. J Prosthet Dent 1988;60:611–6.

[39] Lundh H, Westesson PL, Jisander S, et al. Disk-repositioning onlays in the treatment of temporomandibular joint disk displacement: comparison with a flat occlusal splint and with no treatment. Oral Surg Oral Med Oral Pathol 1988;66:155–62.

[40] Simmons HC 3rd, Gibbs SJ. Recapture of temporomandibular joint disks using anterior repositioning appliances: an MRI study. Cranio 1995;13:227–37.

[41] Davies SJ, Gray RJ. The pattern of splint usage in the management of two common temporomandibular disorders. Part I: the anterior repositioning splint in the treatment of disc displacement with reduction. Br Dent J 1997;183:199–203.

[42] Williamson EH, Rosenzweig BJ. The treatment of temporomandibular disorders through repositioning splint therapy: a follow-up study. Cranio 1998;16:222–5.

[43] Tecco S, Festa F, Salini V, et al. Treatment of joint pain and joint noises associated with a recent TMJ internal derangement: a comparison of an anterior repositioning splint, a full-arch maxillary stabilization splint, and an untreated control group. Cranio 2004;22:209–19.

[44] Lundh H, Westesson PL, Kopp S. A three-year follow-up of patients with reciprocal temporomandibular joint clicking. Oral Surg Oral Med Oral Pathol 1987;63:530–3 [see comments].

[45] Solberg WK. The temporomandibular joint in young adults at autopsy: a morphologic classification and evaluation. J Oral Rehabil 1985;12:303.

[46] Akerman S, Kopp S, Rohlin M. Histological changes in temporomandibular joints from elderly individuals: an autopsy study. Acta Odontol Scand 1986;44:231–9.

[47] Isberg A, Isacsson G, Johansson AS, et al. Hyperplastic soft-tissue formation in the temporomandibular joint associated with internal derangement: a radiographic and histologic study. Oral Surg Oral Med Oral Pathol 1986;61:32–8.

[48] Hall MB, Brown RW, Baughman RA. Histologic appearance of the bilaminar zone in internal derangement of the temporomandibular joint. Oral Surg Oral Med Oral Pathol 1984;58:375–81.

[49] Scapino RP. Histopathology associated with malposition of the human temporomandibular joint disc. Oral Surg Oral Med Oral Pathol 1983;55:382–97.

[50] Solberg WK, Bibb CA, Nordstrom BB, et al. Malocclusion associated with temporomandibular joint changes in young adults at autopsy. Am J Orthod 1986;89:326–30.

[51] Salo L, Raustia A, Pernu H, et al. Internal derangement of the temporomandibular joint: a histochemical study. J Oral Maxillofac Surg 1991;49:171–6.

[52] Blaustein DI, Scapino RP. Remodeling of the temporomandibular joint disk and posterior attachment in disk displacement specimens in relation to glycosaminoglycan content. Plast Reconstr Surg 1986;78:756–64.

[53] Pereira FJ Jr, Lundh H, Westesson PL, et al. Clinical findings related to morphologic changes in TMJ autopsy specimens. Oral Surg Oral Med Oral Pathol 1994;78:288–95.

[54] Pereira FJ Jr, Lundh H, Westesson PL. Morphologic changes in the temporomandibular joint in different age groups: an autopsy investigation. Oral Surg Oral Med Oral Pathol 1994;78:279–87.

[55] Pereira FJ, Lundh H, Eriksson L, et al. Microscopic changes in the retrodiscal tissues of painful temporomandibular joints. J Oral Maxillofac Surg 1996;54:461–8.

[56] Pereira JFJ, Lundh H, Westesson PL. Age-related changes of the retrodiscal tissues in the temporomandibular joint. J Oral Maxillofac Surg 1996;54:55–61.

[57] Kirk WS Jr. Magnetic resonance imaging and tomographic evaluation of occlusal appliance treatment for advanced internal derangement of the temporomandibular joint. J Oral Maxillofac Surg 1991;49:9–12.

[58] Choi BH, Yoo JH, Lee WY. Comparison of magnetic resonance imaging before and after nonsurgical treatment of closed lock. Oral Surg Oral Med Oral Pathol 1994;78:301–5.

[59] Chen CW, Boulton JL, Gage JP. Effects of splint therapy in TMJ dysfunction: a study using magnetic resonance imaging. Aust Dent J 1995;40:71–8.

[60] Tallents RH, Katzberg R, Macher DJ, et al. Use of protrusive splint therapy in anterior disk displacement of the temporomandibular joint: a 1 to 3 year followup. J Prosthet Dent 1990;63:336–41.

[61] Lundh H, Westesson PL. Long-term follow-up after occlusal treatment to correct abnormal temporomandibular joint disk position. Oral Surg Oral Med Oral Pathol 1989;67:2–10.
[62] Lundh H, Westesson PL, Eriksson L, et al. Temporomandibular joint disk displacement without reduction: treatment with flat occlusal splint versus no treatment. Oral Surg Oral Med Oral Pathol 1992;73:655–8.
[63] Vichaichalermvong S, Nilner M, Panmekiate S, et al. Clinical follow-up of patients with different disc positions. J Orofac Pain 1993;7:61–7.
[64] Chung SC, Kim HS. The effect of the stabilization split on the TMJ closed lock. J Craniomandibular Pract 1993;11:95–101.
[65] Tasaki MM, Westesson PL, Isberg AM, et al. Classification and prevalence of temporomandibular joint disk displacement in patients and symptom-free volunteers. Am J Orthod Dentofacial Orthop 1996;109:249–62.
[66] Kai S, Kai H, Tabata O, Shiratsuchi Y, et al. Long-term outcomes of nonsurgical treatment in nonreducing anteriorly displaced disk of the temporomandibular joint. Oral Surg Oral Med Oral Pathol Oral Radiol Endod 1998;85:258–67.
[67] Kurita K, Westesson PL, Yuasa H, et al. Natural course of untreated symptomatic temporomandibular joint disc displacement without reduction. J Dent Res 1998;77:361–5.
[68] Sato S, Takahashi K, Kawamura H, et al. The natural course of nonreducing disk displacement of the temporomandibular joint: changes in condylar mobility and radiographic alterations at one-year follow up. Int J Oral Maxillofac Surg 1998;27:173–7.
[69] Sato S, Goto S, Kawamura H, et al. The natural course of nonreducing disc displacement of the TMJ: relationship of clinical findings at initial visit to outcome after 12 months without treatment. J Orofac Pain 1997;11:315–20.
[70] Sato S, Kawamura H, Nagasaka H, et al. The natural course of anterior disc displacement without reduction in the temporomandibular joint: follow-up at 6, 12, and 18 months. J Oral Maxillofac Surg 1997;55:234–8 [discussion: 238–239].
[71] Sato S, Kawamura H. Natural course of non-reducing disc displacement of the temporomandibular joint: changes in electromyographic activity during chewing movement. J Oral Rehabil 2005;32:159–65.
[72] Minakuchi H, Kuboki T, Maekawa K, et al. Self-reported remission, difficulty, and satisfaction with nonsurgical therapy used to treat anterior disc displacement without reduction. Oral Surg Oral Med Oral Pathol Oral Radiol Endod 2004;98:435–40.
[73] Imirzalioglu P, Biler N, Agildere AM. Clinical and radiological follow-up results of patients with untreated TMJ closed lock. J Oral Rehabil 2005;32:326–31.
[74] Schmitter M, Zahran M, Duc JM, et al. Conservative therapy in patients with anterior disc displacement without reduction using 2 common splints: a randomized clinical trial. J Oral Maxillofac Surg 2005;63:1295–303.
[75] Nicolakis P, Erdogmus B, Kopf A, et al. Effectiveness of exercise therapy in patients with internal derangement of the temporomandibular joint. J Oral Rehabil 2001;28:1158–64.
[76] Cleland J, Palmer J. Effectiveness of manual physical therapy, therapeutic exercise, and patient education on bilateral disc displacement without reduction of the temporomandibular joint: a single-case design. J Orthop Sports Phys Ther 2004;34:535–48.

THE DENTAL
CLINICS
OF NORTH AMERICA

Dent Clin N Am 51 (2007) 105–127

Temporomandibular Disorders: Associated Features

Ronald C. Auvenshine, DDS, PhD[a,b],*

[a]Orofacial Pain Clinic, Michael E. DeBakey VA Hospital, 7505 South Main Street,
#210, Houston, TX 77030, USA
[b]The University of Texas Dental Branch-Houston, Houston, TX, USA

Temporomandibular disorder (TMD) is a collective term that encompasses a number of clinical problems involving the masticatory muscles or the temporomandibular joints. These disorders have been identified as a major cause of nondental pain in the orofacial region, and are considered to be a subclassification of musculoskeletal disorders [1].

Orofacial pain and TMD can be associated with pathologic conditions or with disorders related to somatic and neurologic structures, such as primary headache disorders and neurogenic pain disorders. Primary headache disorders are a group of pain disorders that originate in neuropathology and vascular pathology. Neurogenic pain disorders are conditions resulting from functional abnormalities within the nervous system. When patients present to the dental office with a chief complaint of pain or headaches, it is vital for the practitioner to understand the cause of the complaint and to perform a thorough examination that will lead to the correct diagnosis and appropriate treatment. A complete understanding of the associated medical conditions with symptomology common to TMD and orofacial pain is necessary for a proper diagnosis.

One critical point of understanding for the clinician is the concept of chronic versus acute pain. The International Association for the Study of Pain has defined chronic pain as pain lasting longer than 6 months. Therefore, acute pain refers to pain from onset to 6 months (Fig. 1). The pain pathway has two divisions. One of the divisions travels through the midbrain, to terminate in the posterior aspect of the lateral thalamus (the discriminative system). The other division travels through the medial thalamus to the

* Orofacial Pain Clinic, Michael E. DeBakey VA Hospital, 7505 South Main Street, #210, Houston, TX.
E-mail address: auvenshine244@pol.net

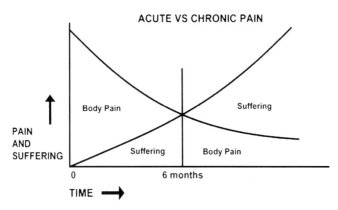

Fig. 1. Time course of change from acute to chronic pain. (*From* Auvenshine RC. Acute vs. chronic pain-an overview. Tex Dent J 2000;117(7):19; with permission.)

hypothalamus and limbic forebrain (the motivational/effective system). The discriminative system allows the brain to properly locate the site and source of pain. The motivational/effective system involves the emotional component of painful experiences [2].

During the first 6 months of pain, the discriminative system dominates the motivational/effective system, allowing the patient to comprehend better the location and duration of his/her pain. The patient can describe the pain more accurately because the brain is better able to localize and isolate it. However, as time progresses, expression of the motivational/effective system gains in strength and begins to play a more dominant role in the pain experience. At 6 months, an inversion of the pain response expression occurs, in which the motivational/effective system now dominates the pain language. Consequently, the pain language used by the chronic pain patient is characterized more by psychologic terms than descriptive terms. As the pain continues without resolution, the pain language becomes so nondescript that it is difficult for the dental practitioner to identify the source and site of the pain. In this situation, the words used to describe the pain can provide only "clues" to diagnosis and treatment. It is vital that the practitioner be aware of the patient's history and any potential conflicts or contributing factors that may play a role in the patient's pain expression [3].

When faced with a patient suffering from pain, the differentiation of acute from chronic pain begins at the initial visit. In history taking, one of the first questions the practitioner must ask is, "How long has this pain been present?"

The most common symptoms of acute pain are headaches, jaw pain, earache, neck pain, muscle soreness, muscle tightness, and teeth pain (Box 1). Conversely, the most common symptoms reported by the chronic pain sufferer are headaches, depression, chronic fatigue, sleep disorders, decreased productivity, feelings of inadequacy, low self-esteem, withdrawal, and mood disorders (Box 2).

Box 1. Symptoms related to acute TMD

- Headaches
- Jaw pain
- Earache
- Neck pain
- Muscle soreness
- Muscle tightness
- Tooth pain

From Auvenshine RC. Acute vs. chronic pain–an overview. Tex Dent J 2000;117(7):19.

Comparison between the symptoms of acute and chronic TMD suggests that the pain language and descriptions of patients who have acute pain are more specific and somatically accurate. Their reported symptoms define location and pain intensity. In contrast, the pain language used by chronic pain sufferers is more vague and less descript. Their pain language becomes wrapped in psychologic terminology, indicating the dominance of the motivational/effective system [2].

Chronic pain continues to be poorly understood and managed. However, research endeavors to broaden our understanding of pain and to contribute valuable insight into pain management. For instance, it is known that nerve signals arising from sites of tissue or nerve injury lead to long-term changes in the central nervous system (CNS) and in the amplification and persistence of pain. These nociceptor activity–induced, neuronal changes, known as central sensitization (CS), have important clinical implications in the

---

Box 2. Symptoms related to chronic TMD

- Headaches
- Depression
- Chronic fatigue
- Sleep disorders
- Decreased productivity
- Feelings of inadequacy
- Low self-esteem
- Withdrawal
- Decreased libido

From Auvenshine RC. Acute vs. chronic pain–an overview. Tex Dent J 2000;117(7):19.

---

development of new approaches to the management of persistent pain and to poorly understood conditions such as oral dysesthesia, burning mouth syndrome, atypical facial pain/atypical odontalgia, common peripheral nerve injury/deafferentation, and phantom tooth syndrome [4].

Historical background

Patients seek help from doctors for symptoms, which are warning signs of impending disease. Symptoms are the expression of a patient's subjective experience in his/her body. Diseases are objectively observable abnormalities in the body. Difficulties arise when the doctor can find no objective changes to explain the patient's subjective experience. When this occurs, these symptoms are referred to as "medically unexplained" or "functional" [5]. Many different functional syndromes have been described. In fact, each medical specialty seems to have at least one. For rheumatologists, prominent muscle pain and tenderness is fibromyalgia (FM); for gastroenterologists, abdominal pain with altered bowel habit is irritable bowel syndrome (IBS); for internal medicine specialists, chronic fatigue and myalgia is a postviral or chronic fatigue syndrome (CFS) (Table 1) [5].

The existence of specific somatic syndromes is said to reflect a tendency of specialists to focus on only those symptoms pertinent to their specialty, rather than on any real differences among patients. Three major questions that can be postulated are:

Table 1
Functional somatic syndromes by specialty

Specialty	Syndrome
Dentistry	Temporomandibular joint disorders
	Atypical facial pain
Neurology	Tension headache
	Migraine
Ear, nose, and throat	Sinusitis
	Ear pain
	Vertigo
	Tinnitus
Allergy	Multiple chemical sensitivity
Internal medicine	Chronic (postviral) fatigue syndrome
Rheumatology	Fibromyalgia
Gastroenterology	Irritable bowel syndrome
	Nonulcer dyspepsia
Gynecology	Premenstrual syndrome
	Chronic pelvic pain
Respiratory medicine	Hyperventilation syndrome
Cardiology	Atypical or noncardiac chest pain/ MVP dysautonomia

1. Do published diagnostic criteria for each specific functional syndrome overlap in their constituent symptoms?
2. Do patients who have one functional somatic syndrome also meet symptom criteria for others?
3. Are there similarities across syndromes and nonsymptom characteristics of sex, coexisting emotional disorders, proposed causes, and prognosis and response to treatment [5]?

Various names have been given to functional somatic syndromes, including somatization, somatoform disorders, and medically unexplained symptoms. Functional somatic syndromes and their symptoms pose a major challenge to medicine and dentistry. These syndromes have symptoms that are common and frequently persistent, and are associated with significant distress and disability. Functional somatic syndromes are not only common, but also clinically important, and can be a major health issue. Most of the current thinking toward these syndromes is focused on medical subspecialties, when, in fact, a review of the literature strongly suggests that these syndromes have much in common. Therefore, they should have a broader definition because several of these syndromes can be present in the same individual. Conventional medical therapy is fairly ineffective for these patients, and results in frustrated physicians and dissatisfied patients with chronic symptoms; it often leads to unnecessary expenditure of medical resources.

Central sensitivity syndrome

In 2000, Yunus [6] reviewed the evidence for CS and functional somatic syndromes. He compared FM-related syndromes, and coined the term "central sensitivity syndrome" (CSS). He stated that CSS comprises a similar and overlapping group of syndromes that lack demonstrable structural pathology and are bound by a common pathway, which leads to CS (Fig. 2). Members of this group include FM syndrome, chronic headaches, IBS, CFS, myofascial pain syndrome, restless leg syndrome, periodic limb movement disorder, TMD, multiple chemical sensitivity (MCS), female urethral syndromes, interstitial cystitis, primary dysmenorrhea/"functional" chronic pelvic pain, posttraumatic stress disorder, and depression [6]. Although proof of CS is lacking in some of the syndromes at this time, Yunus included them, based on clinical presentation.

Yunus [7] first suggested a relationship among these various syndromes in 1981. This controlled study demonstrated an association between IBS, tension type headaches, and migraine. In addition, the presence of overlapping conditions was noted to occur in some patients, with muscle spasms being the common binding symptom [8].

Nearly all chronic pain sufferers complain of depression, despite the current lack of direct evidence linking CS to sensory function in depression.

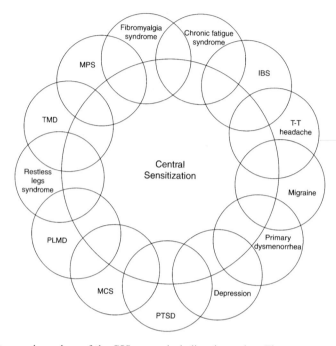

Fig. 2. Proposed members of the CSS group, including depression. The common pathophysiologic binder for the interrelated syndromes is CS. MCS, multiple chemical sensitivity; MPS, myofascial pain syndromes; PLMD, period limb movement disorder; PTSD, posttraumatic stress disorder; T-T headache, tension-type headache. (*From* Yunus MB. The concept of central sensitivity syndromes. In: Wallace DJ, Clauw DJ, editors. Fibromyalgia & other central pain syndromes. Philadelphia: Lippincott Williams & Wilkins. 2005. p. 40; with permission.)

In recent years, Post [9] of the National Institutes of Health has presented arguments suggesting that depression is based on CS. This approach recognizes that most cases of depression follow stressful events, primarily of a psychosocial nature, which initiate various biologic processes, including gene transcription and other neurochemical-hormonal changes. These modifications lead to intracellular changes and subsequent CS [9]. When continued exposure to stress occurs, even of less severity, there is a progressive sensitization of the CNS. Neuronal hyperexcitability then becomes self-sustained, so that, even without discernable stress, depression becomes chronic [9]. A similar model has also been suggested for other psychiatric diseases, such as anxiety disorders [6].

The understanding of CSS is of great value to the dental practitioner. Therefore, emphasis should be placed on training the clinician for recognition, proper treatment, or referral of these distressing disorders. Because these disorders are interrelated and may be expressed in the same individual, knowledge of mutual association is vital for earlier and more accurate diagnosis, thus avoiding unnecessary and expensive investigations. Treatment that is effective by clinical trials in one patient may not be effective in others, but the more that is known about the pathophysiology of CS, the more appropriate will be the treatment rendered and the more positive the outcomes.

Hypothalamic-pituitary-adrenal axis

The hypothalamic-pituitary-adrenal (HPA) axis is known to play a role in the coordinating of the body's physiologic response to physical and emotional stressors. The HPA axis exhibits a circadian rhythm related to night/ day, or sleep/awake, 24-hour cycles. Peak production of cortisol occurs in the early morning hours and decreases steadily to its lowest level in the evening. In addition to normal cortisol production, stress-induced secretion of cortisol can be added to the supply. Regulation of the HPA axis depends on key substances, such as hypothalamic corticotropin-releasing hormone (CRH) acting in synergy with vasopressin. They induce the release of adrenocorticotropic hormone (ACTH) from the anterior pituitary. Release of ACTH results in the production of corticosteroids from the adrenal glands that subsequently exert negative feedback on the hippocampus, the pituitary, and the hypothalamus through mineralocorticoid and glucocorticoid receptors. Other mediators that regulate the HPA axis include serotonin, norepinephrine, substance P, and IL-6 [10,11].

A study recently published by Ulrich-Lai [12] demonstrated a relationship between increased nociceptor sensitivity during chronic pain and alterations in the limbic system, and a disassociation from HPA activation. The limbic system, which integrates behavior, is composed of the limbic forebrain, hippocampus, fornix, amygdala, medial thalamus, mamillary body, hypothalamus, and pituitary. The intimate relationship of the limbic lobe with the hypothalamus, and the inclusion of the neurostructures within the limbic system, have caused many to refer to the limbic system as the *visceral brain* [3]. This system has a close, anatomic, and functional relationship to the hypothalamus. It is concerned intimately not only with emotional expression, but also with the genesis of emotions. In addition to its roles in olfaction and regulation of feeding behavior, the limbic system affects motivation and the expression of fear and rage. It exerts control over the autonomic nervous system by way of the pituitary gland and its target organs.

The close relationship of the limbic lobe to the hypothalamus allows it to influence control over the releasing factors located within the hypothalamus. When released, these factors start a chain of hormonal events that begins with stimulation of the pituitary gland and eventually results in a desired effect on a target organ. For example, stimulation of the pituitary gland causes the release of pituitary hormones that act on target glands to release target gland hormones. Target organs are influenced by the release of target gland hormones, such as cortisone and aldosterone from the adrenal cortex; testosterone, estrogen, and progesterone from the male and female gonads;

thyroxine (T_4) from the thyroid glands; and somatomedin from the liver. These events continue to form a feedback loop as many of the hormones, in turn, affect brain function. The transduction of psychologic events into endocrine changes occurs by way of neuromodulators and neurotransmitters, which regulate the sensitivity of neurons to the stimulation, discharge, and conduction of nerve impulses from one neuron to another across the synaptic clef. Many such substances have been identified in the CNS, including biogenic amines like dopamine, norepinephrine, and serotonin, and acetylcholine, histamine, gamma-aminobutyric acid, and glycine, along with steroid and pituitary hormones and their hypothalamic and inhibiting factors [13].

Chronic pain may be considered a form of chronic stress. Patients experiencing this type of pain often exhibit disturbances in the HPA axis, including abnormal cortisol levels. Chronic pain patients report an increased incidence of depression and anxiety, stress-related disorders that frequently are accompanied by disturbances in the limbic system and in the HPA axis. Despite the fact that the literature supports a strong link between chronic pain, stress disorders, and limbic dysfunctions, the mechanisms underlying the effects of chronic pain on the HPA axis and the limbic system are not understood fully. The HPA axis is hyperactive during depression because of genetic factors or aversive stimuli that may occur during early development or adult life. The functioning of the hypothalamic-pituitary-thyroid axis, on the other hand, is inhibited during depression. Furthermore, a close interaction between the HPA axis and the hypothalamic-pituitary-gonadal axis exists. Organizing effects during fetal life, and activating effects of sex hormones on the HPA axis, have been reported. Such mechanisms may be the basis for a higher prevalence of mood disorders in women, as compared with men [14].

Studies of rats have shown that higher levels of cumulative corticosteroid exposure and extreme chronic stress induce neuronal damage that selectively affects hippocampal structure. The hippocampus has been shown to affect sleep and sleep hygiene dramatically [14].

Because various stressors activate the HPA axis, and because glucocorticoids are the end product of HPA axis activation, these hormones have been viewed as the physical embodiment of stress-induced pathology. It has been suggested that prolonged overproduction of glucocorticoids, whether as a result of ongoing stress or a genetic predisposition to HPA axis hyperactivity, brings about damage to certain brain structures (especially the hippocampus) essential for HPA axis restraint. Such damage, in turn, has been hypothesized to lead to a "feed-forward circuit," in which ongoing stressors drive glucocorticoid production indefinitely. This theory has been called the "glucocorticoid cascade hypothesis" [15].

Despite the popularity of the glucocorticoid cascade hypothesis, increasing data provide evidence that in addition to glucocorticoid excess, insufficient glucocorticoid signaling may play a significant role in the development and expression of pathology in stress-related disorders [15]. Insufficient glucocorticoid signaling is defined as any state in which the signaling capacity of glucocorticoids is inadequate to restrain relevant stress-response systems, either as a result of decreased hormone bioavailability (eg, hypocortisolism) or as a result of weakened glucocorticoid responsiveness (ie, secondary to reduce glucocorticoid receptor sensitivity). As defined, insufficient glucocorticoid signaling implies no specific mechanism or absolute deficiency, but focuses instead on the end point of glucocorticoid activity. A critical function of glucocorticoids is to shape and mobilize immune responses during stress [15]. Virtually all stressors, including infection, physical trauma, and even psychologic insults, are associated with immune activation and release of proinflammatory cytokines such as interleukin-1 (IL-1) and interleukin-6 (IL-6). Because of their inhibitory effects on nuclear factor signaling pathways, glucocorticoids are the most potent anti-inflammatory hormones in the body. They serve to suppress the production and activity of proinflammatory cytokines during stressor exposure and to return the organism back to homeostasis after cessation of the stressor.

The relationship of insufficient glucocorticoid signaling to stress-related disorders has been proposed by Raison [15] as effects stemming from environmental challenges (stress), genetic predisposition, and the influence of interacting systems, including neurotransmitter systems and the endocrine system. Insufficient glucocorticoid signaling is manifested most commonly as either hypocortisolism or impaired glucocorticoid responsiveness. Inadequate glucocorticoid activity, in turn, prevents stress-response systems, including the immune system, the sympathetic nervous system (SNS), and CRH from inhibitory control, which leads to unrestrained stress hyperreactivity. The resulting increased release of proinflammatory cytokines, catecholamines, and CRH leads to health consequences relevant to behavior, CNS function, metabolism, and immune function. Immune activation and cytokine release can then lead to further impairment in glucocorticoid signaling (feed-forward cascade) through direct inhibitory effects on glucocorticoid receptor function (Fig. 3).

Although autoimmunity remains an ongoing risk whenever the immune system is activated, prolonged or repeated exposure to immune stimuli might predispose an individual to reduced glucocorticoid signaling as a means of freeing bodily defenses from inhibitory control in the face of an ongoing infectious threat. Such a release of inflammatory processes might be adaptive under conditions in which recurrent infection is likely and immune readiness is an attendant requirement.

Hypothalamic-pituitary-adrenal axis and sleep

One of the most common symptoms of CSS is sleep deprivation, caused by the effect of the HPA axis on the limbic system (eg, hippocampus and amygdala). The early phase of nocturnal sleep, dominated by extended periods of slow-wave sleep, is the only time of a 24-hour period in which

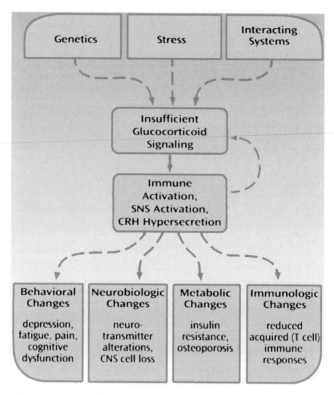

Fig. 3. Insufficient glucocorticoid signaling in the pathophysiology of stress-related disorders. (*From* Raison CL, Miller AH. When not enough is too much: the role of insufficient glucocorticoid signaling in the pathophysiology of stress-related disorders. Am J Psychiatry 2003; 160(9):1561; with permission.)

secretory activity of the HPA axis is subjected to a pronounced and persistent inhibition, resulting in minimum concentrations of ACTH and cortisol. During late sleep, which is predominated by rapid eye movement (REM) sleep, HPA secretory activity reaches diurnal maximum. Born and colleagues [16] demonstrated that early sleep, and in particular slow-wave sleep, is associated with inhibition of pituitary-adrenocortical responsiveness. This association was established by comparing response to administration of exogenous secretions of ACTH in men during sleep and during nocturnal wakefulness. It is presumed that this association is caused by hypothalamic secretion of an as-yet unknown release-inhibiting factor of ACTH. Born also revealed that the pituitary adrenocortical responsiveness during early sleep was disinhibited after administration of correat, which is a selective blocker of mineralocorticoid receptors located primarily in the limbic-hippocampal structures. Hippocampal neuronal networks are known to integrate corticosteroid feedback by way of the mineralocorticoid receptors and the classical corticoid receptors. Born proposed that dysfunction of the identification mode of regulation during early sleep is present in Cushing's disease, in patients who have severe depression, and in aged patients [16]. The proposed connection made by the study strongly suggests that hippocampal dysregulation of sleep alters the production of secretory activity that is prominent during early sleep and does not allow for replenishing of the immune system, making it difficult to meet the stresses of the following day.

Medical conditions with symptoms common to temporomandibular disorders

Temporomandibular disorders

Besides being a potential cause of various headaches, disorders of the temporomandibular joints may contribute to a wide range of other complaints, including jaw, ear, and neck pain. Numerous techniques are available to diagnose TMDs, including imaging techniques and physical examination [1]. Pain in the temporomandibular region appears to be relatively common, occurring in approximately 10% of the population over age 18 [17]. TMDs can be divided into arthralgic TMDs and myalgic TMDs (Box 3). Several medical conditions exist that share various symptoms with TMDs.

Fibromyalgia

FM is a chronic disorder characterized by persistent, widespread pain and abnormal pain sensitivity in response to a wide array of stimuli, such

---

Box 3. Classification of TMDs

Arthralgic TMDs
- Congenital disorder
- Disc derangements
- Fracture
- Dislocation
- Inflammation
- Ankylosis
- Osteoarthritis
- Neoplasia

Myalgic TMDs
- Myofascial pain
- Myositis
- Myospasm
- Local myalgia (unclassified)
- Myofibrotic contracture

as mechanical pressure, cold, heat, and ischemia [18,19]. Individuals with
FM also demonstrate a number of other "medically unexplained" symptoms, including fatigue, sleep disturbances, impairment in attention and
other cognitive functions, stiffness of muscles and joints, and subjective joint
swellings (Box 4). It has been found that patients who have FM are characterized by high levels of psychologic distress. Additional psychosocial factors, such as stressful life events and chronic pain, prompt the FM patient
to seek health care, both conventional and alternative. Consequently,
some health care providers view patients who have FM as being either hy-
pervigilant about common, unpleasant sensory experiences, or as somatizers
who seek to "medicalize" their symptoms [20].

Chronic fatigue syndrome

CFS describes patients who have profound, disabling fatigue, lasting up
to 6 consecutive months. It is not the result of ongoing exertion and is not
alleviated by rest. Patients experiencing CFS report a significant reduction
in activity levels, affecting their occupational, educational, social, and personal lifestyles. CFS patients complain of such symptoms as impairment
of short-term memory or concentration, sore throat, tender cervical and
axillary lymph nodes, myalgia, arthralgia without joint swelling or redness,
headache, unrefreshing sleep, and postexertional fatigue.

Box 4. Symptoms of fibromyalgia

Musculoskeletal
- Pain at multiple sites
- Stiffness
- "Hurt all over"
- Swollen feeling in tissues

Nonmusculoskeletal
- General fatigue
- Morning fatigue
- Sleep difficulties
- Paresthesia
- Dizziness/vertigo
- Tinnitus
- Raynaud's phenomenon
- Anxiety
- Mental stress
- Depression/cognitive dysfunction

Irritable bowel syndrome

IBS is characterized by chronic or recurring abdominal pain associated with altered bowel habits that cannot be explained by biochemical or structural abnormalities. This condition appears to have a female predominance of 2.4:1 [21]. The most prevalent symptoms reported by IBS patients are nausea, bloating, constipation, and extraintestinal symptoms. Several studies have indicated that the menstrual cycle influences gastrointestinal symptoms, which are reportedly increased immediately before and during menses.

Multiple chemical sensitivity syndrome

MCS describes a disorder characterized by a vast array of somatic, cognitive, and affective symptoms, the cause of which is attributed to exposure to low levels of various chemicals. Typically, the physical examination and laboratory findings of patients who have MCS do not exhibit any abnormalities. MCS, as defined by Cullens [22], is an acquired disorder characterized by recurrent symptoms, referable to multiple organ systems, and occurring in response to demonstrable exposure to many chemically unrelated compounds at doses far below those established to cause harmful effects in the general population. MCS is a controversial disorder, with debate over whether it is a nonpsychiatric organ disorder or a psychiatric disorder (such as somatoform disorder), or possibly a combination of both. At present, the exact cause of MCS is unknown; however, the proposed etiologic mechanisms include immunologic dysregulation, "limbic kindling" as described by Bell and colleagues [23], and psychologic dysfunction. Included in the MCS debate are dental amalgam restorations. The controversy over the deleterious health effects of "mercury fillings" has been ongoing since 1970. The potential dangers of using silver-mercury amalgam fillings in dental restorations have been reported primarily by the lay media. It has been purported to produce symptoms similar to FM, chronic fatigue, headaches, cognitive dysfunction, and muscle and joint aches [24]. Although the fears have been heightened in recent years, no convincing evidence currently exists that suggests that removing amalgam restorations from patients will resolve their chemical sensitivities.

Other associated syndromes

Hyperprolactinemia

Hyperprolactinemia is a condition of elevated levels of the serum prolactin, which is produced in the lactotroph cells of the anterior pituitary gland. Secretion is pulsatile [25]. The primary function of prolactin is to stimulate breast epithelial cell proliferation during pregnancy, and to induce lactation. Estrogen stimulates the proliferation of pituitary lactotroph cells, resulting in an increased quantity of these cells in premenopausal women (especially during pregnancy). Although lactation is inhibited by high levels of estrogen and progesterone during pregnancy, the rapid decline of estrogen and progesterone in the postpartum period allows lactation to occur [25]. Prolactin also serves to regulate estrogen and progesterone balance.

Secretion of prolactin is under tonic inhibitory control by dopamine. Prolactin production can be stimulated by the hypothalamic peptides, thyrotropin-releasing hormone, and vasoactive intestinal peptide. Thus, hyperprolactinemia can result from primary hypothyroidism (a high thyrotropin-releasing hormone state) [26].

Hyperprolactinemia is common in men and women. Generally, however, the clinical presentation is more obvious and presents earlier in women, who typically present with oligomenorrhea, amenorrhea, galactorrhea, or infertility. One cause of hyperprolactinemia is a pituitary tumor. If a tumor is present, approximately 90% of the time it is a microadenoma. A complete drug history should be obtained from patients suspected of having hyperprolactinemia because many common medications can cause the disorder [27]. Dopamine receptor antagonist drugs, such as phenothiazine; dopamine-depleting agents such as reserpine; and other drugs, such as tricyclic antidepressants, monoamine antihypertensives, and verapamil, can elevate levels of prolactin when used over an extended period of time [28].

Laboratory tests using hormone assays can help identify hyperprolactinemia. Additionally, thyroid-stimulating hormone (TSH) evaluation is important in detecting hypothyroid conditions in suspected individuals because hypothyroidism can cause prolactin levels to escalate.

If the hyperprolactinemia is caused by a nonadenoid tumor condition, the dopamine-agonist bromocriptine mesylate (Parlodel) is the initial drug of choice. It lowers the prolactin level in 70% to 100% of patients [27].

Mitral valve prolapse dysautonomia

Mitral valve prolapse (MVP) is a common cardiac disorder that may affect 5% to 20% of the general population. It is disproportionately more prevalent among women than men. Symptoms of MVP usually do not present before early teenage years, although adults of any age may be affected. MVP tends to be hereditary [29].

The autonomic nervous system controls the involuntary systems of the body, such as heartbeat, blood pressure, body temperature, intestinal functions, sweating, and so forth. The system is composed of two parts: the SNS (the "accelerator") and the parasympathetic nervous system (the "brakes"). When these two systems are out of balance, it is described as dysautonomia.

Dysautonomia has several categories. When the dysautonomia involves patients who have MVP, the condition is referred to as MVP dysautonomia or MVP syndrome. Symptoms of MVP dysautonomia include anxiety or panic attacks, depression or mood swings, chest discomfort or pain, palpitations or feelings of skipped heartbeats, vertigo, syncope or presyncope, pallor or redness of extremities, weakness, fatigue, headaches, migraines, and numbness or tingling in the extremities [30].

Mechanisms underlying the condition have been shown to include increased adrenergic activity, disturbances in catecholamine regulation, hyperresponsiveness to adrenergic stimulation, anomalous beta-adrenergic receptors, dysfunction of the parasympathetic nervous system, decreased intravascular volume, diminished left ventricular diastolic volume, and abnormal secretion of atrial natriuretic factors. The adrenal glands and the autonomic nervous system coexist and interact, creating a "complex neuroendocrine-cardiovascular process," which may account for many of the symptoms unexplained on the basis of the valvular abnormality alone [31].

Hypothyroidism

Hypothyroidism refers to a metabolic state resulting from a deficiency in thyroid hormone function. It may arise from primary thyroid disease, hypothalamic-pituitary disease, or generalized tissue resistance to thyroid hormone. Early recognition of hypothyroidism remains a challenge, especially when the decline in thyroid function is gradual [32]. Symptoms may be nonspecific in early stages and do not occur necessarily in any sequence. These symptoms may include myalgia, arthralgia, muscle cramps, dry skin, headaches, and dysmenorrhea. The diagnosis of primary hypothyroidism is confirmed by a reduced free-T_4 level and an elevated TSH level. Subclinical hypothyroidism is diagnosed by the demonstration of elevated TSH levels in the setting of normal, free-T_4 levels [33]. The diagnosis of secondary hypothyroidism, resulting from hypothalamic-pituitary dysfunction, can prove more difficult, because TSH levels may be reduced, normal, or even slightly elevated in this condition. Thyroid hormones have two major physiologic effects: they increase protein synthesis in virtually every body tissue, and they increase oxygen consumption by increasing the activity of sodium and potassium ATPase (the sodium pump), primarily in tissues responsible for basal oxygen consumption, such as the liver, kidney, heart, and skeletal muscle. Thyroid hormone regulates both the hypothalamus and the pituitary.

Menstrual migraine

Menstrual migraine typically develops in females during their teenage years around the onset of menstruation, and is most frequent around 40 years of age. It is unique in that it tends to be more severe, last longer, and be less responsive to the medications normally prescribed for migraines experienced during other times of the month [34]. Unlike typical migraine, menstrual migraine commonly occurs without aura. According to the International Classification of Headache Disorders published by the International Headache Society in 2004, menstrual migraine is categorized into two divisions: menstrually related migraine and pure menstrual migraine [35]. Menstrually related migraine differs from pure menstrual migraine in that the headaches do not occur exclusively around the time of menstruation, but are present at other times of the month as well. Only a small number of women experience pure menstrual migraine.

The pathogenesis of menstrual migraine is not well understood. Multiple mechanisms have been proposed that suggest factors such as hormone fluctuation, central serotonin function, abnormal endogenous opioid variation, or decreased melatonin secretion. One of the most widely cited theories centers around the linkage of hormonal interactions triggered by steep drops in estrogen levels just before the onset of bleeding. It has been proposed that this decrease in estrogen may increase blood vessel susceptibility to other factors such as prostaglandins, and this, in turn, can lead to chemical and inflammatory changes in the brain, triggering a headache [34].

The relationship between menstrual migraine and CSS can be seen in the example of a woman who is stressed to the extent of immune system deprivation and sleep deprivation. In this situation, any additional insult to her body may result in an expression of extreme headache. The fact that vascular-type headaches can occur before and around the time of menses strongly suggests a link between menstrual migraines and CSS. Therefore, it is important that the clinician be aware of the associated features of menstrual migraine in the chronic pain sufferer.

The use of antidepressants

Depressed patients who have HPA malfunction respond to antidepressants with changes in both mood and hormones. Two major classes of antidepressant drugs exist: monoamine oxidase inhibitors and monoamine reuptake inhibitors [36]. Monoamine reuptake inhibitors are the most commonly prescribed group of drugs for the treatment of depression. Normalization of a hyperactive HPA system occurs during successful antidepressant pharmacotherapy. One possible mechanism for the success of antidepressants could be an increase in cellular corticosteroid receptor concentration, rendering the HPA system more susceptible to feedback inhibition by cortisol [13]. The inhibitory action of cortisone is exerted by way of receptor sites localized in neurons of the hypothalamus, hippocampus, septum, amygdala, and reticular formation [36]. The inhibitory action of cortisone on the hippocampus is the reason that individuals taking tricyclic antidepressants may enjoy a more restful sleep. By allowing an individual to obtain a more restful sleep, HPA secretory activity can return to its diurnal maximum level. Therefore, the use of certain antidepressants can, in fact, enhance sleep as well as mood, facilitating restoration and normalization of the HPA system.

A new hypothesis put forth by Barden [36] suggests that a primary action of antidepressants could be the stimulation of corticosteroid receptor gene expression, with a resultant decrease in HPA system activity, including reduced expression of CRH. Reduced expression of CRH has been implicated in the pathogenesis of depression. Thus, antidepressants may not only increase the capacity of neurons involved in regulation of the HPA system, but may also have a common mechanism of action at the level of corticosteroid receptor genes.

Clinical management

Medical management of functional somatic syndromes can be broken into six steps, as reported by Barsky [37]:

1. Ruling out the presence of diagnosable medical disease
2. Searching for psychiatric disorders
3. Building a collaborative alliance with the patients
4. Making restoration of function the goal of treatment
5. Providing realistic reassurance
6. Prescribing cognitive behavior therapy for patients who have not responded to the first five steps

Clinicians must uphold their medical mandate with an appropriate search for previously unrecognized medical disorders. However, caution is advised against ordering tests strictly to reassure the patient. If, in fact, the patient is living a "sick role," the clinician must understand the risks of solidifying the patient's conviction that his/her distress has a biomedical cause. It is also helpful to have evidence-based guidelines for appropriate evaluation.

The goal of treatment becomes the identification and alleviation of factors that amplify and perpetuate the patient's symptoms and cause functional impairment. The focus of management should be on coping rather than on curing, and on improving functional status rather than simply eradicating symptoms. Realistic incremental goals should be set and specified in terms of observable behavior. Patients should be encouraged to resume their activities as much as possible and to remain at work if they are at all able to do so [37].

Cognitive-behavioral therapies can be effective in treating persistent distress and disability resulting from functional somatic syndromes, if previous strategies have proved insufficient. Such therapies have been developed for somatoform disorders and some medically unexplained symptoms, such as IBS, FM, CFS, headaches, atypical chest pain, and atypical facial pain. These cognitive-behavioral interventions help patients cope with symptoms by teaching them how to reexamine their health beliefs and expectations, and how to explore the effects of the "sick role," stress, and distress on their symptoms. Cognitive interventions also enable patients to find alternative explanations for their symptoms and to restructure faulty disease beliefs.

Clinical evaluation

The evaluation of a patient who has chronic pain is a complex process. Arriving at a diagnosis is typically insufficient to guide treatment because any given pain diagnosis has a large heterogeneity with respect to symptom causes. Because of this heterogeneity, the most effective treatments can sometimes be elusive. The differential diagnosis of the chronic pain sufferer involves identifying which factors are present in a given individual, to narrow the field of potential somatic disorders.

A complete history and examination remains the most important diagnostic tool. The key to collecting a thorough history is the quality of the patient interview. It is vital that the practitioner listen carefully to the patient and understand what the patient is (or is not) saying. Knowing the right questions to ask is crucial to extracting the correct information. The interviewer should begin with the patient's chief complaint. It is essential to determine the location, onset, quality, frequency, duration, and intensity of the pain; any associated symptoms; precipitating, aggravating, and relieving factors; and prior treatment. Once the clinician has obtained this information, a more accurate diagnosis can be made. Lasagna [38] stated, "The investigator who would study pain is at the mercy of the patient, upon whose ability and willingness to communicate he is dependent."

Clinical studies

38-year-old woman

A 38-year-old woman appeared in the author's office with the chief complaint of chronic, daily headaches with pain localized in the right and left temple area. This pain radiated down the face and into the ears and temporomandibular joints. She stated that she began having headaches several months prior, and waking up in the morning with a "pool of blood" in her mouth. She went to her ear, nose, and throat specialist (ENT), who performed a CT scan of the sinuses. However, the scan appeared normal. She then visited another ENT for a second opinion. This physician told her that he saw no abnormalities in her sinus and to see her dentist for possible TMD. Her dentist referred the patient to the author's office.

The patient reported that she had a history of migraine headaches and recently had changed neurologists in an effort to wean off pain medication, because of fear of rebound headaches. She stated that she had difficulty falling asleep and was a poor sleeper once she did. She reported that she frequently awoke in the middle of the night with head and neck pain, and an awareness that her teeth were clenched together. She also complained of neck stiffness and soreness, and occasional popping of her left temporomandibular joint. She stated that she was taking medication for depression, acid reflux, and IBS, and was also taking a sleep aid. In total, she reported taking nine medications at that time.

Because the patient was treated previously with an intraoral orthotic appliance for nighttime use and desired to reinstitute that treatment, a new appliance was fabricated. She was assured that hers was a complex case involving many factors, largely stress-induced. It was the author's recommendation that she remain under the care of her physician and that they discuss the possibility of behavioral and cognitive counseling to learn coping mechanisms regarding her stress response.

The patient was placed on a 4-week recall and was given instructions to wear the maxillary orthotic appliance on a full-time basis, removing it only to eat and brush her teeth. In addition, palliative instructions were given regarding passive stretching exercises, along with ice, moist heat, and muscle massage with stretching before bedtime. The patient complied with the author's request for behavioral counseling and pursuing other forms of relaxation. Before treatment, she felt as though life was overwhelming and that she had no control over the situation in which she lived. Part of her coping mechanism for the perceived lack of control was to exert control over any portion of her environment where she could. She stated that she would constantly become involved in many projects without completing previous ones. With treatment, she learned to limit the number of projects in which she became involved, and to complete a project before beginning a new one. As she complied with these types of suggestions and care, she was able to eliminate all but two of her medications.

62-year-old man

A 62-year-old male patient presented between recall appointments with the chief complaint of severe, debilitating headaches. He reported that the headaches occurred on waking in the morning and lasted until bedtime. The headaches reached maximum intensity at midday and decreased slowly in intensity until he went to bed. An always underlying level of chronic pain varied from level 4 to as high as 8.5 on a visual analog scale. The patient stated that these headaches began approximately 3 weeks before his visit to the author's office. He had sought help from his primary care physician, who placed him on an analgesic and a muscle relaxant.

The patient was already under long-term care for nocturnal bruxism. He was using a maxillary intraoral orthotic appliance constructed of hard acrylic. He had been instructed to wear the appliance for at least 8 hours at night while sleeping, and was on a 6-month recall. Because he felt that his headaches could be related to his bruxism, he came to the author's office for an evaluation before further testing by his physician.

On examination, heavy wear facets were observed on the appliance. Adjustments were made to the appliance, and a recommendation was given to increase the wearing time from 8 hours to 12 hours in each 24-hour period. He was instructed to place the appliance in his mouth shortly after dinner and wear it until he awakened the next day. Other palliative care was recommended, such as the use of moist heat, soft diet, and so forth. The patient was instructed to return to the author's office in 1 week. He was also encouraged to pursue the tests that his physician had ordered to rule out any catastrophic findings.

The patient returned 1 week later, stating that he had undergone an MRI. The report indicated no significant soft tissue findings. However, it strongly suggested compression at C1 and C2, and a slight bulging of the disc between C3 and C4. He had also undergone a blood test, which revealed no abnormalities. On further evaluation, it was discovered that the patient had retired twice, but was unhappy not working. He had returned to work at a job that required a great deal of travel to foreign countries. He had thought this travel would be enjoyable; however, the current project to which he had been assigned had proven extremely stressful. It had been assigned just 2 weeks before the onset of his severe headaches. He was assured that the next trip he went on would "cost him his job" if it failed. He reported that because of this stress, he had not had a complete night's sleep in weeks.

Based on this information, it was the author's feeling that the patient's stressful occupational situation, his inability to sleep, and his bruxing habit were all leading to cervicogenic headaches. After consulting the patient's physician, the author recommended that the patient be placed on an antidepressant at night, receive physical therapy for the neck and shoulders, and continue the other palliative care recommended previously. Within 3 weeks of this treatment regime, the patient began to experience relief from his headaches and to return to normalization.

10-year-old girl

A 10-year-old girl presented with the chief complaints of continual head pressure and daily headaches. She stated that she would awaken with a headache, which would last throughout the day and still be present when she went to bed. She reported that the headaches began approximately a year before her visit to the author's office; however, the headaches had intensified over the previous 5 weeks to the point where they now included pain in the neck and shoulders. She stated that simply touching the head caused pain throughout her entire body. She was taking adult-strength acetaminophen and Motrin without relief. She preferred to be in a dark room because light intensified her pain. She stated that she had not slept well since the headaches began. She explained that lying down was painful, as was sitting up. She complained of dizziness and of a feeling of weakness because of pain in her legs.

A clinical examination revealed tender points primarily in the anterior temporalis and suboccipital region of the head. The patient was orthodontically skeletal class I with a deep bite and poor anterior tooth contact. She was in mixed dentition.

It was recommended that the patient enter treatment with an intraoral orthotic appliance to add anterior guidance to the functional parameters of the stomatognathic system. It was also recommended that she wear the appliance on a full-time basis for the first 4 to 6 months, removing it only to eat and brush her teeth. In addition to wearing the appliance, the patient was instructed to perform stretching exercises for her jaw and cervical musculature. It was strongly suggested that she visit her primary care physician for a complete evaluation, including imaging.

The results of the diagnostic tests performed by her physician were all negative, including no significant findings from an MRI of the head and neck. The physician placed her on a low dose of amitriptyline and an anti-inflammatory on a "time-contingent" basis. Her physician proposed migraine medication to the patient's parents for her headaches.

During follow-up visits, the patient reported better sleep and that her headaches had begun to improve. At subsequent appointments, it was learned that the headaches began shortly after she and her family moved into a new home in a new neighborhood. The move required her to change schools (which meant new friends and teachers). She was exposed to a difficult teacher who she felt did not understand her. As a result of the demands placed on her at this new school, she became depressed and began to experience vivid dreams, which further impacted her performance in school. Although she had been a straight-A student in her previous school, she was now struggling to deal with her complicated situation. Once her parents learned of the true scope of the problem and took steps to remedy it, the patient began to make dramatic improvements in her pain complaints.

References

[1] Okeson JP. The American Academy of Orofacial Pain. Orofacial pain: guidelines for assessment, diagnosis, and management. Chicago: Quintessence; 1996.

[2] Casey KL. The neurophysiologic basis of pain. In: Bonica JJ, editor. Postgraduate medicine. Minneapolis: McGraw-Hill; 1973. p. 58–63.

[3] Auvenshine RC. Acute vs. chronic pain–an overview. Tex Dent J 2000;117(7):14–20.

[4] Gerschman JA. Chronicity of orofacial pain. Ann R Australas Coll Dent Surg 2000;15: 199–202.

[5] Wessely S, Nimnuan C, Sharpe M. Functional somatic syndromes: one or many? Lancet 1999;354:936–9.

[6] Yunus MB. The concept of central sensitivity syndromes. In: Wallace DJ, Clauw DJ, editors. Fibromyalgia & other central pain syndromes. Philadelphia: Lippincott Williams & Wilkins; 2005. p. 29–43.

[7] Yunus MB, Masi AT, Calabro JJ, et al. Primary fibromyalgia (fibrositis): clinical study of 50 patients with matched normal controls. Semin Arthritis Rheum 1981;11:151–71.

[8] Yunus MB. Primary fibromyalgia syndrome: current concepts. Compr Ther 1984;10:21–8.

[9] Post RM. Transduction of psychosocial stress into the neurobiology of recurrent affective disorder. Am J Psychiatry 1992;149:999–1010.

[10] Pillemer SR, Bradley LA, Crofford LJ, et al. The neuroscience and endocrinology of fibromyalgia. Arthritis Rheum 1997;40:1928–39.

[11] Torpy DJ, Papanicolaou DA, Lotsikas AJ, et al. Responses of the sympathetic nervous system and the hypothalamic-pituitary-adrenal axis to interleukin-6: a pilot study in fibromyalgia. Arthritis Rheum 2000;43:872–80.

[12] Ulrich-Lai YM, Xie W, Meij JT, et al. Limbic and HPA axis function in an animal model of chronic neuropathic pain. Physiol Behav 2006;88(1–2):67–76.

[13] Auvenshine RC. Psychoneuroimmunology and its relationship to the differential diagnosis of temporomandibular disorders. Dent Clin North Am 1997;41(2):279–96.

[14] Swabb DF, Bao AM, Lucassen PJ. The stress system in the human brain in depression and neurodegeneration. Ageing Res Rev 2005;4(2):141–94.

[15] Raison CL, Miller AH. When not enough is too much: the role of insufficient glucocorticoid signaling in the pathophysiology of stress-related disorders. Am J Psychiatry 2003;160(9): 1554–65.

[16] Born J, Fehm HL. Hypothalamus-pituitary-adrenal activity during human sleep: a coordinating role for the limbic hippocampal system. Exp Clin Endocrinol Diabetes 1998;106(3): 153–63.

[17] LeResche L. Epidemiology of temporomandibular disorders: implications for the investigation of etiologic factors. Crit Rev Oral Biol Med 1997;8(3):291–305.

[18] Wolf F, Smythe HA, Yunus MB, et al. The American College of Rheumatology 1990 criteria for the classification of fibromyalgia. Report of the Multicenter Criteria Committee. Arthritis Rheum 1990;33:160–72.

[19] Gibson JJ, Littlejohn GO, et al. Altered heart pain thresholds and cerebral event-related potentials following painful CO_2 laser stimulation in subjects with fibromyalgia syndrome. Pain 1994;58:185–93.

[20] Ciccone DS, Natelson BH. Comorbid illness in women with chronic fatigue syndrome: a test of the single syndrome hypothesis. Psychosom Med 2003;65:268–75.

[21] Chang L, Heitkemper MM. Gender differences in irritable bowel syndrome. Gastroenterology 2002;123:1686–701.

[22] Cullens M. The worker with chemical sensitivities: an overview. Occup Med 1987;2: 655–61.

[23] Bell I, Rossi J, Gilbert M, et al. Testing the neural sensitization and kindling hypothesis for illness from low levels of environmental chemicals. Environ Health Perspect 1997; 105(Suppl. 2):539–47.

[24] Ahlqwist M, Bengtsson C, Furunes B, et al. Number of amalgam tooth fillings in relation to subjectively experienced symptoms in a study of Swedish women. Community Dent Oral Epidemiol 1988;16(4):227–31.

[25] Shenenberger DW, Knee T. Hyperprolactinemia. Available at: http//www.emedicine.com/med/tipic1098.htm. Accessed July 11, 2006.

[26] Lombardi G, Iodice M, Miletto P, et al. Prolactin and TSH response to TRH and metoclopramide before and after l-thyroxine therapy l-thyroxine therapy in subclinical hypothyroidism. Neuroendocrinology 1986;(6):676–8.

[27] Verhelst J, Abs R. Hyperprolactinemia: patholophysiology and management. Treat Endocrinol 2003;2(1):23–32.

[28] Mah PM, Webster J. Hyperprolactinemia: etiology, diagnosis, and management. Semin Reprod Med 2002;20(4):365–74.

[29] Cornell LV. Mitral valve prolapse syndrome: etiology and symptomology. Nurse Pract 1985; 10(4):25–6,29,34.

[30] Vankatesh A, Pauls DL, Crowe R, et al. Mitral valve prolapse in anxiety neurosis (panic disorder). Am Heart J 1980;100(3):302–5.

[31] Boudoulas H, Wooley CF. Mitral valve prolapse syndrome: neuro-endocrinological aspects. Herz 1988;13(4):249–58.

[32] Woeber KA. Update on the management of hyperthyroidism and hypothyroidism. Arch Intern Med 2000;160:1067–71.

[33] Guha B, Krishnaswamy G, Peiris A. The diagnosis and management of hypothyroidism. South Med J 2002;95(5):475–80.

[34] Broner S, Lay C. Menstrual migraine. Chicago: National Headache Foundation; 2005.

[35] Headache Classification Subcommittee of the International Headache Society (HIS). The International Classification of Headache Disorders. 12th edition. Cephalgia 2003;23: 302–8.
[36] Barden N. Implication of the hypothalamic-pituitary-adrenal axis in the physiopathology of depression. J Psychiatry Neurosc 2004;29(3):185–93.
[37] Barsky AJ, Borus J. Functional somatic syndromes. Ann Intern Med 1999;130(11):910–21.
[38] Lasagna L. Clinical measurements of pain. Ann N Y Acad Sci 1960;86:28–37.

THE DENTAL
CLINICS
OF NORTH AMERICA

Dent Clin N Am 51 (2007) 129–144

Temporomandibular Disorders and Headache

Steven B. Graff-Radford, DDS

*The Pain Center, Cedars-Sinai Medical Center, 444 South San Vicente,
#1101 Los Angeles, CA 90048, USA*

Headache is a common symptom, but when severe, it may be extremely disabling. Although the most common headache is tension-type headache, it rarely is severe enough to require medical attention. Migraine is the headache that is seen most commonly by physicians. The disorder affects 28 million Americans, yet only 50% are diagnosed as migraine. Many patients are believed to have tension-type headache and sinus headache. It is assumed that patients who present to dentists with headache often are diagnosed with a temporomandibular disorder (TMD), although many may have migraine. TMD as a collective term may include several clinical entities, including myogenous and arthrogenous components. Pain in the temporomandibular joint (TMJ) may occur in 10% of the population [1], and TMDs have been reported in 46.1% of the United States population [2]. Because headache and TMD are so common they may be integrated or separate entities. Nevertheless, the TMJ and associated orofacial structures should be considered as triggering or perpetuating factors for migraine. Ciancaglini and Radaelli [3] reported that headache occurs significantly more frequently in patients who have TMD symptoms (27.4% versus 15.2%). It is important that the clinician considers peripheral and central processes that may contribute to headache. Often, ignoring the TMJ, muscles, or other orofacial structures as a peripheral trigger results in a poor clinical outcome in managing headache; at the same time, not making the correct diagnosis may lead to unnecessary therapy and poor outcome. The trigeminal nerve is the final conduit of face, neck, and head pain [4]. As a result of the central connections, it is possible for referral to occur between divisions [5]. The management of pain in the first division may be influenced by therapy that is aimed at structures that are innervated

E-mail address: graffs@cshs.org

by the second or third trigeminal division. Therefore, it is important that cause and effect connections between TMD and headache are judged carefully. This article discusses the relationship between the TMJ, muscles, or other orofacial structures and headache.

The teeth and headache

The pathology that is associated with dental disease is not a common cause of headache. Dental disease may be summarized as pulpal or periodontal. Pulpal pain may be characterized as an irreversible pulpitis, where pulpal tissue death is inevitable and results in root canal therapy. Reversible pulpitis may be resolved by eliminating the inciting pathology (eg, caries). Periodontal disorders involve the supporting teeth structures, the bone, periodontal ligament, and cementum. Periodontal disease triggers tissue inflammation, which often produces pain and swelling in the affected site. When acute pain occurs in the dental structures, patients often describe referred pain and tenderness to adjacent structures, including headache. The frequency and epidemiology of headache and tooth pain is unknown. Headache usually is a secondary phenomenon and it does not pose a significant diagnostic dilemma. Pericoronitis may be the most frequent periodontal inflammation that causes headache. Pericoronitis, as its name implies, results from infection or traumatic irritation around a partially erupted tooth, usually a third molar.

These dental problems are managed best with conventional dental therapies, and rarely produce any long-term or significant disability. Chronic dental pains are different, however. Atypical odontalgia (AO) has been linked with headache and described as possible secondary to a migrainous etiology [6,7]. Unfortunately, atypical facial pain has become a wastebasket term for all pains in the face that are not diagnosed readily. Harris [8] first described AO as slightly more specific because it is localized to the tooth site. Graff-Radford and Solberg [9,10] defined AO as pain in a tooth or tooth site where no organic cause is obvious. They emphasized that before making a diagnosis, positive inclusionary criteria are required, rather than arriving at the diagnosis by exclusion. Graff-Radford and Solberg [11,12] suggested a deafferentation mechanism; peripheral, central, or sympathetically maintained pain usually is present when patients are labeled "atypical." The relationship of psychopathology and AO also has been explored by Graff-Radford and Solberg [13], and no positive relationship was found between psychologic diagnosis and the pain. It is most likely that these pains are neuropathic, and follow some neural injury or sensitization; they can be divided into pains that are mediated by the sensory system or the sympathetic system [12]. Therefore, criteria are proposed for defining neuropathic facial pain. The correct term should be "trigeminal deafferentation." The criteria for trigeminal deafferentation include continuous pain that is punctuated with sharp electric pains and requires four of the following:

Known trauma
Presence of neurosensory deficit (numbness)
Allodynia
Hyperalgesia
Temperature change
Block effect (somatic or sympathetic)

Patients who have persistent facial pain may report an increase in their headache frequency. This may result from nociceptive stimuli that trigger migraine or a change in central pain inhibition that lowers the migraine threshold. Nevertheless, headache management may be achieved best by addressing the peripheral trigger and the migraine independently. Medications that are used commonly to manage the neuropathic facial pain also may decrease the migraine frequency; however, patients also should be provided with an acute or abortive migraine-directed medications (eg, triptans).

Migraine and facial pain

Lovshin [14] was the first to describe migraine as a facial pain problem that could occur without pain in the first division of the trigeminal nerve. The pain in facial migraine is described as dull pain, with superimposed throbbing that occurs once to several times per week. Each attack may last minutes to hours. Raskin and Prusiner [15] described ipsilatertal carotid tenderness in facial migraine, a finding that also is seen when migraine occurs in the head. This condition also has been referred to as carotidynia. Treatment of facial migraine is no different from that for migraine that presents in the head. All treatments should include an understanding that the disorder is genetic, and that the goals should be to reduce pain frequency and intensity, restore function, and provide a sense of self-control. Therapy may involve nonpharmacologic and pharmacologic approaches. In general, addressing triggering factors through diet, exercise, and sleep is first-line care. The acute attack is treated by administration of the most effective therapy early. Analgesics, anti-inflammatories, ergots, and triptans are used most commonly. If the headache is frequent, preventative medications may be considered. The groups of medications that may be considered are β-blockers, calcium channel blockers, antidepressants, antiepileptic (membrane-stabilizing) drugs, and antiserotonin drugs [16].

Temporomandibular disorders and headache

Scientific investigation has described the pathways and mechanisms for pain referral from the head to the TMJ and vice versa [17]. Headache may result from temporomandibular structures or pain may be referred to the TMJ, secondary to a primary headache diagnoses. Functional disorders and pain in the anatomic region of the TMJ and associated musculature are referred to as TMDs. This overlap primarily is related to the anatomy and neural innervations. It is essential not to confuse the issue and suggest a cause and effect relationship based on treatment responses. Because the trigeminal nerve is the final pathway for head pain and TMDs, it makes the relationship between TMDs and headache confusing. It is suggested that the two are separate, but may be aggravating or perpetuating factors for each other. Patients who have primary headache can see their pain worsened or triggered when there is a coexisting TMD.

Epidemiology

TMD epidemiology has not differentiated headache from facial pain specifically. In nonpatient population studies, 75% of subjects have at least one joint dysfunction sign (clicking, limited range of motion) and about 33% have at least one symptom (pain, pain on palpation). Out of the 75% of subjects who have a sign or symptom, fewer than 5% require treatment; even fewer have headache as the primary pain location. Headache is referred to often in TMD studies, but few define its etiology. This makes it difficult to determine the relationship of TMD etiology and therapy in specific headache types.

Etiology

Inflammation within the joint accounts for TMD pain, and the dysfunction is due to a disk–condyle incoordination. Muscle pain disorders may include spasm, myositis, muscle splinting, and myofascial pain. Myofascial pain is the most frequent muscle disorder that is included in TMD classification. Although each may be a trigger for headache and they can occur together, they are discussed separately.

Inflammation

Primary inflammatory conditions of the TMJ include capsulitis, synovitis, and the polyarthritides. Polyarthritides are uncommon and are associated primarily with rheumatologic disease. Inflammatory conditions, such as synovitis or capsulitis, frequently occur secondary to trauma, irritation, or infection, and they often accompany other TMDs [18].

Several proinflammatory cytokines have been detected in painful TMDs, which suggests that they may play a role in pain [19]. Capsulitis, an inflammation of the capsule that is related to sprain of capsular ligaments, is clinically difficult, if not impossible, to differentiate from synovitis. The pain that is related to capsulitis increases during all translatory movements and joint distraction, but not usually during clenching, however [20]. Both conditions may be accompanied by a fluctuating swelling (due to effusion) that decreases the ability to occlude on the ipsilateral posterior teeth. Pain that is associated with inflammation is localized to the TMJ capsule and the intracapsular tissues. Typically, the pain is dull achy, but it may be throbbing. It is described frequently as sharp with jaw movements. The pain is continuous, but worsens with jaw function.

Disk derangement disorders

Articular disk displacement is the most common TMJ arthropathy; it is characterized by several stages of clinical dysfunction that involve the disk–condyle relation. The usual direction for displacement is anterior or anteromedial [21,22], although other directions have been described. Pain or mandibular movement symptoms are not specific for disk derangement disorders [23], and disk position may not be related to any presenting symptom [24,25].

The causes of disk displacement are not agreed upon; however, it is postulated that in most cases, stretched or torn ligaments that bind the disk to the condyle permit the disk to become displaced [26] An increased horizontal angle of the mandibular condyle has been associated with more advanced TMJ internal derangement [27,28] Lubrication impairment also has been suggested as a possible etiologic factor of disk displacement [29]. Disk displacement is subdivided into disk displacement with reduction or disk displacement without reduction.

Disk displacement with reduction

Disk displacement with reduction is described when a temporarily misaligned disk reduces or improves its structural relation with the condyle when mandibular translation occurs during opening. This produces a joint noise (sound) that is described as clicking or popping. Disk displacement with reduction usually is characterized by "reciprocal clicking," a reciprocal noise that is heard during the opening movement and again before the teeth occlude during the closing movement. Because disk displacement with reduction is so common, it may represent a physiologic accommodation without clinical significance [30,31]. Clicking in reducing disk displacement is not pathologic, because more than one third of an asymptomatic sample can have moderate to severe derangement, and as many as one quarter of clicking joints show normal or only slightly displaced disk positions. Disk displacement may or may not be a painful condition. If the condition is painful, inflammation of the retrodiskal tissue, the synovial tissues, the capsule or the ligaments, or pressure and traction on the disk attachments are more likely the causes of the pain [32]. TMJ disk displacement with reduction may persist for several years up to decades without progression or complication [33]. de Leeuw and colleagues [33] reported that if clicking in patients who have disk displacement with reduction does not respond to treatment and is still present after 2 to 4 years, it is likely to persist for several decades. Disk displacement with reduction may progress to disk displacement without reduction. This condition is characterized by the sudden cessation of clicking and the sudden onset of restricted mouth opening, and frequently is accompanied by pain.

Disk displacement without reduction

Disk displacement without reduction is a permanently displaced disk that does not improve its relation with the condyle on translation. When acute, it is characterized by sudden and marked limited mouth opening because of a jamming or fixation of the disk secondary to disk adhesion, deformation, or dystrophy. Often, pain is present and is related especially to the patient's attempt to open the mouth. The acute stage is manifested clinically as a straight-line deflection to the affected side on opening, a marked limited laterotrusion to the contralateral side, and a lack of joint noise in the affected joint. As the condition becomes chronic, the pain is reduced markedly from the acute stage to the point of becoming nonpainful in many cases; the opening range may approach normal dimensions over time [34]. If chronic, there usually is a history of joint noise or limitation of mandibular opening [35]; the condition may progress to reveal radiographically visible osteoarthritic changes. Generally, disk displacement is treated with reassurance and education, rest, instructions to avoid loading, control of contributing factors, and mobility exercises within the pain-free range. In the presence of pain, mild analgesics or anti-inflammatory medications are the drugs of choice. Additional management may consist of splint therapy, physical therapy, arthrocentesis, or arthroscopy to restore range of motion. In an acute disk displacement without reduction, one may try to reduce the disk manually and temporarily maintain the disk–condyle relationship with an anterior repositioning splint. This splint holds the lower jaw forward of its resting position, thereby translating it with the objective of keeping the disk in a favorable position. Outcome is poor. When the disk cannot be reduced, a stabilization appliance can be part of the treatment for painful disk displacement with or without reduction. The high degree of spontaneous reduction of symptoms has to be taken into account before recommending any kind of treatment. Surgical treatments, such as arthroscopy and open joint surgeries, may be considered, but only after reasonable nonsurgical efforts have failed and the patient's quality of life is affected significantly [36].

Myofascial pain

Myofascial pain is characterized as a regional muscle pain, described as dull or achy and associated with the presence of trigger points in muscles, tendons, or fascia [37–39]. Myofascial pain is a common cause of persistent regional pain (eg, neck pain, shoulder pain, headaches, orofacial pain) [40]. The major characteristics of myofascial pain include trigger points in muscles and local and referred pain. A trigger point is identified as a localized area of tenderness in a nodule or a palpable taut band of muscle, tendon, or ligament. The trigger points may be active or latent. Active trigger points are hypersensitive and display continuous pain in the zone of reference that can be altered with specific palpation. Latent trigger points display other characteristics of trigger points, such as increased muscle tension or muscle shortening, but do not produce spontaneous pain. Usually, the pain is dull and deep in quality, diffuse in nature, and present in subcutaneous tissues, including muscle and joints.

Myofascial therapy can be directed peripherally or centrally. The emphasis must be on management and controlling perpetuating factors, while enhancing central inhibition. Active relaxation exercises, spray and stretch, acupressure, ultrasound, deep massage, moist heat, electrical stimulation, transcutaneous electrical nerve stimulation, biofeedback, relaxation techniques, cognitive-behavioral techniques, occlusal stabilization appliances, myofascial release, pharmacotherapy (eg, nonsteroidal anti-inflammatory drugs, muscle relaxants, tricyclic antidepressants), needling, and infiltration of taut bands with local anesthetic alone or combined with botulinum toxin have been used [41–44].

Increased tenderness in pericranial muscles is the most prominent clinical finding in patients who have tension-type headache and migraine. The relationship between local tenderness (as seen in trigger points) and general tenderness (as seen in allodynia associated with migraine) must be differentiated. The first indication that there may be a correlation with the muscle tenderness and pain was shown in experiments by Kellgren [45]. He injected an algesic substance (hypertonic saline) into the muscle, and asked the subjects to define the area in which they perceived pain. The subjects who received the hypertonic saline injections mapped out patterns of referral similar to those seen in tension-type headache. Further, he injected local anesthetic into similar areas after the pain was initiated and could abolish the pain. These tender points became known as myofascial trigger points. The question that may be asked is "Under what circumstances could referral take place in the patterns described?".

Mense [46–48] described a hypothesis for muscle pain referral to other deep somatic tissues remote from the original muscle stimulation site. He criticized the convergence-projection pain referral theory because there is little convergence evident at the dorsal horn from deep tissues. Mense's hypothesis adds two new components to the convergence-projection theory. First, the convergent connections from deep tissues to dorsal horn neurons are opened only after nociceptive inputs from muscle are activated. The connections that are opened after muscle stimuli are called silent connections. Second, the referral to muscle, beyond the initially activated site, is due to central sensitization and spread to adjacent spinal segments. The initiating stimulus requires a peripheral inflammatory process (neurogenic inflammation). In the animal model that was described by Mense, the noxious stimulus was bradykinin injected into the muscle. In the work by Kellgren, a hypertonic saline solution was used to trigger the referred pain. This seems to mimic what is seen in the animal model. It is unclear what triggers the muscle referral in the clinical setting where there usually is no obvious inflammation-producing incident. Mense's theory was used by Simons [49] to discuss a neurophysiologic basis for trigger point pain. Simons hypothesized that when the tender area in the muscle is palpated, there is a neurotransmitter release in the dorsal horn (trigeminal nucleus) that results in previously silent nociceptive inputs becoming active. This, in turn, causes distant neurons to produce a retrograde referred pain. This model accounts for most of the clinical presentation and therapeutic options that are seen in myofascial pain, but it does not account for what initiates the peripheral tenderness that must be present to activate the silent connections. Perhaps a central nervous system–activated neurogenic inflammation, similar to migraine, stimulates nociceptors in muscle, rather than around the blood vessel. Calcitonin gene–related peptide, neurokinin A, and substance P have been used to demonstrate their contribution in myofascial pain [50]. Fields [51] described a means whereby the central nervous system may switch on nociception. He described the presence of "on" cells, which, when stimulated, may produce activation of trigeminal nucleus nociceptors.

In 1991, Olesen and Jensen [52] were the first to suggest a relationship between myofascial pain and tension-type headache. They proposed a vascular-supraspinal-myogenic model for headache pain. This model hypothesizes that perceived pain (headache) intensity is modulated by the central nervous system. In tension-type headache, the inputs primarily are myofascial, whereas in migraine these inputs are vascular. This model helps to explain why the clinical presentation and treatment options often are similar for migraine and tension-type headache, and why there is only temporary relief with peripheral treatments (eg trigger point injections). The resultant hyperalgesia or trigger point sensitivity in myofascial pain may represent a peripheral sensitization to serum levels of serotonin. Ernberg and colleagues [53] showed a significant correlation between serum serotonin levels and allodynia that is associated with muscular face pain. Based on this information, it is proposed that in patients who present with dull aching head pain and related muscle tenderness, the cause may be myofascial pain. In other words, myofascial pain and tension-type headache may be associated with the same or similar mechanisms. Bendtsen [54] hypothesized that central neuroplastic changes may affect the regulation of peripheral mechanisms that lead to increased pericranial muscle activity or release of neurotransmitters in the muscle tissues. By these mechanisms, the central sensitization can be maintained even after the initial eliciting factors are gone. This may account for conversion of episodic headache into chronic tension-type headache.

Treating headache by targeting temporomandibular disorders

Because there are believed to be several etiologic factors involved in TMDs, it is to be expected that there are several therapeutic approaches.

Unfortunately, most of the literature concerning the treatment of TMDs consists of uncontrolled observations; less than 5% of treatment studies have been controlled clinical trials [55]. Even these are sometimes compromised by weaknesses in their design. Thus, only general conclusions can be drawn regarding treatment effectiveness. When the effects of different treatments are compared, the results seldom reveal major advantages of one method over another. Elimination of the cause would be the most effective treatment; however, if the cause cannot be identified, symptomatic treatment has to be provided. The goals of treatment are to decrease pain, decrease adverse loading, and restore normal function. Because the signs and symptoms of TMDs can be transient and self-limiting, simple and reversible treatments have to be preferred over complicated and irreversible procedures.

Nonsurgical treatment

In an uncontrolled study, 33 patients who had TMDs were treated with occlusal splint (OS) therapy [56]. Following 4 weeks of therapy, 64% of patients reported a decrease in the number of weekly headaches; 30% showed a complete remission of headache. Patients who had a high frequency of headaches (≥ 4 per week) seemed to respond more favorably to OS therapy.

In another uncontrolled study with patients who had TMDs, changes in headache were followed 1 year after the start of TMD treatment [57]. The treatment consisted of OSs, therapeutic exercises for masticatory muscles, or occlusal adjustment—most often combinations of these measures. Seventy percent of the patients reported less frequent headaches than 1 year earlier. Forty percent reported less severe head pain. The results achieved seemed to be lasting at a 2.5-year follow-up [58]. These studies, however, did not control for the placebo effect, and the type of headache being treated was not stated clearly. Furthermore, one cannot know what part of the treatment was necessary.

Vallon and coworkers [59–61] assessed the effects of occlusal adjustment on headache in patients who had TMDs. Fifty patients were assigned randomly to a treatment group or a control group that received counseling only. The treatment outcome was evaluated after 1, 3, and 6 months and 2 years by a blinded examiner. No significant differences were found regarding changes in frequency of headache. The problem with the study was the significant drop-out of patients, which ranged from 20% at the 3-month follow-up to 66% at 2 years.

A new form of splint therapy has been suggested to manage headache effectively. Shankland [62] suggested an intraoral Nociceptive Trigeminal Inhibition Tension Suppression System (NTI-tss) device for the reduction of frequency and severity of tension-type and migraine headaches, as compared with the known efficacy of the noncommercially available full-coverage OS. A multicenter open-labeled trial was conducted to determine the response in patients who had migraine. The NTI-tss is a small intraoral device that is fitted over the two maxillary central incisors; it has a dome-shaped protrusion that extends lingually. The dome is customized by the provider to act as single-point contact at the incisal embrasure of the two mandibular central incisors, thereby preventing posterior or canine tooth contact. Following a 4-week pretreatment baseline observation, patients were instructed to insert and wear their device during sleep—and as required during perceived stressful times during the day—for eight consecutive weeks. A control device—mandibular full-coverage OS—was used. Ninety-four patients were studied and randomized to the NTI-tss (n = 43) or full coverage OS (n = 51). Although this was a migraine study, it seems that patients had chronic tension-type headache. The statistical analysis is confusing, because no information is given on pretreatment days of headache and outcome is reported as the number of headaches reduced. As with many other intraoral appliance studies, it is difficult to correlate outcome with pharmacologic studies of prevention, because the patient selection, outcome criteria, and statistical analyses are confusing. This is not to detract from the concept that managing a TMD in a patient who has migraine may reduce headache frequency.

Because TMDs are believed to have a multifactorial etiology, it is assumed that the best treatment results are achieved by using several treatment methods to eliminate as many predisposing and perpetuating factors as possible. This assumption was addressed in a randomized, controlled study that compared the effects of occlusal equilibration with other forms of TMD therapy in patients who had signs and symptoms of TMDs, including headache [63]. The TMD therapy consisted of OSs as well as muscle exercises and minor occlusal adjustment in some cases, whereas the comparison group received only occlusal equilibration therapy. The reductions in the symptoms of TMD and the frequency and intensity of headache were significantly greater in the group that received combined therapy.

Some studies that focused on signs and symptoms that are attributable to TMDs have been performed on patients who have a variety of diagnoses. In a series of studies, 100 patients who had recurrent headache and were referred for neurologic examination were invited for a functional examination of the stomatognathic system [64]. In total, 55 patients displayed pain that was caused by a TMD. The pain was determined to be of myogenous origin in 51 patients and of arthrogenous origin in 4 patients. The 55 patients were divided randomly into two groups [65]. One group was treated by the neurologist with conventional headache treatment regimes; the other group was treated with stabilization splints for 6 weeks, and, in some cases, with physical therapy. Headache frequency decreased in 56% of the patients who received treatment for TMDs (compared with 32% of the patients who received neurologic treatment). There also were significant differences in the reduction of headache intensity and in the use of symptomatic medication to abort a headache at the time of onset. Thus, the clinical result of TMD therapy exceeded the results of the neurologic treatment in patients in whom headache was assumed to be related to TMD. The confounding factor is that the group that received treatment for a TMD had a much greater exposure to the treating clinician, which could account, in part, for the difference.

A randomized, controlled trial by Forssell and colleagues [66] evaluated the effect of occlusal adjustment versus a mock adjustment on tension-type headache using a double-blind study design. The subjects included 56 patients who had tension headaches (20 of them also had migraine [ie, combination headache]) from a neurologic clinic. Most of them reported subjective symptoms of TMD, and signs of TMD were registered in all patients. Patients were assigned randomly to active and placebo groups, and after a 4- to 8-month follow-up period a neurologist evaluated the treatment outcome. The headache frequency and intensity were reduced in 80% and 47%, respectively, of patients who had active treatment (50% and 16%, respectively with placebo). Some of the patients who received placebo and had moderate to severe TMD symptoms were treated with occlusal therapy afterwards [67]. A significant reduction in headache frequency also was observed in these patients. Except for the possible confounder that the same clinician performed both treatments (active and placebo) unblinded, this study again supports the value of TMD treatment for tension-type headache that is associated with TMD signs and symptoms.

Contradictory results were reported by Quayle and coworkers [68] in an uncontrolled study of patients who had headache and were treated with soft OSs for 6 weeks. Many patients who had migraine-type headache improved, but most patients who suffered from tension headache failed to benefit from splint therapy. The small number of patients (n = 9) in the group that had tension headache may reduce the significance of the result.

In the double-blind trial by Karppinen [69], 44 patients who sought treatment for chronic headache and neck and shoulder pain received a routine battery of physical therapy. In addition, 23 of the patients were allocated randomly to occlusal adjustment and 21 received mock adjustment. Patients were followed up at 6 weeks and 12 months. The short-term response to physical therapy was good and was not associated with the type of occlusal treatment. At 12 months, the effects of treatment began to subside in the group that received mock adjustment, but further improvement was evident in the group that had occlusal adjustment. A statistically significant decrease in the occurrence of headache was observed with the real adjustment compared with the mock adjustment. In a qualitative systematic review of randomized controlled trials of analysis of occlusal therapies for TMD, Forssell and colleagues [70] concluded that there was insufficient evidence to support the use of occlusal adjustments, and suggestive evidence for splint therapy.

Because several controlled clinical trials seem to suggest that TMD treatment can be effective for headache, the question arises whether some special features could, in practice, help to single out patients whose headache is related to TMD. Reik and Hale [71] suggested that patients who had continuous unilateral headache had a TMD. This was not supported by Schokker and colleagues [72], who found that headaches that were responsive to TMD treatment mainly were bilateral and showed only a tendency to be present permanently. In that study, patients who had headaches that were linked to TMD showed a greater difference between passive and active mouth opening recorded before treatment. This is considered to be a sign of myogenous origin of TMD. Another study showed that patients who had reported pain while chewing responded more favorably in terms of headache reduction following TMD therapy [73]. Pain while chewing is one of the most common subjective symptoms of TMD.

Several investigators who performed systematic reviews of the TMD literature concluded that there is evidence to support the use of stabilization splints in patients who have more severe TMDs, but weak evidence to support their use with mild TMDs. Care should be taken to avoid repositioning therapy of partial coverage therapy because it may result in significant changes to the occlusion [74–76].

Surgical treatment

TMJ surgery is considered to be useful treatment for certain TMDs. There are few studies that examined surgery and response to headache. Vallerand and Hall [77] reported on 50 patients who were diagnosed with internal TMJ derangements, myalgia, and headaches who had not responded to nonsurgical management. The surgical procedures that they underwent included disk repositioning, repair of disk perforation, disk recontouring, lysis of adhesions, and diskectomy. In the retrospective evaluation, most patients reported decreases in headache as well as decreases in joint pain and noise. The surgeons suggested that the change in head pain is a secondary result of decreasing joint pain, which allowed the patients to cope better with other pains. In another study, Montgomery and colleagues [78] reported significant changes in TMJ and ear, neck, and shoulder pains, whereas headaches were changed less consistently following arthroscopy of the TMJ.

Summary

Much can be learned by trying to identify and understand pain mechanisms and apply current therapeutic options based on these concepts. This allows a broad approach to an often complex and challenging problem. Our primary goal must be to alleviate the pain and suffering that our patients who have head, neck, and facial pain experience. Therefore, we are obliged to approach pain management using all of the therapies at our disposal, with specific care not to worsen the situation. Sometimes, therapy can be aimed specifically at the source of nociception; however, in chronic situations, dealing with behavior and suffering may be more important than altering the nociception. To this end, all clinicians are encouraged to understand the mechanisms that cause pain, and to remember that attached to every joint and nerve is a human being.

References

[1] Glass EG, McGlynn FD, Glaros AG, et al. Prevalence of temporomandibular disorder symptoms in a major metropolitan area. Cranio 1993;11:217–20.
[2] Le Resche L. Epidemiology of temporomandibular disorders: implications for the investigation of etiologic factors. Crit Rev Oral Biol Med 1997;8:291–305.
[3] Ciancaglini R, Radaelli G. The relationship between headache and symptoms of temporomandibular disorders in the general population. J Dent 2001;29:93–8.
[4] Piovesan EJ, Kowacs PA, Tatsui CE, et al. Referred pain after painful stimulation of the greater occipital nerve in humans: evidence of convergence of cervical afferents on trigeminal nuclei. Cephalalgia 2001;21(2):107–9.
[5] Bartsch T, Goadsby PJ. Increased responses in trigeminocervical nociceptive neurons to cervical input after stimulation of the dura mater. Brain 2003;126:1801–13.
[6] Brooke RI. Periodic migrainous neuralgia: a cause of dental pain. Oral Surg Oral Med Oral Pathol 1978;46:511–5.
[7] Sicuteri F, Nicolodi M, Fusco BM, et al. Idiopathic headache as a possible risk factor for phantom tooth pain. Headache 1991;31:577–81.
[8] Harris M. Psychosomatic disorders of the mouth and face. Practitioner 1975;214:372–4.
[9] Graff-Radford SB, Solberg WK. Atypical odontalgia. J Calif Dent Assoc 1986;14:27–31.
[10] Graff-Radford SB, Solberg WK. Atypical odontalgia. J Craniomandib Disord Oral Facial Pain 1992;6:260–6.
[11] Graff-Radford SB, Solberg WK. Differential neural blockade in atypical odontalgia. Cephalalgia 1991;Suppl 11(2):289–91.
[12] Graff-Radford SB. Facial pain. Curr Opin Neurol 2000;13:291–6.
[13] Graff-Radford SB, Solberg WK. Is atypical odontalgia a psychological problem? Oral Surg Oral Med Oral Pathol 1993;75:579–82.
[14] Lovshin LL. Carotidynia. Headache 1977;17:192–5.
[15] Raskin NH, Prusiner S. Carotidynia. Neurology 1977;27:43–6.
[16] Silberstein SD. Practice parameter. Evidence-based guidelines for migraine headache: report of the Quality Standards Subcommittee of the American Academy of Neurology. Neurology 2000;55:754–62.
[17] Cairns BE, Sessel BJ, Hu JW. Evidence that excitatory amino acid receptors within the temporomandibular joint region are involved in the reflex activation of jaw muscles. J Neurosci 1998;18:8056–64.
[18] Schille H. Injuries of the temporomandibular joint: classification, diagnosis and fundamentals of treatment. In: Kruger E, Schilli W, editors. Oral and maxillofacial traumatology, vol. 2. Chicago: Quintessence Publishing Co.; 1986.
[19] Takahashi T, Kondoh T, Fukuda M, et al. Proinflammatory cytokines detectable in synovial fluids from patients with temporomandibular disorders. Oral Surg Oral Med Oral Pathol Oral Radiol Endod 1998;85:135–41.
[20] Okeson JP. Diagnosis of temporomandibular disorders. In: Okeson JP, editor. Temporomandibular disorder and occlusion. 4th edition. St. Louis (MO): Mosby; 1998. p. 310–51.
[21] Isberg-Holm AM, Westesson PL. Movement of the disc and condyle in temporomandibular joints with clicking: An arthrographic and cineradiographic study on autopsy specimens. Acta Odontol Scand 1982;40:151–64.
[22] Farrar WB, McCarty WL. A clinical outline of the temporomandibular joint diagnosis and treatment. Edited by NS Group, Montgomery, 1983. p. 19.
[23] Tallents RH, Hatala M, Katzberg RW, et al. Temporomandibular joint sounds in asymptomatic volunteers. J Prosthet Dent 1993;69:298–304.

[24] Kozeniauskas JJ, Ralph WJ. Bilateral arthrographic evaluation of unilateral temporomandibular joint pain and dysfunction. J Prosthet Dent 1988;60:98–105.
[25] Davant TS, Greene CS, Perry HT, et al. A quantitative computer-assisted analysis of disc displacement in patients with internal derangement using sagittal view magnetic resonance imaging. J Oral Maxillofac Surg 1993;51:974–9.
[26] Stegenga B, de Bont LG, Boering G, et al. Tissue responses to degenerative changes in the temporomandibular joint: a review. J Oral Maxillofac Surg 1991;49:1079–88.
[27] Westesson PL, Bifano JA, Tallents RH, et al. Increased horizontal angle of the mandibular condyle in abnormal temporomandibular joints. A magnetic resonance imaging study. Oral Surg Oral Med Oral Pathol 1991;72:359–63.
[28] Nilner M, Petersson A. Clinical and radiological findings related to treatment outcome in patients with temporomandibular disorders. Dentomaxillofac Radiol 1995;24:128–31.
[29] Nitzan DW. The process of lubrication impairment and its involvement in temporomandibular joint disc displacement: a theoretical concept. J Oral Maxillofac Surg 2001;59:36–45.
[30] Scapino RP. The posterior attachment: its structure, function, and appearance in TMJ imaging studies. Part 1. J Craniomandib Disord 1991;5:83–95.
[31] Scapino RP. The posterior attachment: its structure, function, and appearance in TMJ imaging studies. Part 2. J Craniomandib Disord 1991;5:155–66.
[32] Dolwick MF. Intra-articular disc displacement. Part I: Its questionable role in temporomandibular joint pathology. J Oral Maxillofac Surg 1995;53:1069–72.
[33] de Leeuw R, Boering G, Stegenga B, et al. Clinical signs of TMJ osteoarthrosis and internal derangement 30 years after nonsurgical treatment. J Orofac Pain 1994;8:18–24.
[34] Stegenga B, de Bont LG, Dijkstra PU, et al. Short-term outcome of arthroscopic surgery of temporomandibular joint osteoarthrosis and internal derangement: a randomized controlled clinical trial. Br J Oral Maxillofac Surg 1993;31:3–14.
[35] Choi BH, Yoo JH, Lee WY. Comparison of magnetic resonance imaging before and after non-surgical treatment of closed lock. Oral Surg Oral Med Oral Pathol 1994;7:301–5.
[36] de Bont LG, Dijkgraaf LC, Stegenga B. Epidemiology and natural progression of articular temporomandibular disorder. Oral Surg Oral Med Oral Pathol 1997;83:72–6.
[37] Rivner MH. The neurophysiology of myofascial pain syndrome. Curr Pain Headache Rep 2001;5:432–40.
[38] Gerwin RD. Classification, epidemiology, and natural history of myofascial pain syndrome. Curr Pain Headache Rep 2001;5:412–20.
[39] Simons DG, Travell JG, Simons LS. The trigger point manual, vol. 1. 2nd edition. Baltimore (MD): Lippincot Williams and Wilkins; 1998.
[40] Fricton JR. Masticatory myofascial pain: an explanatory model integrating clinical, epidemiological and basic science research. Bull Group Int Rech Sci Stomatol Odontol 1999;41:14–25.
[41] Graff Radford SB, Reeves JL, Jaeger B. Management of chronic head and neck pain: effectiveness of altering factors perpetuating myofascial pain. Headache 1987;27(4):186–90.
[42] Solberg WK. Temporomandibular disorders: masticatory myalgia and its management. Br Dent J 1986;160:351–6.
[43] Dao TT, Lavigne GJ, Charbonneau A, et al. The efficacy of oral splints in the treatment of myofascial pain of the jaw muscles: a controlled clinical trial. Pain 1994;56:85–94.
[44] Cheshire WP, Abashian SW, Mann JD. Botulinum toxin in the treatment of myofascial pain syndrome. Pain 1994;59:65–9.
[45] Kellgren JH. Observations on referred pain arising from muscle. Clin Sci 1938;3:175–90.
[46] Mense S. Referral of muscle pain: new aspects. Pain Forum 1994;3(1):1–9.
[47] Mense S. Considerations concerning the neurobiological basis of muscle pain. Can J Physiol Pharmacol 1991;9:610–6.
[48] Mense S. Nociception from skeletal muscle in relation to clinical muscle pain. Pain 1993;54:241–89.

[49] Simons DG. Neurophysiological basis of pain caused by trigger points. APS Journal 1994; 3(1):17–9.

[50] Pedersen-Bjergaard U, Nielsen LB, Jensen K, et al. Calcitonin gene related peptide, neurokinin A and substance P on nociception and neurogenic Inflammation in human skin and temporal muscle. Peptides 1991;12:333–7.

[51] Fields HL, Heinricher M. Brainstem modulation of nociceptor-driven withdrawal reflexes. Ann N Y Acad Sci 1989;563:34–44.

[52] Olesen J, Jensen R. Getting away from simple muscle contraction as a mechanism of tension-type headache. Pain 1991;46:123–4.

[53] Ernberg M, Hadenberg-Magnusson B, Alstergren P, et al. Pain, allodynia, and serum serotonin level in orofacial pain of muscular origin. J Orofacial Pain 1999;13:56–62.

[54] Bendtsen L. Central sensitization in tension-type headache- possible pathophysiological mechanisms. Cephalalgia 2000;20(5):486–508.

[55] Antczak-Bouckoms A. Epidemiology of research for temporomandibular disorders. J Orofacial Pain 1995;9:226–34.

[56] Kemper JT, Okeson JP. Craniomandibular disorders and headaches. J Prosthet Dent 1983; 49:702–5.

[57] Magnusson T, Carlsson GE. Changes in recurrent headache and mandibular dysfunction after various types of dental treatment. Acta Odontol Scand 1980;38:311–20.

[58] Magnusson T, Carlsson GE. A 2.5-year follow-up of changes in headache and mandibular dysfunction after stomatognathic treatment. J Prosthel Dent 1983;49:398–402.

[59] Vallon D, Ekberg EC, Nilner M, et al. Short-term effect of occlusal adjustment on craniomandibular disorders including headaches. Acta Odontol Scand 1991;49:89–96.

[60] Vallon D, Ekberg EC, Nilner M, et al. Occlusal adjustment in patients with craniomandibular disorders including headaches. A 3- and 6-month follow-up. Acta Odontol Scand 1995; 53:55–9.

[61] Vallon D, Nilner M. A longitudinal follow-up of the effects of occlusal adjustment in patients with craniomandibular disorders. Swed Dent J 1997;21:85–91.

[62] Shankland WE. Nociceptive trigeminal inhibition—tension suppression system: a method of preventing migraine and tension headaches. Compend Contin Educ Dent 2002;23:105–8.

[63] Wenneberg B, Nyström T, Carlsson G. Occlusal equilibration and other stomatognathic treatment in patients with mandibular dysfunction and headache. J Prosthel Dent 1988; 59:478–83.

[64] Schokker RP, Hansson TL, Ansink BJJ. Craniomandibular disorders in headache patients. J Craniomandib Disord Facial Oral Pain 1989;3:71–4.

[65] Schokker RP, Hansson TL, Ansink BJJ. The results of treatment of the masticatory system of chronic headache patients. J Craniomandib Disord Facial Oral Pain 1990;4:126–30.

[66] Forssell H, Kirveskari P, Kangasniemi P. Changes in headache after treatment of mandibular dysfunction. Cephalalgia 1985;5:229–36.

[67] Forssell H, Kirveskari P, Kangasniemi P. Response to occlusal treatment in headache patients previously treated by mock occlusal adjustment. Acta Odontol Scand 1987;45:77–80.

[68] Quayle AA, Gray RJM, Metcalfe RJ, et al. Soft occlusal splint therapy in the treatment of migraine and other headaches. J Prosth Dent 1990;18:123–9.

[69] Karppinen K. Purennan hoito osana kroonisten pää-, niska- ja hartiakipujen hoitoa [doctoral dissertation]. Universim of Turku, Finland: Annales Universitatis Turkuensis; 1995.

[70] Forssell H, Kalso E, Koskela P, et al. Occlusal treatments in temporomandibular disorders: a qualitative systematic review of randomized clinical trials. Pain 1999;83:549–60.

[71] Reik L, Hale M. The temporomandibular joint pain-dysfunction syndrome: a frequent cause of headache. Headache 1981;21:111–6.

[72] Schokker RP, Hansson TL, Ansink BJJ. Differences in headache patients regarding their response to treatment of the masticatory system. J Craniomandib Disord Facial Oral Pain 1990;4:228–32.

[73] Forssell H, Kirveskari P, Kangasniemi P. Distinguishing between headaches responsive and irresponsive to treatment of mandibular dysfunction. Proc Finn Dent Soc 1986;82:219–22.
[74] Kreiner M, Betancor E, Clark GT. Occlusal stabilization appliances. Evidence of their efficacy. J Am Dent Assoc 2001;132(6):770–7.
[75] Forssell H, Kalso E, Koskela P, et al. Occlusal treatments in temporomandibular disorders: a qualitative systematic review of randomized controlled trials. Pain 1999;83(3):549–60.
[76] Al-Ani MZ, Davies SJ, Gray RJ, et al. Stabilisation splint therapy for temporomandibular pain dysfunction syndrome. Cochrane Database Syst Rev 2004;(1):CD002778.
[77] Vallerand WP, Hall MB. Improvement in myofascial pain and headaches following TMJ surgery. J Craniomandib Disord Facial Oral Pain 1991;5:197–204.
[78] Montgomery MT, Van Sickels JE, Harms SE, et al. Arthroscopic TMJ surgery: effects on signs, symptoms, and disc position. J Oral Maxillofac Surg 1989;47:1263–71.

ELSEVIER
SAUNDERS

THE DENTAL
CLINICS
OF NORTH AMERICA

Dent Clin N Am 51 (2007) 145–160

Psychological Factors Associated with Orofacial Pains

Charles R. Carlson, PhD[a,b],*

[a]Department of Psychology, 106 Kastle Hall, University of Kentucky, Lexington,
KY 40506-0044, USA
[b]Department of Oral Health Science, 106 Kastle Hall, University of Kentucky, Lexington,
KY 40506-0044, USA

This article develops the case for why trigeminal pain is a unique and challenging problem for clinicians and patients alike, and provides the reader with insights for effective trigeminal pain management based on an understanding of the interplay between psychologic and physiologic systems. There is no greater sensory experience for the brain to manage than unremitting pain in trigeminally mediated areas. Such pain overwhelms conscious experience and focuses the suffering individual like few other sensory events. Trigeminal pain often motivates a search for relief that can drain financial and emotional resources. Therefore, it is not uncommon for individuals to spend hundreds, if not thousands, of dollars in the quest for quieting trigeminal pain. In some instances, the search is rewarded by a treatment that immediately addresses an identifiable source of pain (eg, appropriate endodontic treatment for an infected tooth). In other cases, however, it can stimulate never-ending pilgrimages from one health provider to another in the hopes of finding some relief for unrelenting trigeminal pain. Ongoing trigeminal pain demands attention and can prevent an individual from living any semblance of a normal life.

When trigeminal pain is present, it is difficult for the individual to imagine why pain could ever be a "good thing." In fact, it is not uncommon for practitioners and patients alike to view trigeminal pain, or any pain for that matter, as the enemy; it is something to be fought against and abolished by excision, ablation, medication, or someday perhaps, even gene therapy. There are some people, however, who suffer greatly because they do not

* Department of Psychology, 106 Kastle Hall, University of Kentucky, Lexington, KY 40506-0044.
  E-mail address: ccarl@uky.edu

have the ability to experience pain. Individuals who live with leprosy must learn to deal with life without the benefit of pain sensations from peripheral tissues. The bacillus that causes this infection that much of the world knows as "Hansen's disease," destroys the nervous tissue that is responsible for transmitting nociceptive information to the brain. A person who has leprosy does not have access to normal pain sensations to tell her/him that a wrinkle in the leather of a sandal is rubbing a blister on the sole of the foot with each footstep. It was not too long ago that health care providers learned that the digit loss that often is associated with leprosy came from rodents gnawing at exposed fingers and toes while the sleeping person was unaware of noxious sensory experience, and not from the leprous disease process itself. Life without pain sensations can present its own special challenges.

A few years ago, Dr. Paul Brand, MD, an English orthopedic surgeon, obtained a research grant to develop an artificial "pain" glove for persons with leprosy so that they could protect themselves from exposure to excessive tissue-damaging pressures while they worked with their hands. After much effort to develop the appropriate algorithms for combining force of pressure and duration of pressure together, the research group perfected an artificial glove system that signaled when excessive pressure over time was being applied and there was danger for tissue damage. What surprised the researchers was that those using the artificial gloves would ignore the audible signals and persist in performing an activity even though they knew what they were doing was tissue damaging. In hopes of rectifying the situation, the researchers redesigned the signaling system so that instead of using an audible warning, the gloves were fixed to send a small electrical impulse to the axilla region, one of the more sensitive areas of the human body. The researchers found that when the persons who had leprosy were engaged in work that created the potential for tissue damage, they turned this modified signaling system off, rather than changed their work habits. This experience challenged Brand's research group, and reminded them that pain is an important biologic signal. It is not surprising that access to the pain "off" button is difficult to obtain. It is, however, conceivable that if one had the capacity to turn natural pain systems off, it likely would lead to personal harm rather than benefit, because the pain system would be shut down in pursuit of reward from work, even though the excessive usage might cause personal injury.

Given the importance of pain signaling systems, it is now useful to focus on the psychologic issues that are associated with trigeminal pain systems so that the reader can develop an appreciation for why trigeminal pain can be such a management challenge for practitioners and patients alike. Several unique features of trigeminally mediated pain will be integrated with recent scientific findings. The intent of the remainder of this article is to develop a broad framework for understanding the psychologic issues that may be present in those who seek help for trigeminal pain, and use this understanding to guide the development of more effective treatments.

Several research groups have identified the frequency with which psychiatric disorders have been diagnosed among persons who have orofacial pain. For example, Korszun and colleagues [1] found that 28% of patients who have chronic pain meet criteria for the diagnosis of depression. Kight and colleagues [2] noted that 31% of patients who had orofacial pain were experiencing anxiety disorders. Consideration of psychologic distress, therefore, is an important factor to consider in the initial evaluation of a patient who has orofacial pain. Rugh and colleagues [3] suggested that general practitioners could use two screening questions—"How depressed are you?" and "Do you consider yourself more tense than calm or more calm than tense?"—to identify patients who have orofacial pain and ought to be referred to a mental health provider for further evaluation. Any response that indicates awareness of depression or more tension than calmness indicates a need for further psychologic evaluation.

An alternative to brief screening questions is to use standardized psychometric instruments to take advantage of the use of actuarial information-gathering strategies. These actuarial strategies enable the clinician to compare an individual patient's results with standardized normative data and make judgments based on statistical inferences rather than clinical observation alone. The Research Diagnostic Criteria (RDC) Axis II [4] uses the somatization and depression scales of the Symptom Checklist 90 revised (SCL-90R) [5] to assist the clinician in evaluating the role that psychologic factors may play in a patient's ongoing experience with pain. At the University of Kentucky Orofacial Pain Center, the entire SCL-90R is used to provide a comprehensive review of psychologic symptoms for individual patients who have orofacial pain, in addition to gathering the data needed for RDC decisions. For pain assessment, the MultiDimensional Pain Inventory [6] can provide the clinician with a comprehensive review of the intensity and impact of pain for the individual patient. Alternatively, the RDC makes use of a 0 to 10 linear pain scale and the Graded Chronic Pain Scale to index pain severity and pain-related life interference. The important point here is that there are many means by which to evaluate carefully the psychologic status of patients who have orofacial pain, and systematic attempts should be made to assess psychologic status as the standard of care with every patient.

One of the interesting psychologic findings that is emerging recently is the extent to which persons who have orofacial pain may be carrying the marks of exposure to trauma [7]. Several years ago, Curran and colleagues [8] found that a significant number (67%) of patients who had orofacial pain reported on an anonymous survey that they had experienced physical or sexual abuse. Sherman and colleagues [7] conducted comprehensive diagnostic interviews among patients who had orofacial pain. They found that one in four patients met criteria for the lifetime experience of posttraumatic stress disorder (PTSD). Diagnostic criteria for PTSD include (1) exposure to threat to self or others with a response of fear, helplessness or horror; (2) persistent re-experiencing of the traumatic event through memories, dreams, flashbacks, or symbolic events; (3) persistent avoidance of stimuli that remind one of the trauma and numbing of general responsiveness; (4) persistent symptoms of increased arousal that include sleep dysfunctions, anger outbursts, and hypervigilance; and (5) the symptoms have a duration of greater than 1 month and cause significant distress and impairment of functioning. PTSD has an inordinately high co-occurrence with orofacial pain conditions; the clinician needs to be sensitive to the possibility that it may be interfering with a patient's ability to manage an orofacial pain condition.

Several years ago, Gatchel's research group reported that almost one of every three patients who have orofacial pain and present in an orofacial pain clinic have a diagnosable personality disorder [2]. A personality disorder is an enduring pattern of behavior that does not conform to normal standards. For example, the person who has an antisocial personality disorder does not believe that the rules of society apply to her/him. The person who has borderline personality disorder struggles with establishing and maintaining adequate boundaries. In the orofacial pain practice, this can be seen in a situation where a patient is overly reliant on late night phone calls to the health care provider and seems not to be aware of their intrusive nature. Although it is difficult to diagnose personality disorders without an extensive structured clinical interview, the orofacial pain clinician should be sensitive to the possibility that difficult patients may be difficult because of enduring personality issues that can interfere with the effective delivery of care.

Biopsychosocial model and features of orofacial pain

The interplay between psychologic and physical functioning is communicated by the biopsychosocial model. This perspective provides for a broad understanding of the biologic, psychologic, and sociologic contexts that are associated with a person who is experiencing a physical or emotional disorder [9]. The biopsychosocial perspective takes into account the interplay among these various systems and helps to provide an organizing construct for the multiple information sources that are relevant to understanding a pain condition. Complex orofacial pain conditions generally do not represent a simple, linear cause and effect model. Rather, these conditions, particularly when chronic, demonstrate the complex interplay among biologic and behavioral systems that are constantly in a state of change. Therefore, the orofacial pain clinician must take into account the multiple interacting factors that influence a patient's ongoing pain state. The biopsychosocial model is a tool that helps the clinician to implement this perspective.

Foremost within the biopsychosocial perspective is appreciating the biologic factors that contribute to the pain experience. These factors include, among other things, genetics, fitness level, nutritional status, autonomic balance, and allostatic load. Allostatic load refers to the physical stress on an individual from repeated physiologic activation and inhibition that comes from responding to life stressors. Pain can be influenced by a variety of biologically based variables; the pain clinician needs to ensure a careful review of biologic factors during the initial evaluation. Biomedical assessment strategies that include a physical examination, laboratory tests, and diagnostic imaging are important tools for the clinician to use in developing a biologic perspective on the patients who present complaints.

It also is important to review behaviors or psychologic factors that may be contributing to the pain experience as well. Ohrbach [10] has rightly noted that treatments that fail to take into account the behavioral and psychologic factors that are associated with orofacial pains likely will not work reliably. Therefore, behavioral factors that include principles of learning (eg, reinforcement, punishment, modeling, discrimination), interpersonal processes, inhibitory control (eg, relaxation skills, delay of gratification), and cognitive regulatory strategies (eg, goals, expectations, plans) need to be assessed as a part of the initial evaluation. The treatment plan must take into account the multiple biologic and behavioral (biobehavioral) systems that can contribute to the development and maintenance of orofacial pains. Therefore, the astute clinician will use a careful psychosocial interview and diagnostic psychologic questionnaires to help form the database for comprehensive behavioral assessments of patient behaviors that may be contributing to the presenting complaints.

It is helpful to keep in mind that the assessment of pain in the trigeminal area needs to be informed by the importance that is attached to the meaning of pain in this region. Because the head region contains structures that are necessary for survival (eg, mouth, nose), pain in this region can be perceived as a threat to survival. Further, these orofacial structures also are conduits for giving and receiving pleasure. Pain in orofacial structures can limit an individual's ability to receive pleasurable stimuli or to deliver such stimuli. It is not uncommon for patients to eschew kissing or any form of touching in the face when trigeminal pain is active. The same structures represent a prime communication system and pain can threaten an individual's ability to communicate. Therefore, pain in the orofacial region may involve unique psychologic interpretations that the clinician needs to be sensitive to and account for in treatment planning and delivery.

There are excitatory and inhibitory factors in pain modulation that should inform the diagnosis and treatment of orofacial pain conditions. Excitatory factors, or those factors that can enhance pain sensitivity, include attention, expectancies for pain (eg, "this pain is something you'll have for the rest of your life"), anxiety, fear, and anger. Recently, a graduate student in the author's research laboratory conducted a functional MRI study of how anger and fear influence activation in brain centers that are responsible for trigeminal pain experience [11]. His results indicated that pain, anger, and fear are processed in similar regions in the brain; anger, especially, increases the activity of brain regions that are responsible for processing trigeminal pain. It is not unusual for patients who have orofacial pain to report significant levels of anger. The clinician must be willing to explore the nature of a patient's anger experience if an effective treatment plan is to be developed and implemented. The astute clinician is aware that attention, expectancies, and ongoing emotional states can increase an individual's awareness and self report of pain.

Conversely, pain sensitivity can be reduced by such factors as confidence, self-efficacy (beliefs about one's ability to manage pain successfully), assurance, distraction, relaxation, and positive emotional states. Several years ago, the author's laboratory, for example, published data indicating that positive emotional states (eg, happiness) and brief relaxation procedures could reduce pain sensitivity in individuals who were exposed to a standard pain stressor [12]. Furthermore, there is ample evidence that relaxation strategies, including progressive relaxation training, postural relaxation, and breathing entrainment, can be used effectively to manage orofacial pain conditions [13]. It is important to recognize and incorporate strategies that can mitigate pain experience in the development of a comprehensive pain management program.

It is said often that patients who have pain are "just more sensitive to painful stimulation" than are pain-free individuals. Although there are data suggesting that patients who have pain are more sensitive to painful stimulation in trigeminal regions [14] and to ischemic pain stimulation in the forearm [15], it is also true that patients who have pain are no more sensitive than are pain-free individuals when experiencing pressure pain in nontrigeminal areas (eg, hand) [16]. It would be a mistake to conclude that patients who have pain generally are more sensitive than are pain-free individuals, but it also would be incorrect to say that patients who have trigeminal pain are not more sensitive to certain kinds of sensory stimulation, particularly in trigeminal areas. It is well known that pain heightens sensitivity in painful regions and can cause reflexive modifications in function to protect the individual from further provocation from pain and tissue damage that are associated with inappropriate movements. The orofacial pain clinician needs to be aware of heightened pain sensitivity, but should be careful not to ascribe that sensitivity to inherent mental or physical deficiencies in the individual patient.

Fatigue is one of the common symptoms that is reported by many patients who have pain. In fact, the pain–fatigue–sleep disturbance triad is represented in most individuals who seek care for chronic orofacial pain conditions. Fatigue can be viewed as the perception of tiredness, rather than as the true inability to do work. When it is not possible to perform physical work because the muscles will not carry out the required actions, the problem typically is described as "peripheral fatigue." Central fatigue, on the other hand, is a perception of tiredness that may not necessarily be accompanied by physical fatigue in the working muscles. It is interesting to speculate on the role that the perception of fatigue may play among patients who have orofacial pain. The author and colleagues [14,17] have found that patients who have orofacial pain report greater fatigue than do those who are not in pain. Although the nature of this fatigue (central or peripheral) is not clear for patients who have orofacial pain, many patients report experiencing debilitating levels of fatigue; strategies to address this problem should be discussed in the treatment plan.

It is natural to consider the importance of sleep variables at this point in the discussion. Most patients who have pain report disturbed sleep at some level [14,18]. The nature and extent of disturbed sleep can be assessed quantitatively using the Pittsburgh Sleep Quality Index [19]. This instrument provides a psychometrically sound method for assessing sleep onset, duration, and quality. Because sleep typically is initiated when brain activity diminishes, one way to conceptualize sleep disturbances in patients who have pain is failure of the brain to quiet to the point that sleep is initiated. Moreover, frequent awakenings that are reported by patients who have pain suggest that arousal regulatory mechanisms are disturbed. Lavigne and colleagues [20] discussed the role of sleep disturbance in orofacial pain and recommended that treatments to restore sleep be a part of a comprehensive pain management plan. Recently, an National Institutes of Health consensus panel concluded that relaxation training is useful in helping patients who have chronic pain to initiate and maintain sleep [21]. These findings are consistent with conceptualizing the sleep problems for patients who have pain as a failure of the brain to quiet (lack of inhibitory control). Thus, patients who have orofacial pain may obtain significant sleep benefits from learning specific relaxation skills.

Persistent stressors—and certainly, unremitting pain can be considered a persistent stressor—involve prolonged activation of the reticular formation in the brain and subsequent regulatory control of glucose and ATP availability, oxygen and carbon dioxide levels, motor unit recruitment to perform work, and release of endogenous opioids (eg, β endorphin) for compensatory inhibitory control. When these systems experience long-term demands, effective function may be compromised and inefficient anaerobic metabolism may develop; respiratory changes may lead to subtle alterations in blood pH that can affect axonal excitability and sympathetic nervous system activation; myoelectric frequency shifts in muscle activity occur as motor units fatigue; and endogenous opioids have diminished effectiveness for quieting physiologic systems. These changes can lead to dysregulation of the autonomic nervous system and heighten the experience of pain, sleep disruptions, and negative affect (anxiety, fear, anger) that are common in chronic orofacial pain conditions.

Although increased autonomic activation is a normal adaptive mechanism for managing life stressors, heightened emotional and physical responsivity is characteristic of a chronic defense reaction in the presence of relentless stressors [22,23]. Prolonged stimulation from nociception, for example, is known to be one of the most significant activators of the sympathetic nervous system; it can be viewed as an important endogenous stressor itself [24]. Recent evidence showed that when primary nociceptors are stimulated by tissue damage, activity by collateral nonnociceptive peripheral neurons further increases the rate of activity from those nociceptors [25,26]. Even in nonpain situations, anxiety-induced autonomic activity that alters carbon dioxide levels may cause ectopic impulses to be generated from dense receptive fields within the trigeminal region [27]. Under conditions that promote central sensitization, sympathetic activity from a variety of stimuli may have significant effects on nociceptive interpretation or subsequent pain reports [28]. Therefore, management of dysregulated autonomic activity can be regarded as an important treatment goal for persons who have pain disorders, although it may not be clear whether the altered autonomic activity is a causative factor or a consequence of the pain experience [29].

Recently, it was noted that the complex integration of central and autonomic nervous system functioning can be indexed by vagally mediated heart rate variability (HRV) [30,31]. The HRV measure serves as a marker for the negative feedback that is conveyed to the heart by way of the vagus nerve that is important for self-regulation and efficient cardiovascular performance through control of cardiac rate and electrical conduction speed. The vagus nerve primarily exerts tonic inhibitory control of the cardiovascular system [31]. Although HRV represents the changes in beat-to-beat interval over time, it is evaluated commonly by spectral analyses whereby heart rate data are transformed from the time domain (beat-to-beat intervals) to the frequency domain (oscillations). Typically, these transformations are done with Fast Fourier analyses, such that the high-frequency (0.15–0.4 Hz) component of the power spectrum density of HRV reflects primarily parasympathetic activity linked to respiration rate (respiratory sinus arrhythmia), the low-frequency component (0.05–0.15 Hz) is a combination of sympathetic and parasympathetic activity, and a very low–frequency component (0.005–0.05 Hz) relates to sympathetic mediation of vascular tone and body temperature [32–34]. Moreover, the ratio of the low-frequency to high-frequency components of HRV data is believed to represent primarily sympathetic activity, although there is not uniform agreement on this interpretation. The meanings of HRV measures and the complexity of cardiac regulatory processes are still being elaborated. Porges [35] for example, noted that autonomically mediated modulatory controls are not always similar to tonic autonomic controls, as is illustrated by the uncoupling in cardiac regulation that occurs during the orienting reflex when there is a vagally controlled decrease in heart rate accompanied by a pause in respiratory sinus arrhythmia.

In normal individuals, HRV is high and an indication of positive health status, with well-regulated sympathetic and parasympathetic functioning [31]. Reduced HRV, however, has been associated with a broad range of dysfunctional states, including heart disease, obesity, gastrointestinal esophageal reflux disease, irritable bowel syndrome, mood disorders, and anxiety disorders [31,36,37]. It also has been shown that HRV can be enhanced by behavioral strategies that include relaxation and paced breathing [38–40]. Recently, John Schmidt [41] conducted a study in the author's laboratory that compared HRV measures during rest and recall of a personally relevant stressor between patients who had orofacial pain and matched normal controls. He found that patients who had orofacial pain demonstrated an increase in sympathetic tone and less HRV than did matched controls; however there are no known studies of HRV after treatment, in persons who have orofacial pain conditions. Further examination of this potentially important physiologic variable in a population that has orofacial pain may shed light on its usefulness as an index of allostatic load, as well as treatment outcome.

Sustained activation of autonomic and hypothalamic–pituitary–adrenal (HPA) axis functioning may have significant negative consequences. With an increase in HPA axis functioning under acute stress, the principal stress hormone that is released—in addition to epinephrine and norepinephrine—is cortisol. Cortisol is secreted by the adrenal cortex as a result of release of adrenocorticotropin hormone from the pituitary gland [24]. Cortisol is known to influence glucose metabolism, immune function, and tissue repair. Recent evidence indicated that persons who experience rheumatoid arthritis [42], primary fibromyalgia syndrome [43], PTSD [44], and chronic pain [45] have decreased cortisol levels, presumably as a consequence of prolonged physiologic activation. These findings have been interpreted to suggest that normal HPA function is disrupted under conditions of prolonged stress within certain patient groups.

Generally, cortisol levels demonstrate substantial fluctuation during the course of a 24-hour period, and for women there also are changes over the 28-day menstrual cycle. It has been shown, however, that the increase in cortisol levels within the 60 minutes after awakening follows a highly reliable pattern for most individuals that is not related to age, weight, smoking, sleep duration, time of awakening, and alcohol usage [46,47]. The "free cortisol response to awakening" is assessed by sampling salivary cortisol levels immediately after waking and at 15-minute intervals for the first hour after awakening. This measure has demonstrated reliability as a biologic marker for adrenocortical activity. Geiss and colleagues [45], for example, found that persons who had persistent back and leg pain had lower overall cortisol concentrations and a blunted free cortisol response to awakening as compared with healthy pain-free controls. Moreover, they found that the concentration of interleukin-6, a proinflammatory cytokine, was increased in the group that had chronic pain. Recent data from the author's laboratory indicate that patients who have chronic orofacial pain also exhibit blunted free cortisol responses to awakening [48]. These data are consistent with the hypothesis that chronic pain conditions alter HPA function in a manner that may impede tissue repair and recovery, as well as promote heightened sensitivity to environmental challenges or stimuli, whether generated from the outside environment or internally, by the individual.

One common view among patients and practitioners is that orofacial pain conditions, particularly those that involve muscles of mastication, are accompanied by increased muscle activity in those muscle groups. In fact, several research teams have identified low levels of increased muscle activity as characterizing individuals who have masticatory muscle pain conditions [49]. There is alternative evidence, however, to suggest that excessive muscle activity does not characterize muscle pain conditions in the orofacial region [14,16,50]. Although it can be demonstrated that pain alters muscle function, it is not wise to make a generalization to an individual patient without objective data that quantify the nature of the muscle activity.

There are data, however, suggesting that the physiologic overactivity in patients who experience chronic muscle pain in the muscles of mastication can alter two measurable parameters [14]. These parameters include resting diastolic blood pressure and end-tidal carbon dioxide levels. These findings suggest that chronic muscle pain, at least, may lead to decreased diastolic blood pressure because of pooling in vascular capillary beds. It is well known in the cardiovascular literature that chronic stress can result in poor venous return because of the capillary pooling. The finding that patients who have chronic muscle pain have decreased diastolic blood pressure is consistent with a chronic stress hypothesis.

The lower end-tidal carbon dioxide levels in patients who have pain, as compared with matched controls, also can be explained based on a chronic stress reaction. Respiration rate and depth can change automatically when there is a stress reaction. In the case of chronic pain, because there typically is limited physical activity when the respiration rate increases as a natural response to the sympathetic activation from the pain, the ventilation of carbon dioxide occurs without compensatory production of carbon dioxide in body tissues. Therefore, the concentration of carbon dioxide decreases in the serum. Because carbon dioxide levels in the blood are directly proportional to the concentration of carbon dioxide in expired air, there are lower end-tidal carbon dioxide levels at rest in patients who have pain than in matched normal controls.

The implications of lower end-tidal carbon dioxide levels in patients who have pain are potentially far-reaching. Carbon dioxide is necessary to maintain blood pH through the bicarbonate buffer. Lowered concentrations of carbon dioxide can result in slightly elevated pH levels (7.5–7.6) from the body's normal level of 7.4. Such increases can result in further increases in sympathetic tone, increased neuronal excitability, reduced peripheral blood flow, and impaired dissociation of oxygen from hemoglobin [51]. Thus, restoration of normal carbon dioxide levels in serum is a potentially important behavioral intervention target to achieve in patients who have chronic orofacial pain.

Biobehavioral approaches to orofacial pain management

The remainder of this article is devoted to introducing behaviorally based strategies for helping patients develop better management of their pain. The phrase "management of their pain" was selected intentionally because it underscores the importance of using pain as an important biologic signal that "something is disturbed." The basic premise is that when pain is perceived, there is a physiologic disturbance that needs attention, whether it be in peripheral tissues or in the brain itself. Unless the physiologic disturbance is attended to, the pain will remain. Importantly, the patient's pain is interpreted as real. It is not something that is "manufactured," but rather represents an important reflection of an individual's perception. When a health provider accepts the reality of another's perception it builds trust in the therapeutic relationship and fosters the working alliance. The management approach also focuses on the reality that pain of a chronic nature often is not "cured" or taken away permanently. Rather, pain is managed effectively so that an individual can engage life to the fullest.

The management approach often requires an individual to change. The process of change can be difficult, yet understanding how people change is important for the orofacial pain provider. There is a five-step process of change that has been developed in the literature [52]. The first step in the process is described as precontemplation. In the precontemplation phase the individual is not aware of a need for change, but when an awareness is developed s/he has moved to the stage of contemplation. During this phase an individual is weighing the costs and benefits of change for themselves. The third stage of change is preparation for taking action. The individual is taking the steps necessary to make a successful attempt at change. The fourth step is action, whereby the individual implements the new behaviors. The fifth change stage is maintenance, during which the individual is doing those things that are necessary to continue with the changes that were implemented in the fourth stage. Consideration of each of these stages of change helps the orofacial pain clinician appreciate the challenges that a patient faces when confronted with information that suggests s/he may need to change in some way to obtain pain relief.

One of the important messages of behavioral research over the past several decades is that helping individuals change is fostered by brief interventions and change talk. There are many examples of the effectiveness of brief interventions. For instance, Holroyd and colleagues [53] developed an effective approach to migraine headache treatment that involves minimal therapist contact and primarily home-based interventions. Similarly, Chapman and Huygens [54] demonstrated that brief therapy for alcoholics was just as effective as was a long-term (6 weeks) intensive treatment program for reducing drinking behavior. In orofacial pain, brief interventions also were shown to be effective in reducing pain for significant periods of time [13,55]. The Physical Self Regulation (PSR) program that was developed jointly by scientist-practitioners at the University of Kentucky and the National Naval Dental Center provides skills training for orofacial pain management during two 50-minute training sessions. These sessions target proprioceptive re-education, relaxation skills, criterion-based diaphragmatic breathing, increased physical activity, sleep hygiene instructions, and fluid/nutrition management as areas for change. These treatment domains were based upon laboratory research findings [14,50] and were shown to provide significant relief of pain (average of 69% reduction in self-report of pain) and improved jaw functioning immediately after training and at 6-month follow-up evaluations [13]. The effectiveness of the PSR training has resulted in it becoming the standard baseline treatment for many patients who have chronic orofacial pain. The bottom line for this discussion is that important and meaningful change can occur following brief interventions. Elaborate and lengthy interventions are not necessary for significant change to take place in the lives of individuals who are ready to change.

The clinician can help the patient to change by encouraging her/him to engage in "change talk." Typically, change talk involves three components. The first component is enabling the individual to speak about the disadvantages of his/her current status. The second component is to have the individual speak about the advantages of making a change. Finally, the third component of change talk is helping the individual to express specific intentions to change. The clinician who fosters change talk will discover that an individual becomes much more willing to begin the process of change and will persist in efforts to change until old habits have been altered. When change talk is accompanied by a clinician's use of empathic listening where a patient feels like s/he is truly understood, a patient's capacity to mobilize resources for change is engaged most fully.

Ideally, specific biobehavioral strategies for orofacial pain conditions should follow a stepped approach to self-regulation training. This stepped approach is patterned after the stepped-care strategies that are used to address common medical conditions (eg, hypertension). The first, or foundational step, is ensuring basic skills in PSR or self-care strategies. The basic protocol for PSR establishes a foundation for understanding and regulating behaviors that can contribute to trigeminally mediated pain conditions. There are many individuals for whom home PSR training alone provides the necessary skills for effective pain management. Advanced progressive relaxation or biofeedback strategies can build upon this basic foundation as the second level of biobehavioral training. Training in progressive relaxation techniques [56] or specific biofeedback modalities (ie, electromyography for muscle relaxation, end-tidal carbon dioxide training to control carbon dioxide levels in the blood, hand temperature training to increase blood flow to peripheral areas) can augment basic self-regulation abilities that are obtained through PSR training. The third level, or step, of biobehavioral training can be engaging in specific cognitive-behavioral psychotherapies to address issues, such as depression, PTSD, or other psychologic concerns, that may be interfering with normal functioning and contributing to the maintenance of a chronic pain state. The use of a stepped approach in bio-behavioral strategies can maximize the efficiency with which persons in pain develop the resources that are needed to improve their ability to manage their pain experience more effectively.

When the orofacial pain clinician recognizes the need for referral to other health professionals for biobehavioral training that s/he cannot provide, it is important to develop a strategy for making the transition to another health provider successfully. Often when a dental practitioner makes a referral to a psychologist for biobehavioral training, unless the dental practitioner exercises care in what is said, the patient can misconstrue the intentions of the dental practitioner. It is not uncommon for patients to infer from the referral that the dentist "thinks my pain is not real and it is all in my head." To reduce the likelihood for this to occur, it may be helpful to use the words "stress management" when talking about the need for a biobehavioral consultation with a patient. Most persons are more comfortable with the idea of seeing another health provider for a "stress management consultation" than because there are questions about one's psychologic status. There are times, however, if the dental clinician has a significant concern about the level of depression or anxiety, that direct communication with the patient about concerns for her/his welfare as the reasons for the referral to another health provider will be most effective in helping that patient make a successful transition to the new health provider. It is useful if the dentist take the initiative to set the appointment and helps to ensure that the patient follows through with the visit to the biobehavioral training specialist. Successful referrals for biobehavioral training require an adroit dental practitioner who has established strong working relationships with competent specialists who are skilled in delivering biobehavioral interventions.

Summary

This article has provided a broad overview of the unique psychologic and physiologic issues that are associated with the management of orofacial pain conditions in general. Trigeminal pain problems can be vexing challenges for patient and clinician alike. Even the most skilled clinicians can be put to the test with unusual trigeminal pain presentations. Fortunately, many acute orofacial pains can be managed in a straightforward manner and full remission of the pain symptoms can be achieved. There are, however, some chronic orofacial pains that result in a varying clinical course, particularly when the underlying cause is unknown. The biobehavioral perspective can be an important guide in helping patients who have chronic pain presentations come to understand their conditions and learn to manage them more effectively while they are receiving competent dental care. The ideal professional model is for the biobehavioral approach to be an essential component of the standard care that a patient who has orofacial pain receives. The intent of this article is to lay a foundation for dental practitioners to integrate biobehavioral perspectives routinely into their delivery of orofacial pain interventions.

References

[1] Korszun A, Hinderstein B, Wong M. Comorbidity of depression with chronic facial pain and temporomandibular disorders. Oral Surg Oral Med Oral Pathol Oral Radiol Endod 1996;82: 496–500.
[2] Kight M, Gatchel RJ, Wesley L. Temporomandibular disorders: evidence for significant overlap with psychopathology. Health Psychol 1999;18:177–82.
[3] Rugh JD, Woods BJ, Dahlstrom L. Temporomandibular disorders: assessment of psychological factors. Adv Dent Res 1993;1993:127–36.
[4] Dworkin SF, LeResche L. Research diagnostic criteria for temporomandibular disorders: review, criteria, examinations and specifications, critique. J Craniomandib Disord 1992;6: 301–55.
[5] Derogatis LR. SCL-90R manual: administration, scoring, and procedures. Towson (MD): Clinical Psychometric Research; 1992.
[6] Kerns RD, Turk DC, Rudy TE. The West Haven-Yale Multidimensional Pain Inventory (WHYMPI). Pain 1985;23:345–56.
[7] Sherman JJ, Carlson CR, Wilson JF, et al. Post-traumatic stress disorder among patients with orofacial pain. J Orofac Pain 2005;19:309–17.
[8] Curran SL, Sherman JJ, Cunningham LC, et al. Physical and sexual abuse among orofacial pain patients: linkages with pain and psychological distress. J Orofac Pain 1995;10: 141–50.
[9] Dworkin SF. Psychosocial issues. In: Lavigne GJ, Lund JP, Dubner R, et al, editors. Orofacial pain: from basic science to clinical management. Chicago: Quintessence; 2001. p. 115–27.
[10] Ohrbach R. Biobehavioral therapy. In: Laskin DM, Greene CS, Hylander WL, editors. Temporomandibular disorders: an evidence-based approach to diagnosis and treatment. Chicago: Quintessence Publishing; 2006. p. 391–402.
[11] Davis CE. Functional magnetic resonance imaging of pain and emotion [doctoral dissertation]. Lexington (KY): University of Kentucky; 2003.
[12] Bruehl S, Carlson CR, McCubbin JA. An evaluation of two brief interventions for acute pain. Pain 1993;54:29–36.
[13] Carlson CR, Bertrand PM, Ehrlich AD, et al. Physical self-regulation training for the management of temporomandibular disorders. J Orofac Pain 2001;15:47–55.
[14] Carlson CR, Reid KI, Curran SL, et al. Psychological and physiological parameters of masticatory muscle pain. Pain 1998;76:297–307.
[15] Maixner W, Fillingim R, Booker D, et al. Sensitivity of patients with painful temporomandibular disorders to experimentally evoked pain. Pain 1995;63:341–51.
[16] Curran SL, Carlson CR, Okeson JP. Emotional and physiological responses to laboratory challenge: temporomandibular disorder patients versus matched controls. J Orofac Pain 1995;9:141–50.
[17] de Leeuw R, Studts JL, Carlson CR. Fatigue and fatigue-related symptoms in TM pain patients. Oral Surg Oral Med Oral Pathol Oral Radiol Endod 2005;99:168–74.
[18] Yatani H, Studts J, Cordova M, et al. Comparison of sleep quality and clinical and psychologic characteristics in patients with temporomandibular disorders. J Orofac Pain 2002;16: 221–8.
[19] Buysse DJ, Reynolds CF, Monk TH, et al. The Pittsburgh Sleep Quality Index: a new instrument for psychiatric practice and research. Psychol Res 1989;28:193–213.

[20] Lavigne GJ, Brousseau M, Montplaisir J, et al. Pain and sleep disturbances. In: Lund JP, Lavigne GJ, Dubner R, et al, editors. Orofacial pain: from basic science to clinical management. Chicago: Quintessence; 2001. p. 139–50.

[21] National Institutes of Health. Integration of behavioral and relaxation approaches into the treatment of chronic pain and insomnia. NIH Technology Assessment Panel on Integration of Behavioral and Relaxation Approaches in to the Treatment of Chronic Pain and Insomnia. JAMA 1996;276:313–8.

[22] Boscarino JA. Posttraumatic stress disorder, exposure to combat and lower plasma cortisol among Vietnam veterans: findings and clinical implications. J Consult Clin Psychol 1996;64: 191–201.

[23] McEwen BS. Protective and damaging effects of stress mediators. N Engl J Med 1998;338: 171–9.

[24] Guyton AC, Hall JE. Textbook of medical physiology. 9th edition. Philadelphia: W.B. Saunders; 1997.

[25] Devor M, Wall PD. Cross-excitation in dorsal root ganglia of nerve-injured and intact rats. J Neurophys 1990;64:1733–46.

[26] Lisney SJ, Devor M. After discharge and interactions among fibers in damaged peripheral nerve in the rat. Brain Res 1987;415:122–36.

[27] Macefield G, Burke D. Paraesthesiae and tetany induced by voluntary hyperventilation. Increased excitability of human cutaneous and motor axons. Brain 1991;114:527–40.

[28] Dubner R, Ruda MA. Activity-dependent neuronal plasticity following tissue injury and inflammation. Trends Neurosci 1992;15:96–103.

[29] Sessle BJ, Hu WJ. Mechanisms of pain arising from articular tissues. Can J Physiol Pharmacol 1991;69:617–26.

[30] Thayer JF, Siegle GJ. Neurovisceral integration in cardiac and emotional regulation. IEEE Eng Med Biol Mag 2002;21:24–9.

[31] Thayer JF, Lane RD. A model of neurovisceral integration in emotion regulation and dysregulation. J Affect Disord 2000;61:201–16.

[32] Pagani M, Malliani A. Interpreting oscillations of muscle sympathetic nerve activity and heart rate variability. J Hypertens 2000;18:1709–19.

[33] Lehrer PM, Vaschillo E, Vaschillo B. Resonant frequency biofeedback training to increase cardiac variability: rationale and manual for training. Appl Psychophysiol Biofeedback 2000;25:177–91.

[34] Heart rate variability: standards of measurement, physiological interpretation, and clinical use. Task Force of the European Society of Cardiology and the North American Society of Pacing and Electrophysiology. Circulation 1996;93:1043–65.

[35] Porges SW. Orienting in a defensive world: mammalian modifications of our evolutionary heritage. A Polyvagal theory. Psychophysiology 1995;32:301–18.

[36] Schwartz AR, Gerin W, Davidson KW, et al. Toward a causal model of cardiovascular responses to stress and the development of cardiovascular disease. Psychosom Med 2003;65: 22–35.

[37] Friedman BH, Thayer JF. Autonomic balance revisited: panic anxiety and heart rate variability. J Psychosom Res 1998;44:133–51.

[38] Lehrer PM, Vaschillo E, Vaschillo B, et al. Heart rate variability biofeedback increases baroreflex gain and peak expiratory flow. Psychosom Med 2003;65:796–805.

[39] Sakakibara M, Hayano J. Effect of slowed respiration on cardiac parasympathetic response to threat. Psychosom Med 1996;58:32–7.

[40] Sakakibara M, Takeuchi S, Hayano J. Effect of relaxation training on cardiac parasympathetic tone. Psychophysiology 1994;31:223–8.

[41] Schmidt J. A comparison of heart rate variability between orofacial pain patients and matched controls [doctoral dissertation]. Lexington (KY): University of Kentucky; 2006.

[42] Hedman M, Nilsson E, de la Torre B. Low blood and synovial fluid levels of sulpho-conjugated steroids in rheumatoid arthritis. Clin Exp Rheumatol 1992;10:25–30.

[43] Griep EN, Boersma JW, Lentjes EG, et al. Function of hypothalamic-pituitary-adrenal axis in patients with fibromyalgia and low back pain. J Rheumatol 1998;25:1374–81.

[44] Heim C, Ehlert U, Hellhammer DH. The potential role of hypocortisolism in the pathophysiology of stress-related bodily disorders. Psychoneuroendocrinology 2000;25:1–35.

[45] Geiss A, Varadi E, Steinbach K, et al. Psychoneuroimmunological correlates of persisting sciatic pain in patients who underwent discectomy. Neurosci Lett 1997;237:65–8.

[46] Pruessner JC, Wolf OT, Hellhammer DH, et al. Free cortisol levels after awakening: a reliable biological marker for the assessment of adrenocortical activity. Life Sci 1997;61:2539–49.

[47] Wust S, Federenko I, Hellhammer DH, et al. Genetic factors, perceived chronic stress, and the free cortisol response to awakening. Psychoneuroendocrinology 2000;25:707–20.

[48] Venable VV. Cortisol awakening response in masticatory muscle pain patients: evidence of hypocortisolism [doctoral dissertation]. Lexington (KY): University of Kentucky; 2003.

[49] Ohrbach R. Stress reactivity, adaptation, and response specificity in individuals with chronic muscle pain [doctoral dissertation]. Buffalo (NY): State University of New York at Buffalo; 1996.

[50] Carlson CR, Okeson JP, Falace D, et al. A comparison of psychological and physiological functioning between patients with masticatory muscle pain and matched controls. J Orofac Pain 1993;7:15–22.

[51] Fried R. The psychology and physiology of breathing. New York: Plenum; 1993.

[52] Prochaska JO, DiClemente CC, Norcross JC. In search of how people change. Applications to addictive behaviors. Am Psychol 1992;47:1102–14.

[53] Holroyd KA, Holm JE, Hursey KG, et al. Recurrent vascular headache: home-based behavioral treatment versus abortive pharmacological treatment. J Consult Clin Psychol 1988;56: 218–23.

[54] Chapman PL, Huygens I. An evaluation of three treatment programmes for alcoholism: an experimental study with 6- and 18-month follow-ups. Br J Addict 1988;83:67–81.

[55] Dworkin SF, Huggins KH, Wilson L, et al. A randomized clinical trial using research diagnostic criteria for temporomandibular disorders-Axis II to target clinical cases for a tailored self-care TMD treatment program. J Orofac Pain 2002;16:48–63.

[56] Carlson CR, Okeson JP, Falace D, et al. Stretch-based relaxation training and the reduction of EMG activity among masticatory muscle pain patients. J Craniomandib Disord 1991;5: 205–12.

ELSEVIER
SAUNDERS

THE DENTAL
CLINICS
OF NORTH AMERICA

Dent Clin N Am 51 (2007) 161–193

Temporomandibular Disorders, Head and Orofacial Pain: Cervical Spine Considerations

Steve Kraus, PT, OCS, MTC

2770 Lenox Road, Suite 102, Atlanta, GA 30324, USA

Head and orofacial pain originates from dental, neurologic, musculoskeletal, otolaryngologic, vascular, metaplastic, or infectious disease and is treated by many health care practitioners, such as dentists, oral surgeons, and physicians, who specialize in this pathology. This article's focus relates to the nonpathologic involvement of the musculoskeletal system as a source of head and orofacial pain. The areas of the musculoskeletal system that are reviewed include the temporomandibular joint (TMJ) and muscles of mastication—collectively referred to as temporomandibular disorders (TMDs) and cervical spine disorders [1].

Often, conservative treatment is recommended for most patients who experience TMDs and cervical spine disorders [1,2]. Physical therapists offer conservative treatment in rehabilitation of TMDs and cervical spine disorders. The American Physical Therapy Association (APTA) defines physical therapy as " … the care and services provided by or under the direction and supervision of a physical therapist… " [3]. The position of the APTA is " … only physical therapists provide or direct the provision of physical therapy" [4]. The most valuable contribution that physical therapists make regarding the management of TMDs and cervical spine disorders is in the proper identification of the components in the musculoskeletal system that contribute to a patient's symptoms and functional limitations. This is done by collecting a detailed history from the patient and conducting an appropriate physical assessment based on the history [4]. A properly performed evaluation by a physical therapist determines the type of treatment offered, and results in optimal and meaningful functional outcomes.

Consequently, the validity of research that investigates physical therapy interventions for TMDs and head and orofacial pain should be questioned

E-mail address: stevekraus@mindspring.com

0011-8532/07/$ - see front matter © 2007 Elsevier Inc. All rights reserved.
doi:10.1016/j.cden.2006.10.001

when it is unclear if a physical therapist participated in the evaluation of the patient or provided physical therapy treatment. Referring to physical therapy as only a modality is misleading, and conclusions made about the therapeutic value of physical therapy may be inaccurate [5,6]. The objective of this article is to demonstrate the extent to which a physical therapist who is trained in the specialty of TMDs and cervical spine disorders contributes to the successful management of this condition.

The first part of this article highlights the role of physical therapy in the treatment of TMDs. The second part discusses cervical spine considerations in the management of TMDs and head and orofacial symptoms. The article concludes with an overview of the evaluation and treatment of the cervical spine.

Physical therapy management of temporomandibular disorders

TMD is divided into arthrogenous disorders, which involve the TMJ, and myogenous disorders, which involve the muscles of mastication [1]. An extensive subclassification for arthrogenous and myogenous disorders exists [1]. The common arthrogenous and myogenous disorders that are seen clinically by physical therapists, dentists, oral surgeons, and physicians are addressed in this article (Box 1). The diagnostic criterion for each of the common TMD conditions that follows is referenced in the literature and is not covered in this article [1,7–9]. The objective of this portion of the article is to highlight physical therapy treatment for common TMDs.

Box 1. Common temporomandibular disorders with corresponding *International Classification of Diseases, Ninth Revision* (ICD-9) codes

TMD arthrogenous
  Inflammation 524.62
  Hypermobility 830.1
  Fibrous adhesions 524.61
  Disc displacements 524.63
    Disc displacement with reduction
    Disc displacement without reduction
    Chronic disc displacement without reduction

TMD myogenous
  Masticatory muscle pain 728.85

Temporomandibular disorders: arthrogenous

Inflammation

Inflammation can originate from TMJ tissues, such as the capsule, medial, and lateral collateral ligaments, TMJ ligament, or posterior attachment. TMJ tissue inflammation can result from blunt trauma and microtrauma that are caused by parafunctional activity. Parafunctional activity is nonfunctional activity, which, when in the orofacial region, includes nail biting, lip or cheek chewing, abnormal posturing of the jaw, and bruxism [1]. Bruxism is diurnal or nocturnal clenching, bracing, gnashing, and grinding of the teeth [1] Inflammation also can result from arthritic conditions.

Physical therapy treatment for TMJ inflammation involves patient education regarding dietary and oral habits [9]. Iontophoresis, phonophoresis, and interferential electric stimulation are therapeutic modalities that are used to decrease TMJ inflammation [10–12]. Patients who are diagnosed with TMJ inflammation may have altered mandibular dynamics that are due to intracapsular swelling and resultant joint pain. Physical therapists teach patients range of motion exercises that maintain functional mandibular dynamics during the rehabilitation phase without causing more inflammation.

Hypermobility

Hypermobility is excessive translation of the mandibular condyle during opening of the mouth [13]. With condylar hypermobility, the condyle translates anteriorly during opening following the slope of the articular eminence past the articular crest onto the articular tubercle [13]. Hypermobility that occurs unilaterally may be associated with deviation of the mandible, which is observed during mouth opening. Deviation is the mandible moving away from midline, but returning to midline at the end of opening [9]. Although hypermobility may cause disc displacement of the TMJ, the cause and effect relationship has not been established [14,15]. Hypermobility is a common, and, frequently, benign, condition.

Patients who exhibit hypermobility without pain do not require treatment [14]. Controlling hypermobility is necessary only when other TMJ conditions exist. If the patient has TMJ inflammation, hypermobility may perpetuate the inflammation when the patient opens his/her mouth wide during yawning. In the presence of TMJ inflammation, full mouth opening, regardless of whether hypermobility exists, needs to be avoided.

Dislocation of the condyle can result from uncontrolled hypermobility. Diagnosis of condylar dislocation is made if a patient complains that his or her jaw catches on closing from a full, open mouth position. Hypermobility also may be accompanied by palpable joint noises. Palpable joint noises are noises that are heard by the patient and felt by the clinician while palpating over the TMJ during opening and closing movements of the mandible. Joint noises that are associated with hypermobility need to be differentiated from joint noises that are associated with a disc displacement. Although the patient may not have pain with jaw movement, the experience of joint noise, the feeling of a condyle catching on closing, and an awareness of deviation of the mandible on opening are events that are disconcerting to the patient.

The most important aspect regarding treatment for hypermobility is patient education. Physical therapists should inform their patients that noises and deviations of the jaw are not necessarily signs of significant pathology, and that they can be controlled with proper muscular re-education strategies. When mouth closing is associated with catching, the amount of mouth opening needs to be controlled through neuromuscular coordination exercises that are taught by a physical therapist who is knowledgeable in exercise interventions for TMJ hypermobility [9].

Disc displacement

Disc displacement can be classified into three stages: disc displacement with reduction, disc displacement without reduction, and chronic disc displacement without reduction [16]. Not all disc displacements are painful or interfere with functional movements of the mandible. Treatment is necessary when a patient experiences pain with or without functional limitations of the jaw [17]. Treatment choices for disc displacements that are painful or interfere with function consist of repositioning the disc to the condyle or allowing the disc to remain displaced while improving the function and decreasing the pain in the intra-articular and associated periarticular/myofascial tissues about the TMJ.

When choosing to reposition the disc to the condyle, the options are arthrotomy or an anterior-repositioning appliance. Because of the progressive nature of disc displacement, which is accompanied by increasing pathologic changes in the disc itself and its peripheral attachments, restoring a satisfactory functional disc–condyle relationship may be difficult [17]. Consequently, arthrotomy and anterior-repositioning appliances have led to mixed results in maintaining a normal long-term disc–condyle relationship [18–22].

Arthrotomy is a treatment choice for patients who do not respond to conservative care. Conservative care consists of physical therapy, medication, and a full-coverage acrylic appliance that does not reposition the mandible [23].

An anterior-repositioning appliance, which repositions the mandible, is the most controversial treatment option for repositioning the disc to the condyle [24]. The controversy relates to whether the anterior-repositioning appliance actually recaptures the disc [24]. During the use of an anterior-repositioning appliance, the absence of joint noises and pain with functional mouth opening does not necessarily indicate that the disc has been recaptured [20,24]. Studies using pre- and post-CT and well as MRI showed that permanent long-term disc recapture using an anterior-repositioning appliance was noted in only 10% to 30% of the patients [20]. When an anterior-repositioning appliance is discontinued, some patients may require orthodontics and possible orthognathic surgery. For the most part, an anterior-repositioning appliance should be considered on a case-by-case basis, and only should be used as an infrequent treatment option for repositioning disc displacements [24].

If the choice is not to reposition the disc to the condyle, the treatment options are arthroscopy (in its simplest format involving lavage/lysis), arthrocentesis, and physical therapy. The therapeutic value common to arthroscopy, arthrocentesis, and physical therapy interventions relates to the facilitation of adaptive responses of the articular tissues to the disc displacement. The human TMJ can adapt or remodel in response to articular disc displacement, regardless of the type of intervention, and often best when there is no intervention. For example, the posterior attachment of the disc (superior and inferior stratum and retrodiscal pad) becomes a pseudo disc that can withstand loading of the condyle during function [17,25]. Restoring a normal disc position is not a necessary component for treating pain and functional resolution [17]. Nonpainful disc displacements are so prevalent in patient and nonpatient populations that they may be considered a normal anatomic variability [26–28]. Because adaptive responses of the articular tissues within the TMJ are common secondary to disc displacement—and in most cases lead to pain-free and functional outcomes—perhaps the most therapeutic intervention should be the least invasive (ie, physical therapy).

Disc displacement without reduction

An article that has reviewed the literature comparing arthrocentesis, arthroscopic surgery, and physical therapy for the treatment of disc displacement without reduction has demonstrated no significant difference in the effects of maximum mandibular opening, pain intensity, or mandibular function [29]. The decision to perform arthroscopy or arthrocentesis instead of physical therapy should be based upon an evidence-based evaluation as well as the needs of the informed patient. When noninvasive treatment is recommended, physical therapy that is performed by a licensed physical therapist with an orthopedic specialty—and preferably a subspecialty in TMDs—should be the first choice in the treatment of disc displacements without reduction.

Physical therapy procedures may be successful in the treatment of pain and limited mouth opening that are associated with disc displacement without reduction [30–33]. Using various active and passive jaw exercises, as well as intraoral mobilization techniques, physical therapists may restore functional mandibular dynamics without pain when the disc is displaced. Inflammation that results from the disc displacement or that coexists with the disc displacement may be treated as identified previously. An oral appliance that is fabricated by a dentist also may facilitate the reduction of inflammation, especially if the patient bruxes. If physical therapy and the use of an oral appliance have not reduced pain to a satisfactory level or regained functional movements of the jaw after 4 to 12 weeks, the patient should consult with an oral surgeon to discuss surgical options.

Disc displacement with reduction and chronic disc displacement without reduction. Patients who experience a disc displacement with reduction or a chronic disc displacement without reduction may have functional movements of the mandible without pain [17]. The first goal of physical therapy consists of educating the patient on the cause of his or her joint noises (ie, reciprocal click or crepitus), so that he or she is aware of the aggravating factors of the condition. If the patient has TMJ pain that is due to inflammation, the goal of physical therapy is to reduce pain and improve mandibular function through manual therapy and exercise interventions, despite the disc displacement. An oral appliance that is fabricated by a dentist also may facilitate the reduction of inflammation, especially if the patient bruxes. A patient who has joint inflammation that does not respond to an oral appliance or 4 to 12 weeks of physical therapy may be referred to an oral surgeon to discuss surgical options.

A physical therapist may attempt to eliminate or decrease joint noises that are associated with a disc displacement with reduction. Clinically, the goal of physical therapy treatment is to have functional mandibular dynamics without pain and without noises, despite the disc being displaced permanently. The following criteria are used for patient selection:

Joint noises are disturbing to the patient
Patient experiences intermittent catching/locking with or without pain during mouth opening
Patient understands that the treatment may (a) cause joint pain or (b) cause limited mouth opening, or (c) result in having TMJ surgery because (a) or (b) could not be resolved.
Patient has consulted with a dentist or oral surgeon previously

Exercises and intraoral manual procedures for treating a reducing disc are not the same as exercises and intraoral manual procedures for increasing limited mouth opening that is associated with a nonreducing disc and fibrous adhesions. Progressing a reducing disc to a nonreducing disc involves the application of exercises and intraoral manual procedures that prevent the disc from reducing on opening. Preventing the disc from reducing on opening elongates the posterior attachment. Once sufficient elongation of the posterior attachment occurs, the patient can achieve functional opening without popping with the disc remaining displaced [9,34,35]. The patient may go through a short period with limited opening and possible pain. In the author's experience, 4 to 12 weeks is a sufficient time to achieve functional mandibular dynamics without pain and with an absence of joint noises with the disc displaced permanently.

Fibrous adhesions

Fibrous adhesions may appear in the capsular-ligament tissues and in the upper joint space of the TMJ [36]. Fibrous adhesions can result from chronic inflammation, blunt trauma, postoperative healing of a capsular incision, or immobility that occurs with intermaxillary fixation or from limited opening that is associated with a disc displacement without reduction. The physiologic changes that are associated with fibrous adhesions are documented in the literature [37–40]. Physical therapy procedures and modalities for the treatment of fibrous adhesions are similar, but not identical, to those that are used for treating a disc displacement without reduction. Treating fibrous adhesions involves applying an intraoral mobilization technique that is referred to as "lateral glide." A lateral glide passive intraoral mobilization procedure may be performed at the same time that the patient opens his or her mouth actively. Clinically, this passive/active mobilization force targets the restrictions in the lateral aspect of the capsular–ligament complex of the TMJ. The clinical decisions that are necessary to determine the duration, intensity, frequency, and progression of exercise intervention strategies require skill and experience. The effectiveness of a mobilization technique is related to proper patient selection, appropriate choice of technique, effective execution of the procedure, and making adjustments that are based on tissue response and patient feedback. Inappropriate management of a mechanical dysfunction of the TMJ by untrained personnel may lead to an exacerbation of symptoms and a worsening of the condition.

Temporomandibular disorders: myogenous

Masticatory muscle pain

Masticatory muscle pain is a common clinical finding in patients who experience head and orofacial pain [41]. The relationship between bruxism and masticatory pain is unclear [42]; however, parafunctional activity, such as bruxism, may be a predisposing, precipitating, or perpetuating factor of masticatory muscle pain [43,44]. The common treatment for managing bruxism/masticatory pain is an oral appliance [1]. Oral appliances have been shown to be effective in the treatment of masticatory pain [45,46].

Physical therapists may provide treatments that offer symptomatic relief in masticatory muscle pain through modalities and therapeutic procedures. Modalities, such as iontophoresis, ultrasound, and electric muscle stimulation, may help to reduce muscle pain [9]. Intraoral and extraoral soft tissue mobilization to the muscles of mastication also may provide symptomatic relief [9]. Therapeutic exercises to the mandible that consist of isometric, isotonic, and eccentric contraction have been observed clinically to reduce masticatory muscle pain [30]. Patient education strategies that are related to oral modifications and enhancing self-awareness about aggravating factors also have been shown to provide relief in masticatory muscle pain [47]. Oral modifications consist of diet changes as well as eliminating or limiting oral habits, such as gum chewing and nail, lip, or cheek biting. Self-awareness strategies also include instructing the patient on the proper rest position of the tongue and mandible. Patients who take an active role in making oral modifications and performing neuromuscular exercises may achieve satisfactory daytime relief from masticatory muscle pain. Decreasing the cumulative loading during the day also may provide relief in nighttime pain that is associated with bruxism. Nocturnal bruxism is more difficult to treat, even when the patient wears an oral appliance. Physical therapists can assist in reducing nocturnal bruxism by addressing head and neck positioning while sleeping. Instructing the patient on proper selection and usage of pillow support that is appropriate for their cervical spine alignment and motion function may help to lessen the tendency for bruxism at night by enabling a more restful mandibular position. Cervical spine disorders that may contribute to bruxism are covered in a later section.

Cervical spine considerations in the management of temporomandibular disorders and head and orofacial pain

The coexistence of neck pain and TMD is common [48–61]. One study found that neck pain is associated with TMD 70% of the time [55]. There also is a high occurrence of neck pain in patients who have facial pain. A study was conducted on 200 consecutive female patients who were referred to a university facial pain clinic. The patients were asked to mark all painful sites on sketches that showed contours of a human body in the frontal and rear views [62]. An analysis of the pain distribution according to the arrangements of dermatomes revealed three distinct clusters of patients: (1) those with pain restricted to the region innervated by the trigeminal nerve (n = 37); (2) those with pain in the trigeminal dermatomes and any combination involving the spinal dermatomes C2, C3, and C4, but no other dermatomes (n = 32); and (3) those with pain sites involving dermatomes in addition to those listed in (1) and (2) (n = 131).

In summary, the pain distribution of the 200 patients who had facial pain is more widespread than commonly assumed [62]. One hundred and sixty-three of 200 patients had pain that extended outside of the head and face to areas that included the C2, C3, and C4 dermatomes [62]. Other studies also have concluded that patients who have head and orofacial pain often experience widespread pain in the neck and shoulder areas [63,64].

A systematic review of the association between cervical posture and TMDs has been conducted [65]. The review examined 12 studies that satisfied the same inclusion criteria for participants. It concluded that an association between TMDs and cervical posture is unclear. The uncertainty of the association between TMDs and cervical posture was related to poor methodologic quality of the 12 studies [65]. Determining the typical resting posture of the head and neck for a study that evaluates upper body positional relationships is difficult, because all individuals assume many different head and neck postures during the course of a day's activities. Perhaps future studies that investigate cervical spine and TMD relationships should account for the dynamics of the cervical spine, instead of focusing on rest positions. The relationship of mandibular dynamics and the cervical spine needs to be analyzed in future studies by using reliable clinical instrumentation to compare active movements of the cervical spine to mandibular opening and closing or masticatory muscle pain.

The following section highlights cervical spine considerations in the management of TMD; it is followed by a discussion on cervical spine considerations for head and orofacial pain.

Cervical spine considerations with temporomandibular disorders–arthrogenous involvement

The TMJ is a load-bearing joint [1]. TMJ inflammation may be perpetuated by bruxism that loads the joint excessively [66,67]. An oral appliance helps to control bruxism [24]; however, not all patients respond favorably to an oral appliance that is designed to control bruxism. Many variables can contribute to bruxism, which is why an oral appliance may not always be therapeutic in controlling bruxism. One variable is cervical spine involvement. Decreasing the intensity and duration of bruxism by managing cervical spine disorders may reduce pain that originates from arthrogenous involvement. Cervical spine involvement as a cause of masticatory muscle pain or bruxism is discussed later in this article.

Typically, full mouth opening is accompanied by extension of the head, whereas mouth closing typically is accompanied by flexion of the head [68]. A frequently observed abnormal posture involves an extended head–neck position which is a component of "forward head posture." The forward head posture may facilitate wider mouth opening during functional activities, such as yawning and eating a large sandwich. Increasing patient awareness of forward head posture and instruction in correcting forward head posture during sitting, standing, and walking may control excessive mouth opening that is associated with hypermobility; it should be a part of the conservative management program for every patient who has a TMD.

On the other hand, if the objective is to facilitate mouth opening, physical therapists may position the patient's head and neck in slight extension during procedures (eg, intraoral mobilization and static–dynamic jaw exercises) that increase mouth opening. When the patient stands for mouth-opening exercises, the patient is instructed to allow his or her head to extend slightly while opening.

Patients often believe that their head and orofacial pain are due entirely to their disc displacement. Many patients believe that the only way to feel better is to have the disc "put back into place." This may be true, however, in only a small percentage of patients who have a disc displacement. Often, the source of the patient's pain is independent of the disc displacement. Instead, it originates from TMJ inflammation, overactive masticatory muscles, and irritation of the pain-sensitive structures of the cervical spine. Cervical spine involvement as a source of head and orofacial pain is discussed later.

Cervical spine considerations with temporomandibular disorders–myogenous involvement

Bruxism is more common in patients who have myofascial pain in the masticatory and cervical spine muscles [51]. Patients who have TMDs report neck symptoms more frequently than do patients who do not have TMDs; patients who have neck pain report more signs and symptoms of TMDs than do healthy controls [58]. Neck and shoulder pain is more prevalent in patients who have a TMD with a myogenous component than in patients who have a TMD with an arthrogenous component [56]. Therefore, the prevalence of neck pain coexisting with masticatory pain may be more than a coincidence. Cervical spine involvement as a predisposing, precipitating, or perpetuating variable to masticatory muscle pain or bruxism is highlighted in the following three theories.

Theory one

The first theory is that afferent input that is associated with neck pain converges onto trigeminal motor neurons in the trigeminocervical nucleus, which results in an increase in masticatory muscle hyperactivity and pain. Motor activity of trigeminal-innervated muscles of mastication increases when tissues that are innervated by upper cervical spine segments are irritated experimentally [69–73]. Little information on human subjects is available regarding the influence of experimental pain in the neck and shoulder muscles on motor activity in the orofacial region. One study was done to clarify the effects of experimental trapezius muscle pain on pain spread and on jaw motor function [74]. Experimental pain was induced in the superior border of the trapezius muscle of 12 subjects, aged 25 to 35 years of age, by injecting 0.5 mL of hypertonic (6%) saline. Results showed pain spread over a wide area to include the temporomandibular region, with pain referral accompanied by a reduction of mouth opening [74]. Afferent nociceptive input from the neck muscles may excite efferent (motor) neurons of cranial V, which results in contraction of masticatory muscles [75,76]. Similar convergences and central excitation phenomena—as seen with cervical and trigeminal sensory neurons—also may exist for trigeminal motor neurons [77,78].

Theory two

The second theory is that masticatory muscles contract in response to the contraction of cervical spine muscles. A neurophysiologic interplay exists that involves a synergistic relationship between the cervical spine and the muscles of mastication under normal circumstances [79–85]. Synergistic co-contraction can be observed with jaw and neck muscles during activities involving chew, talk, and yawn. Reciprocal innervations of opposing muscles has been demonstrated [82]. The cervical spine muscles and the muscles of mastication can be viewed as agonistic and antagonistic to one another [83]. In overt motor patterns, such as walking, augmentation and diminution of antagonistic muscles contracting concurrently (co-contraction) with agonist muscles contracting has been demonstrated [84,85].

Sometimes common daily events may cause the muscles of mastication to disproportionately contract in response to cervical muscles contracting. Head, neck, shoulder girdle, and upper extremity posture must be positioned precisely during eye–hand coordination activities, such as writing, painting, computer work, and driving. A task that involves a specific head and neck posture requires a constant low-level contraction of the cervical spine muscles. The longer that a subject spends on maintaining a specific head–neck posture, the more likely an exaggerated contraction of the muscles of mastication will occur in response to cervical spine muscles contracting.

Isometric, isotonic, or eccentric contractions of cervical spine muscles occur during lifting, carrying, pushing, pulling, and reaching activities. When cervical spine muscles perform repetitive activity, under load, and over a long duration, the more likely it is that the muscles of mastication will disproportionately contract.

Theory three

The third theory is that the patient bruxes in response to neck pain. Patients start to brux or the intensity and frequency of their bruxing may be exacerbated by their response to acute or chronic neck pain.

Thus, a neurophysiologic interplay exists between the muscles of mastication and the cervical spine, which needs to be addressed in the thorough management of the patient who has a TMD. Although these three theories need further clinical research, physical therapists observe that treating cervical spine pain often decreases masticatory muscle pain. Consequently, neck pain should be added to the list of factors that contribute to bruxism and masticatory muscle pain.

Cervical spine considerations with oral appliances

Common treatments for masticatory muscle pain are medication and application of an oral appliance, both of which can be offered by a dentist or oral surgeon [24]. Physical therapists should be familiar with the different structural designs of splints as well as be able to explain the rationale and therapeutic benefits for oral appliance use [46,86,87].

One common feature of the use of oral appliances and postural re-education/manual therapy intervention of cervical spine dysfunction is that both treatment strategies influence the rest position of the mandible. Rest position of the mandible determines the initial path of closure into tooth-to-tooth contact or teeth contact onto an appliance [88]. The design of an oral appliance influences the vertical and horizontal positions of the mandibular rest position; this changes the path of mandibular closure and affects how the teeth and oral appliance make contact [89].

Conversely, head and neck posture also influences the vertical and horizontal positions of the mandibular rest position, which subsequently alters the path of closure into teeth-to-teeth contact [90–98]. Mohl [90] stated, "if the rest position is altered by a change in head position, the habitual path of closure of the mandible must also be altered by such a change." Clinically, physical therapists have recognized that cervical spine motion restrictions and forward head posture affect mandibular closure, which, in turn, alters how the teeth and oral appliance make contact.

Patients may complain that they do not "hit," "bite," or "make contact" evenly on their appliance. If the patient's complaint cannot be explained by interferences that are caused by the appliance design, the dentist should consider a mechanical disorder within the cervical spine that affects the path of closure of the mandible onto the appliance. Patients who do not to respond to an oral appliance in a 4-week period may not need more time wearing the appliance or a change in the design of the appliance [1]. Another alternative is to have a physical therapist evaluate the cervical spine to assess for possible dysfunctions that might be interfering with the effectiveness of the oral appliance. Clinically, cervical spine dysfunction with respect to abnormal posture or motion impairment can be treated before, during, or after the use of an oral appliance. Favorable outcomes are more likely to be achieved when cervical spine treatment is rendered concurrently with the use of an oral appliance, according to physical therapists who are experienced in managing masticatory muscle pain.

Cervical spine considerations with head and orofacial pain

Symptoms that originate from the cervical spine and require immediate medical attention secondary to spinal pathology include gross mechanical instability that may affect spinal cord function, primary bone tumor, metastatic disease, infections, fracture, and dislocation [99]. Symptoms also may be referred to the cervical spine from visceral pathology [100]. "Red flags" that suggest a visceral pathology should alert the clinician to a nonmusculoskeletal origin of the patient's pain (Box 2). Imaging studies and erythrocyte sedimentation rates can help in detecting whether an underlying pathology is present [101].

Most cervical spine–related symptoms are not caused by spinal or visceral pathology [102]. Nonpathologic symptoms may originate from disc disorders, nerve root irritation, spinal cord compromise secondary to spinal stenosis, facet joint dysfunction, and myofascial pain. Common medical diagnoses for each cervical spine tissue are listed in Box 3. Patients

---

Box 2. Pathologic conditions are suspected with the following "red flags"

Fever
Unexplained loss of weight
History of inflammatory arthritis
History of malignancy
Osteoporosis
Vascular insufficiency
Blackouts
History of drug abuse, AIDS, or other infection
Immunosuppression
Lymphadenopathy
Severe trauma
Minor trauma or strenuous lifting in an older patient
Increasing or unremitting pain

Data from Jarvik J, Deyo R. Diagnostic evaluation of low back pain with emphasis on imaging. Ann Intern Med 2002;137:586–97.

---

frequently have more than one cervical spine–related tissue that is the source of their cervical spine–related symptoms. Multiple cervical spine tissue involvement can be referred to collectively as cervical spine disorders. Cervical spine disorders can cause pain or functional limitations of the cervical spine in which symptoms vary with physical activity or static positioning, which may develop gradually or follow trauma.

The prevalence of nonpathologic neck pain is high. Seventy percent of the general population is affected with neck pain at some time in their lives [103]. Fifty-four percent of the general population has experienced neck pain in the last 6 months [104]. The general population has a point prevalence of neck pain that varies between 9.5% and 22% [105].

Box 3. Common sources of neck symptoms with corresponding *International Classification of Diseases, Ninth Revision* (ICD-9) codes

Disc: 722.6, degeneration; 722.2, herniation
Nerve root: 723.4, cervical radiculopathy
Spinal cord: 721.1, cervical myelopathy
Facet joint: 719.5, hypomobility
Muscle: 728.5, muscle spasm; 729.1, myalgia

Head and orofacial pain of cervical spine origin

The International Headache Society has created a list of 144 different headache types that fall into one of 13 categories (Box 4) [106]. The cervical spine is listed as a possible causative factor for headaches and is reported as "neck" in classification 11, subclassification 11.2.

The literature is clear that cervical spine tissues refer pain to the head and orofacial areas [77,107]. The neuroanatomic mechanism that explains the referred pain is the convergence between trigeminal afferents and afferents of the upper three cervical nerves [108]. This convergence occurs in an area that is referred to as the trigeminocervical nucleus [109]. The trigeminocervical nucleus is located in the upper cervical spinal cord within the pars caudalis portion of the spinal nucleus of the trigeminal nerve (Fig. 1) [110,111].

Box 4. Classification and diagnostic criteria for headache disorders, cranial neuralgias, and facial pain

1. Migraine headache
2. Tension-type headache
3. Cluster headache and chronic paroxysmal hemicrania
4. Miscellaneous headache, unassociated with structural lesion
5. Headache associated with head trauma
6. Headache associated with vascular disorders
7. Headache associated with nonvascular intracranial disorders
8. Headache associated with substances or withdrawal
9. Headache associated with noncephalic infection
10. Headache associated with metabolic disorder
11. Headache or facial pain associated with disorder of cranium, neck, eyes, ears, nose, sinuses, teeth, mouth, or other facial or cranial structures
    11.1 Cranial bones including the mandible
    11.2 Neck
    11.3 Eyes
    11.4 Ears
    11.5 Nose and sinuses
    11.6 Teeth and related oral structures
    11.7 Temporomandibular joint
    11.8 Masticatory muscles
12. Cranial neuralgias, nerve trunk pain, and deafferentation pain
13. Headache not classified

Adapted from International Headache Society, Classification Committee. Classification and diagnostic criteria for headache disorders, cranial neuralgias and facial pain. Cephalalgia 1998;8(Suppl 7):9–96.

Primary sources of head and orofacial pain that originate from the cervical spine lie in the structures that are innervated by C1 to C3 spinal nerves [111]. The lower segmental levels, C4 thru C7, also may contribute to head and orofacial pain through the trigeminocervical nucleus [112]. Box 5 lists the tissues with sensory innervations from the upper three cervical nerves that contribute to referred symptoms to the head and orofacial areas [111].

The greater occipital nerve (GON) branches off from the C2 nerve root [113]. GON cutaneous branches and their innervations are:

Medial branch: innervates the occipital skin
Lateral branch: innervates the region above the mastoid process and be-
    hind the pinna (the projecting part of the ear lying outside of the head)
Intermediate branches: run rostrally and ventrally across the top of the
    skull as far as the coronal suture. Anastomosis of the GON to the

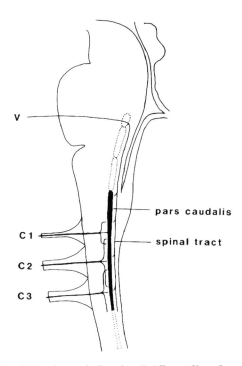

Fig. 1. A sketch of the "trigeminocervical nucleus." Afferent fibers from the trigeminal nerve (V) enter the pons and descend in the spinal tract to upper cervical levels, sending collateral branches into the pars caudalis of the spinal nucleus of the trigeminal nerve and the gray matter of the C1 to C3 spinal cord segments. Afferent fibers from the C1, C2, and C3 spinal nerves ramify in the spinal gray matter at their segment of entry and at adjacent segments. That column of gray matter that receives trigeminal and cervical afferents constitutes the trigeminal nucleus (*black*). (*From* Bogduk N. Cervical causes of headache and dizziness. In: Grieve G, editor. Modern manual therapy. 2nd edition. Edinburgh (UK): Churchill Livingstone; 1986. p. 317, with permission.)

Box 5. Sensory innervations from the upper three cervical nerves

C1 sensory innervation
  Suboccipital tissues and muscles
  Atlantoccipital and atlantoaxial facet joints
  Paramedian dura of the posterior cranial fossa and dura
    adjacent to the condylar canal
  Upper prevertebral muscles (longus capitis and cervicis
    and the rectus capitis anterior and lateralis)

C2 sensory innervation
  Skin of the occiput
  Upper posterior neck muscles; semispinalis capitis,
    longissimus capitis and splenius capitis, the
    sternocleidomastoid, trapezius, and prevertebral muscles
  Atlantoaxial facet joint
  Paramedian dura of the posterior cranial fossa
  Lateral walls of the posterior cranial fossa

C3 sensory innervation
  Multifidus, semispinalis capitis, sternocleidomastoid,
    trapezius, and prevertebral muscles
  Suboccipital skin
    C2/3 facet joint
  Cervical portion and intracranial branches of the vertebral
    artery

---

supraorbital nerve, which is a trigeminal branch, occurs at the coronal suture.

Trauma or suboccipital muscle tightness may involve the GON, referred to as occipital neuralgia [114]. Symptoms that are associated with occipital neuralgia refer to the occipital area, top of the skull, TMJ area, and in or around the ear [115,116].

Cervicogenic headache

The term "cervicogenic headache" was used first in 1983 by Sjaastad and colleagues [117]. Cervicogenic headache refers to head and orofacial pain that originates from the cervical spine tissues. Cervicogenic headache can be a perplexing pain disorder [118]. The following is a clinical presentation of cervicogenic headache as described by Sjaastad et al [117]:

> The pain is usually unilateral but when severe can be felt on the opposite side. It is a head pain and not just a neck pain. The main manifestation

of the headache is in the temporal, frontal, and ocular areas. It has fluctuating long-term course with remissions and exacerbations; some patients have a continuous basal headache, others do not. During the headache attack, there may be the following accompanying phenomena; ipsilateral blurring and reduced vision, a "migrainous" phenomena like nausea and loss of appetite; there may even be vomiting. Phonophobia and photophobia occur frequently. Some patients complain of dizziness and of difficulty swallowing during symptomatic periods. Even between attacks, patients may feel stiffness and reduced mobility of the neck.

Prevalence of cervicogenic headache

Cervicogenic headache is one of the three large headache groups; the other two are tension-type headache and common migraine without aura [119]. Cervicogenic headache accounts for 15% to 35% of all chronic and recurrent headaches [119–121].

Although cervicogenic headache has been diagnosed more frequently over recent years, it also has been misdiagnosed because of the considerable overlap in symptoms with more popular causes of headache (tension-type and migraine) [117,122,123]. Cervical pain and muscle tension are common symptoms of a migraine [124,125]. In a study of 50 patients who had migraine, 64% reported neck pain or stiffness associated with their migraine, with 31% experiencing neck symptoms during the prodrome, 93% experiencing neck symptoms during the headache phase, and 31% experiencing neck symptoms during the recovery phase [124]. Other studies show that neck pains often coexist with migraine headaches [126,127]. In addition, cervical muscles may play a role in the pathogenesis of migraine headaches [128]. Patients often suffer several headache types concurrently [129]. Patients may require medications for migraine, application of an oral appliance for tension headache, and physical therapy for cervicogenic headache. In summary, many patients are misdiagnosed to have migraine or tension type headaches, when in fact these patients actually have headaches of cervical origin. Therefore, the appropriate treatment should be targeted to mechanical dysfunction or muscle tension in the cervical spine.

Dizziness

Dizziness and vertigo refer to a false sensation of motion of the body, which patients describe as a spinning or swaying feeling [130,131]. They are synonymous terms that are used to describe spinning, swaying, the subjective accompaniments of ataxia, and a variety of other colloquially described sensations. Dizziness may result from involvement of the eyes, the parietal and temporal lobes, and cerebellum—most commonly as a result of disease affecting the labyrinth or the vestibular nuclei [132,133]. In the absence of disease, the vestibular nuclei can be affected by disorders of the neck in two ways: through ischemic processes or disturbances of neck proprioceptors [133]. Disturbance of the vestibular nuclei secondary to dysfunctional neck proprioceptors are addressed for this discussion.

Afferent input from neck proprioceptors (ie, facet joints and muscles) is believed to affect the vestibular nuclei activity, which results in a variety of motor and subjective abnormalities [133]. Cervical facet joints and muscles may produce a generalized ataxia, with symptoms of imbalance, disorientation, and motor incoordination [134–139]. Vertigo, ataxia, and nystagmus were induced in animals and man by injecting local anesthetic into the neck [140]. The injections presumably interrupted the flow of afferent information from joint receptors and neck muscles to the vestibular nuclei. Vertigo following a whiplash injury (an extension/flexion movement of the head and neck) may be due to afferent excitation that originates from cervical muscles, ligaments, facet joints, and sensory nerves [141]. Patients who do not respond to treatments for dizziness that is believed to be originating from the eye, inner ear, or sinus should be suspected of having cervicogenic vertigo. Patients who experience cervicogenic vertigo may complain of pain, stiffness, and tightness in the neck; they are good candidates for physical therapy intervention that focuses on the cervical spine [142,143].

Subjective tinnitus and secondary otalgia

Objective tinnitus is characterized by physiologic sounds and represents only 1% of cases of tinnitus. Subjective tinnitus is an otologic phenomenon of phantom sounds. Although 10% of the population suffers from subjective tinnitus, its cause is unknown [144].

Subjective tinnitus has been related to cervical spine involvement. The sensory upper cervical dorsal roots and the sensory components of four cranial nerves (V, VII, IX, X) converge on a region of the brain stem that is known as the medullary somatosensory nucleus [145]. Subjective tinnitus is a neural threshold phenomenon and cervical muscle contraction alters the neural activity that is responsible for tinnitus [146]. One hundred and fifty patients were tested with a series of head and neck maneuvers to assess whether any of the maneuvers changed their subjective tinnitus. Eighty percent of patients had increased tinnitus during the test [146]. A similar study tested 120 patients who had subjective tinnitus and 60 subjects who did not have tinnitus [147]. The findings showed that forceful head and neck contractions, as well as loud sound exposure, were significantly more likely to modulate ongoing auditory perception in people who had tinnitus than in those who did not have tinnitus [147]. This study supports the concept that subjective tinnitus has a neural threshold [147].

Secondary otalgia (ie, earache not caused by primary ear pathology) is common in patients who are suffering from earache [148]. In a standardized examination and interview of 100 subjects, 91 subjects had secondary otalgia and 9 had primary otalgia [149]. An epidemiologic study investigated subjects who had secondary otalgia during a 2-year follow-up period [150].

Subjects who had secondary otalgia had pain with palpation over the masticatory muscles and TMJ, and reported neck and shoulder pain more frequently than did the individuals who did not have secondary otalgia [150]. Kuttila and colleagues [149] investigated whether secondary otalgia is associated with cervical spine disorder, TMDs, or both [149]. Most of the subjects who reported secondary otalgia also had signs and symptoms of cervical spine and TMD involvement. An examination of the cervical spine and TMD is recommended as a routine diagnostic process for patients who have secondary otalgia.

Cervical spine examination

History

Orthopedic-related cervical spine problems are suspected first during the history. Primary symptoms of cervical spine disorders are neck, shoulder, and upper extremity pain and headaches (cervicogenic). Cervicogenic headaches are described by patients as pain that projects from the neck to the forehead, orbital region, temples, vertex, or ears. The symptoms for cervicogenic headaches as identified by the International Headache Society criteria for cervicogenic headache are listed in Box 6 [151]. Symptoms, such as dizziness, ear pain (secondary), and subjective tinnitus, also may have a cervicogenic origin. A complete list of cervical spine–related symptoms in shown in Box 7 [152].

The patient's symptoms can be quantified by documenting frequency, intensity (visual analog scale), and duration of symptoms. This information can be used to monitor the patient's response to treatment. The Copenhagen Neck Functional Disability Scale or the Functional Rating Index can be used to document improvement [153,154]. Duration of sleeping and sitting as well as the patient's ability to reach, pull, and lift are documented in a measurable manner. Change in medication intake also can be used to monitor the patient's response to treatment.

Physical examination

A physical examination of the cervical spine involves tests that incriminate nerve involvement. Often, neurologic signs are the result of nerve root compromise and are referred to as cervical radiculopathy, whereas spinal cord compromise is referred to as cervical myelopathy. Aside from physical tests that evaluate nerve function (manual muscle tests, sensory tests, reflex responses, and nerve tension tests), the physical therapy examination assesses for motion impairments of the cervical spine that influence gross range of motion or result in abnormal segmental vertebral motion that corresponds to the patient's symptoms and functional limitations. Palpatory tests evaluate for myofascial pain and dysfunction with respect to tenderness, and tightness. Pain also can be accessed upon

---

Box 6. International Headache Society criteria for cervicogenic headache

A. Pain localized in the neck and occipital region. May project to the forehead, orbital region, temples, vertex, or ears.
B. Pain is precipitated or aggravated by special neck movements or sustained neck posture.
C. At least one of the following occurs:
   a. Resistance to or limitation of passive neck movements
   b. Changes in neck muscle contour, texture, tone or response to active and passive stretching and contraction
   c. Abnormal tenderness in neck muscles

D. Radiologic examination reveals at least one of the following:
   a. Movement abnormalities in flexion/extension
   b. Abnormal posture
   c. Fractures, congenital abnormalities, bone tumors, rheumatoid arthritis, or other distinct pathology (not spondylosis or osteochondrosis)

Adapted from International Headache Society. Classification and diagnostic criteria for headache disorders, cranial neuralgias and facial pain. Cephalalgia 1998;8(Suppl 7):9–96.

---

contraction of the muscle. Manual muscle and neuromotor tests are used to assess strength and coordination. A postural analysis is included to evaluate for possible areas of stress concentration. Physical therapists often determine the patient's response to manual traction during the initial examination to evaluate the need for mechanical cervical traction treatment. Physical examination procedures are listed in Box 8. Imaging studies may be needed if the history and physical examination findings are questionable or vague.

Treatment strategies for cervical spine and related symptoms

Invasive procedures

Treatment guidelines, such as the Scientific Monograph of the Quebec Task Force on Whiplash-Associated Disorders and Evidence-based Practice Guidelines for Interventional Techniques in the Management of Chronic Spinal Pain, recommend a noninvasive approach in the treatment of cervical spine symptoms with or without neurologic signs [152,155]. Only after unsuccessful conservative treatment should invasive procedures be considered [156]. Invasive procedures include epidural injections, nerve root

---

Box 7. Symptoms that may originate from cervical spine disorders

Neck/shoulder pain
Reduced/painful neck movements
Numbness, tingling or pain in arm or hand
Reduced/painful jaw movement
Headaches
Dizziness/unsteadiness
Nausea/vomiting
Difficulty swallowing
Ringing in the ears
Vision problems
Numbness, tingling, or pain in leg or foot
Lower back pain
Memory problems
Problems concentrating

Data from Spitzer WO, Skovron ML, Salmi LR, et al. Scientific monograph of the Quebec Task Force on Whiplash-Associated Disorders: redefining "whiplash" and its management. Spine 1995;20(8 Suppl):1S–73S.

---

injections, facet joint denervation, myofascial trigger point injections, and surgery (ie, cervical fusion).

Unless neurologic signs suggest otherwise, patients who have symptoms of radiculopathy or myelopathy should be considered for surgery after conservative care has failed. Three studies examined the effects of surgery and conservative care on pain for sensory loss and weakness in patients who had minimal to moderate cervical radiculopathy or myelopathy. Two studies were prospective, randomized studies that evaluated a total of 130 patients; the other study was a randomized study that involved 68 participants [157–159]. No differences were found in sensation or motor strength between the patients who were treated surgically and those who were managed conservatively in follow-up examinations at 24 and 36 months. Therefore, patients need to be informed that the long-term outcomes for conservative treatment of minimal to moderate cervical radiculopathy or myelopathy may be the same as having surgical intervention, and in some cases, the only reason for selecting a surgical approach may be to achieve faster pain relief.

Conservative care

Patients who have neck pain can choose from several complementary/alternative treatments that may be part of a physical therapist's knowledge

---

Box 8. Procedures used to diagnose cervical spine disorders (disc, nerve root, spinal cord, facet joint, and muscle)

Neurologic testing for nerve function
  Deep tendon reflex
  Sensation
  Strength
  Spurlings test
  Hoffman's reflex
  Lhermitte's test
  Nerve tension tests

Active range of motion

  Passive range of motion
  Cardinal plane movement
  Intersegmental movement

Muscle contraction (isometric/isotonic/eccentric)

Palpation
  Muscles
  Facet joints
  Greater occipital nerve

Manual traction

Posture

---

and skill base. Complementary and Alternative Medicine (CAM) is a diverse group of health-related professionals that have not documented the therapeutic value of their alternative treatments (eg, magnet therapy, crystal application) through randomized clinic trials [160]. Physical therapy, however, is not CAM. Physical therapists offer evidence-based treatments for TMDs and cervical spine disorders with data that are well documented in peer-reviewed journals [161–167]. Physical therapists follow evidence-based guidelines using a multimodal conservative treatment approach for cervical spine symptoms that consists of manual therapy, exercise, patient education, and mechanical cervical traction.

A multicenter, randomized, controlled trial with unblinded treatment and blinded outcome measures was conducted to investigate the efficacy of physical therapy management of cervicogenic headache [168]. A group of 200 participants who met the diagnostic criteria for cervicogenic headache was randomized into four treatment groups: manipulative therapy, exercise therapy, combined therapy, and no treatment. The primary outcome measured was a change in headache frequency. Other outcomes evaluated included changes in headache intensity and duration, improvement in the Northwick Park Neck Pain Index, reduction in medication intake, and patient satisfaction. The physical outcomes evaluated included pain on neck movement, upper cervical joint tenderness, a craniocervical flexion muscle test, and a photographic measure of posture. The treatment period was 6 weeks with follow-up assessment after treatment, then at 3, 6, and 12 months. At the 12-month follow-up assessment, manipulative therapy and specific exercise had reduced headache frequency and intensity and neck pain significantly, and effects were maintained ($P < .05$ for all). In summary, manipulative therapy and specific therapeutic exercise reduce the symptoms of cervicogenic headache in the short and long term [168].

Manual therapy

Manual therapy techniques consist of a continuum of skilled passive movements to joints or related soft tissues that are applied at varying speeds and amplitudes, including a small-amplitude/high-velocity therapeutic movement [169]. Mobilization (nonthrust) or manipulation (thrust), when used with exercise, is effective for alleviating persistent pain and improving function when compared with no treatment. When compared with each other, neither mobilization nor manipulation is superior [161]. The psychologic, neurophysiologic, and mechanical benefits of manual therapy have been covered adequately in the literature [170,171].

Exercise

Exercises may be effective in treating and preventing neck pain [172]. Specific exercises combined with manual therapy may be effective in the treatment of subacute and chronic neck pain, with or without headache, in the short and long term [155,173]. Physical therapists can identify muscles of the cervical, shoulder, and thoracic areas that are tight, weak, and have difficulty in regulating tension levels. Physical therapists instruct patients in exercise programs that consist of stretching, strengthening, conditioning, and coordination that are specific to the patient's needs. Modification of the exercise program frequently is necessary after re-evaluation of the patient, and is dependent upon the changes in the patient's signs and symptoms. A successful home exercise program is a function of proper patient performance and diligence. The skill of the physical therapist in teaching correct exercise form, making modifications in the exercises based on patient's response, and motivating the patient to perform his or her home program are critical in obtaining an optimal outcome.

Patient education

Patient education focuses on many elements of patient care, and often involves instructing the patient on proper sitting and sleep postures. Support and encouragement of patients also is important to help them overcome fear, anxiety, and misconceptions about their condition. Frequently, well-meaning advice from friends or family members may interfere with recovery because of misbeliefs or incorrect information. In some cases, incorrect information is being received from online computer resources that the patient has read. Frequently, physical therapists must dispel myths that the patient may have obtained from different sources to alleviate anxiety-fear and manage pain [174,175].

Patients are educated about the meaning of their diagnosis by physical therapists because physical therapists typically spend more time with the patient than do medical professionals. Patients often perceive that "something is wrong" (ie, irreversible) from a medical diagnosis, such as degenerative joint disease, when degenerative joint disease in itself is neither predictive of, nor strongly correlated with, the patient's symptoms. In this way, a medical diagnosis may enhance the feelings of fear and anxiety, which can intensify symptoms and lead the patient to believe that a cure is not available [176]. Patients can become preoccupied with their diagnosis and often seek invasive treatment in an attempt to "fix" the condition.

The health practitioner must understand that a patient's fear, misunderstanding, and beliefs about the meaning of pain may determine whether he or she progresses from acute to chronic neck pain [177]. A patient is less likely to develop a chronic pain mentality when he or she is educated about the condition secondary to the knowledge obtained about the medical diagnosis and symptoms. The physical therapist plays a major role in reducing patient anxiety and fear by keeping the patient focused to functional goals.

Mechanical cervical traction

Traction is a treatment that is based on the application of a longitudinal force to the axis of the spinal column. Medically accepted uses for spinal traction include soft tissue tightness, joint stiffness, cervical radiculopathy, and cervical myelopathy that are caused by disc degeneration or disc herniation [178]. The therapeutic value of traction was demonstrated in a trial of 30 patients who had unilateral C7 radiculopathy [179]. Patients were assigned randomly to a control group or an experimental group. The application of cervical traction, combined with electrotherapy and exercise, produced an immediate improvement in the hand-grip function in patients who had cervical radiculopathy compared with the control group that received electrotherapy/exercise treatment [179]. Although this is only one study that provides support for the use of mechanical traction, it does demonstrate its potential for radicular signs and symptoms.

The benefits of neck traction are optimal when performed with the patient in a supine position. The traction unit should not pull through the mandible, but only through the base of the skull/mastoid process areas. Guidelines are available that recommend angle of pull, poundage, and duration of pull [178]. A physical therapist considers the patient's signs and symptoms to adjust the force and duration of stretch to get the desired results.

Summary

Physicians, dentists, oral surgeons, and physical therapists need to work together to achieve the best outcomes for patients who experience TMDs and head and orofacial pain. Physical therapists play an important role in the conservative care of TMDs and cervical spine disorders that cause head and orofacial pain. Physicians and dentists should keep in mind that not all physical therapists have specialty practices that focus on TMDs and cervical spine disorders. Therefore, referral to an orthopedic physical therapist who specializes in TMDs and cervical spine disorders is important for the appropriate management of the patient.

Physical therapists treat TMDs that are secondary to inflammation, hypermobility, disc displacements, fibrous adhesions, and masticatory muscle pain and bruxism. Studies have shown that masticatory muscle pain and bruxism may be perpetuated by cervical spine involvement. Research evidence suggests a neurophysiologic interplay between the muscles of mastication and the cervical spine muscles. The cervical spine should be evaluated and treated when patients' TMD symptoms do not respond to medication and an oral appliance.

Often, cervical spine involvement is a misdiagnosed or unrecognized source of head and orofacial pain (ie, headache), dizziness, subjective tinnitus, and secondary ear pain. Head and orofacial pain that originates from the cervical spine is referred to as cervicogenic headache. Cervicogenic headache symptoms can be similar to other common headache disorders, such as migraine or tension-type headache.

Cervical spine disorders that are treated by physical therapists using evidence-based interventions, such as manipulation/mobilization and therapeutic exercise, can decrease the protracted course of costly treatment and reduce the patient's pain. Physical therapists, therefore, have an important role in the management of head-neck and orofacial pain. Patients who present with TMD and cervical spine disorders many times can be effectively treated by a physical therapist that has specialized skills and experience. Consequently, physical therapists should be an important member of the group of health practitioners who work with patients who have head, neck, and orofacial pain.

References

[1] Differential diagnosis and management considerations of temporomandibular disorders. In: Okeson JP, editor. Orofacial pain; guidelines for assessment, diagnosis, and management. Carol Stream (IL): Quintessence Publisher Co., Inc.; 1996. p. 45–52.

[2] Hoving JL, Gross AR, Gasner D, et al. A critical appraisal of review articles on the effectiveness of conservative treatment for neck pain. Spine 2001;26(2):196–205.

[3] A guide to physical therapist practice. Volume I: A description of patient management. Phys Ther 1995;75:70756.

[4] APTA House of Delegates Policies HOD #06–93–22–43. Alexandria (VA): American Physical Therapy Association; 1996.

[5] Clark G, Seligman D, Solberg W, et al. Guidelines for the treatment of temporomandibular disorders. J Craniomandib Disord 1990;4:80–8.
[6] Feine J, Widmer C, Lund J. Physical therapy: a critique. Presented at the National Institutes of Health Technology Assessment Conference on Management of Temporomandibular Disorders. Bethesda (MD), April 29–May 1, 1996.
[7] McNeill C, editor. Temporomandibular disorders. Guidelines for classification, assessment and management. 2nd edition. Carol Stream (IL): Quintessence Publishing Co., Inc; 1993.
[8] Dworkin S, LeResche L. Research diagnostic criteria for temporomandibular disorders: review, criteria, examination and specifications critique. J Craniomandib Disord 1992;6: 301–55.
[9] Kraus SL. Temporomandibular disorders. In: Saunders HD, Saunders Ryan R, editors. Evaluation, treatment and prevention of musculoskeletal disorders, vol. 1 - Spine. 4th edition. Chaska (MN): The Saunders Group, Inc.; 2004. p. 173–210.
[10] Schiffman E, Braun B, Lindgren J, et al. Temporomandibular joint iontophoresis: a double-blind randomized clinical trial. J Orofac Pain 1996;10:157–65.
[11] Shin S-M, Choi J-K. Effect of indomethacin phonophoresis on relief of TMJ pain. J Craniomandibular Pract 1997;15(4):345–8.
[12] Watson T. The role of electrotherapy in contemporary physiotherapy practice. Man Ther 2000;5(3):132–41.
[13] Dijkstra PU, de Bont LGM, Leeuw R, et al. Temporomandibular joint osteoarthrosis and temporomandibular joint hypermobility. J Craniomandibular Pract 1993;11:268–75.
[14] Westling L, Mattiasson A. General joint hypermobility and temporomandibular joint derangement in adolescents. Ann Rheum Dis 1992;51:87–90.
[15] Dijkstra PU, de Bont LGM, Stegenga B, et al. Temporomandibular joint osteoarthrosis and generalized joint hypermobility. J Craniomandibular Pract 1992;10:221–7.
[16] Moffett BC. Definitions of temporomandibular joint derangements. In: Moffett BC, Westesson P-L, editors. Diagnosis of internal derangements of the temporomandibular joint, vol 1. Double-contrast arthrography and clinical considerations. Proceedings of a Continuing Dental Education Symposium. Seattle, 1984.
[17] Milam S. Pathophysiology of articular disk displacements of the temporomandibular joint. In: Fonseca RJ, editor. Oral & maxillofacial surgery: temporomandibular disorders, vol. 4. 1st edition. Philadelphia: W.B. Saunders Company; 2000. p. 46–72.
[18] Montgomery MT, Gordon SM, Van Sickels JE, et al. Changes in signs and symptoms following temporomandibular joint disc repositioning surgery. J Oral Maxillofac Surg 1992; 50(4):320–8.
[19] Assael LA. Arthrotomy for internal derangements. In: Kaplan AS, Assael LA, editors. Temporomandibular disorders: diagnosis and treatment. Philadelphia: W.B. Saunders Company; 1991. p. 663–79.
[20] Orenstein ES. Anterior repositioning appliances when used for anterior disk displacement with reduction—a critical review. J Craniomandib Pract 1993;11(2):141–5.
[21] Chen CW, Boulton J, Gage JP. Splint therapy in temporomandibular joint dysfunction: a study using magnetic resonance imaging. Aust Dent J 1995;40(2):71–8.
[22] de Leeuw R. Clinical signs of TMJ osteoarthrosis and internal derangement 30 years after nonsurgical treatment. J Orofac Pain 1994;8:18–24.
[23] Bays R. Surgery for internal derangement. In: Fonseca RJ, editor. Oral & maxillofacial surgery: temporomandibular disorders, vol. 4. 1st edition. Philadelphia: W. B. Saunders Company; 2000. p. 275–300.
[24] Sollecito T. Role of splint therapy in treatment of temporomandibular disorders. In: Fonseca RJ, editor. Oral & maxillofacial surgery: temporomandibular disorders, vol. 4. 1st edition. Philadelphia: W. B. Saunders Company; 2000. p. 145–60.
[25] Blaustein DI, Scapino RP. Remolding of the temporomandibular joint disc and posterior attachment in disc displacement specimens in relation to glycosaminoglycan content. Plast Reconstr Surg 1986;79:756–64.

[26] Turell J, Ruiz HG. Normal and abnormal findings in temporomandibular joints in autopsy specimens. J Craniomandib Disord 1987;1:257–75.

[27] Kircos LT, Ortendahl DA, Mark AS, et al. Magnetic resonance imaging of the TMJ disc in asymptomatic volunteers. J Oral Maxillofac Surg 1987;45:852–4.

[28] Westesson PL, Eriksson L, Kurita K. Reliability of a negative clinical temporomandibular joint examination: prevalence of disk displacement in asymptomatic temporomandibular joints. Oral Surg Oral Med Oral Pathol 1989;68:551–4.

[29] Kropmans TJ, Dijkstra PU, Stegenga B, et al. Therapeutic outcome assessment in permanent temporomandibular joint disc displacement. J Oral Rehabil 1999;26:357–63.

[30] Kraus SL. Physical therapy management of temporomandibular disorders. In: Fonseca RJ, editor. Oral & maxillofacial surgery: temporomandibular disorders, vol. 4. 1st edition. Philadelphia: W. B. Saunders Company; 2000. p. 161–93.

[31] Segami N, Murakami K-I, Iizuka T. Arthrographic evaluation of disk position following mandibular manipulation technique for internal derangement with closed lock of the temporomandibular joint. J Craniomandib Disord 1990;4:99–108.

[32] Van Dyke AR, Goldman SM. Manual reduction of displaced disk. J Craniomandib Pract 1990;8:350–2.

[33] Minagi S, Nozaki S, Sato T, et al. A manipulation technique for treatment of anterior disk displacement without reduction. J Prosthet Dent 1991;65:686–91.

[34] Scapino RP. The posterior attachments: its structure, function, and appearance in TMJ imaging studies: Part 1. J Craniomandib Disord 1991;5(2):83–94.

[35] Scapino RP. The posterior attachments: its structure, function, and appearance in TMJ imaging studies: Part 2. J Craniomandib Disord 1991;5(3):155–66.

[36] Holmlund AB. Arthroscopy. In: Fonseca RJ, editor. Oral & maxillofacial surgery: temporomandibular disorders, vol. 4. 1st edition. Philadelphia: W. B. Saunders Company; 2000. p. 255–74.

[37] Hardy MA. The biology of scar formation. Phys Ther 1989;69(12):22–32.

[38] Akeson WH, Amiel D, Woo S. Immobility effects of synovial joints the pathomechanics of joint contracture. Biorheology 1980;17:17–95.

[39] Salter RB. The biologic concept of continuous passive motion of synovial joints: the first 18 years of basic research and its clinical application. Clin Orthop Relat Res 1989;242: 12–25.

[40] Frank C, Akeson WH, Woo SL, et al. Physiology and therapeutic value of passive joint motion. Clin Orthop Relat Res 1984;185:113–25.

[41] Moss R, Rum M, Sturgis E. Oral behavioral patterns in facial pain, headache, and non-headache populations. Behav Res Ther 1984;6:683–97.

[42] Dao TTT, Lund JP, Lavigne GJ. Comparison of pain and quality of life in bruxers and patients with myofascial pain of the masticatory muscles. J Orofac Pain 1994;8:350–6.

[43] Faulkner KDB. Bruxism: a review of the literature. Part I. Aust Dent J 1990;35:266–76.

[44] Faulkner KDB. Bruxism: a review of the literature. Part II. Aust Dent J 1990;35:355–61.

[45] Boero RP. The physiology of splint therapy: a literature review. Angle Orthod 1989;59(3): 165–80.

[46] Al-Ani MZ, Davies SJ, Gray RJM, et al. Stabilisation splint therapy for temporomandibular pain dysfunction syndrome. Cochrane Database Syst Rev 2004;(1):CD002778.

[47] Molina OF, Santos JD, Mazzetto M, et al. Oral jaw behavior in TMD and bruxism: a comparison study by severity of bruxism. J Craniomandib Pract 2001;19:114–22.

[48] Clark GT. Examining temporomandibular disorder patients for craniocervical dysfunction. J Craniomandib Pract 1984;2:56–63.

[49] Clark GT, Green EM, Doman MR, et al. Craniocervical dysfunction levels in a patient sample from a temporomandibular joint clinic. J Am Dent Assoc 1987;115:251–6.

[50] Kirveskari P, Alanen P, Karskela V, et al. Association of functional state of stomatognathic system with mobility of cervical spine and neck muscle tenderness. Acta Odont Scand 1988; 46:281–6.

[51] Isaccsson G, Linde C, Isberg A. Subjective symptoms in patients with temporomandibular joint disc displacement versus patients with myogenic craniomandibular disorders. J Prosthet Dent 1989;61:70–1.

[52] Cacchiotti DA, Plesh O, Bianchi P, et al. Signs and symptoms in samples with and without temporomandibular disorders. J Craniomandib Disord 1991;5:167–72.

[53] Braun BL, DiGiovanna A, Schiffman E, et al. A cross-sectional study of temporomandibular joint dysfunction in post-cervical trauma patients. J Craniomandib Disord 1992;6:24–31.

[54] De Laat A, Meuleman H, Stevens A. Relation between functional limitations of the cervical spine and temporomandibular disorders [abstract]. J Orofac Pain 1993;1:109–10.

[55] Padamsee M, Mehta N, Forgione A, et al. Incidence of cervical disorders in a TMD population [abstract]. J Dent Res 1994;186.

[56] Lobbezoo-Scholte AM, De Leeuw JRJ, Steenks MH, et al. Diagnostic subgroups of craniomandibular disorders. Part 1: self-report data and clinical findings. J Orofac Pain 1995;9: 24–36.

[57] de Wijer A, Steenks A, de Leeuw MH, et al. Symptoms of the cervial spine in temporomandibular and cervical spine disorders. J Oral Rehabil 1996;23(11):742–50.

[58] de Wijer A, de Leeuw JRJ, Steenks MH, et al. Temporomandibular and cervical spine disorders: self-reported signs and symptoms. Spine 1996;21:1638–46.

[59] De Laat A, Meuleman H, Stevens A, et al. Correlation between cervical spine and temporomandibular disorders. Clin Oral Investig 1998;2:54–7.

[60] Ciancaglini R, Testa M, Radaelli G. Association of neck pain with symptoms of temporomandibular dysfunction in the general adult population. Scand J Rehab Med 1999;31: 17–22.

[61] Visscher CM, Lobbezzo F, de Boer W, et al. Clinical tests in distinguishing between persons with or without craniomandibular or cervical spinal pain complaints. Eur J Oral Sci 2000; 108:475–83.

[62] Turp JC, Kowalski CJ, O'Leary N, et al. Pain maps from facial pain patients indicate a broad pain geography. J Dent Res 1998;77(6):1465–72.

[63] Hagberg C, Hagberg M, Koop S. Musculoskeletal symptoms and psychological factors among patients with craniomandibular disorders. Acta Odontol Scand 1994; 52:170–7.

[64] Sipila K, Ylostalo P, Joukamaa M, et al. Comorbidity between facial pain, widespread pain, and depressive symptoms in young adults. J Orofac Pain 2006;20:24–30.

[65] Olivo SA, Bravo J, Magee DJ, et al. The association between head and cervical posture and temporomandibular disorders: a systematic review. J Orofac Pain 2006;20(1): 9–23.

[66] Molina OF, dos Santos J, Nelson SJ, et al. Prevalence of modalities of headache and bruxism among patients with craniomandibular disorders. J Craniomandib Pract 1997;15: 314–25.

[67] Trenouth MJ. The relationship between bruxism and temporomandibular joint dysfunction as shown by computer analysis of nocturnal tooth contact patterns. J Oral Rehabil 1979;6:81–7.

[68] Eriksson PO, Zafar H, Nordh E. Concomitant mandibular and head-neck movements during jaw opening-closing in man. J Oral Rehab 1998;25:859–70.

[69] Hu JW, Yu XM, Vernon H, et al. Excitatory effect on neck and jaw muscle activity of inflammatory irritant applied to cervical paraspinal muscles. Pain 1993;55:243–50.

[70] McCouch G, Deering I, Ling T. Location of receptors for tonic neck reflexes. J Neurophysiol 1951;14:191–6.

[71] Sumino R, Nozaki S, Katoh M. Trigemino-neck reflex. In: Kawamura Y, Dubner R, editors. Oral-facial sensory and motor functions. Tokyo: Quintessence Books Publishing Co Inc.; 1981. p. 81–8.

[72] Wyke BD. Neurology of the cervical spinal joints. Physiotherapy 1979;65:72–6.

[73] Funakoshi M, Amano N. Effects of the tonic neck reflex on the jaw muscles of the rat. J Dent Res 1973;52:668–73.

[74] Komiyama O, Arai M, Kawara M, et al. Pain patterns and mandibular dysfunction following experimental trapezius muscle pain. J Orofac Pain 2005;19:119–26.

[75] Svensson P, Arendt-Nielsen L. Muscle pain modulates mastication: an experimental study in humans. J Orofac Pain 1998;12:7–16.

[76] Komiyama O, Arai M, Kawara M, et al. [Effects of experimental pain induced in trapezius muscle on mouth opening]. J Jpn Soc TMJ 2003;15:173–7 [in Japanese].

[77] Sessle BJ, Hu JW, Amano M, et al. Convergence of cutaneous, tooth pulp, visceral, neck and muscle afferents onto nociceptive and nonnociceptive neurons in trigeminal subnucleus caudalis and its implications for referred pain. Pain 1986;27:219–35.

[78] Carlson CR, Okeson JP, Falace DA, et al. Reduction of pain and EMG activity in the masseter region by trapezius trigger point injection. Pain 1993;55:397–400.

[79] Clark GT, Browne PA, Nakano M, et al. Co-activation of sternocleidomastoid muscles during maximum clenching. J Dent Res 1993;72:1499–502.

[80] Ehrlich R, Garlick D, Ninio M. The effect of jaw clenching on the electromyographic activities of 2 neck and 2 trunk muscles. J Orofac Pain 1999;13:115–20.

[81] Eriksson PO, Haggman-Henrikson B, Nordh E, et al. Co-ordinated mandibular and head-neck movements during rhythmic jaw activities in man. J Dent Res 2000;79: 1378–84.

[82] Sherrington CS. The integrative action of the nervous system. 2nd edition. New Haven (CT): Yale Press; 1906.

[83] Kapandji IA. The physiology of the joint. The Trunk and Vertebral Column 1974;3: 170–251.

[84] Ralston HJ, Libet B. The question of tonus in skeletal muscle. Am J Phys Med 1953;32: 85–92.

[85] Smith AM. The coactiviation of antagonist muscles. Can J Physiol Pharmacol 1981;59: 733–47.

[86] Major PW, Nebbe B. Use and effectiveness of splint appliance therapy: review of literature. J Craniomandibular Pract 1997;15:159–66.

[87] Clark GT. A critical evaluation of orthopedic interocclusal appliance therapy: design, theory and overall effectiveness. J Am Dent Assoc 1984;108:359–64.

[88] Posselt U. Studies on the mobility of the human mandible. Acta Odontol Scan 1952;10: 1–50.

[89] Lawrence ES, Razook SJ. Nonsurgical management of mandibular disorders. In: Kraus SL, editor. Temporomandibular disorders. 2nd edition. New York: Churchill Livingstone Inc.; 1994. p. 125–60.

[90] Mohl N. Head posture and its role in occlusion. New York State Dent J 1976;42:17–23.

[91] McLean LF. Gravitational influences on the afferent and efferent components of mandibular reflexes [doctoral dissertation]. Philadelphia: Thomas Jefferson University of Philadelphia; 1973.

[92] Lund P, Nishiyama T, Moller E. Postural activity in the muscles of mastication with the subject upright, inclined, and supine. Scand J Dent Res 1970;78:417–24.

[93] Eberle WR. A study of centric relation as recorded in a supine position. J Am Dent Assoc 1951;42:15–26.

[94] Mclean LF, Brenman HS, Friedman MGF. Effects of changing body position on dental occlusion. J Dent Res 1973;52:1041–5.

[95] Goldstein DF, Kraus SL, Williams WB, et al. Influence of cervical posture on mandibular movement. J Prosthet Dent 1984;52:421–6.

[96] Darling DW, Kraus SL, Glasheen-Wray MB. Relationship of head posture and the rest position of the mandible. J Prosthet Dent 1984;52:111–5.

[97] Root GR, Kraus SL, Razook SJ, et al. Effect of an intraoral appliance on head and neck posture. J Prosthet Dent 1987;58:90–5.

[98] Mohl ND. The role of head posture in mandibular function. In: Solberg WK, Clark GT, editors. Abnormal jaw mechanics diagnosis and treatment. Chicago (IL): Quintessence Publishing; 1984. p. 97–111.

[99] Mausner JS, Kramer S. Screening in the detection of disease. In: Mausner, Baum, editors. Epidemiology: an introductory text. Philadelphia: WB Saunders Co.; 1985. p. 214–37.

[100] Ness TJ, Gebhart GF. Visceral pain: a review of experimental studies. Pain 1990;41: 167–234.

[101] Jarvik J, Deyo R. Diagnostic evaluation of low back pain with emphasis on imaging. Ann Intern Med 2002;137:586–97.

[102] Spitzer WO, LeBlanc FE, Dupuis M, et al. Scientific approach to the assessment and management of activity- related spinal disorders. A monograph for Clinicians Report of the Quebec Task Force on Spinal Disorders. Spine 1987;12:S4–59.

[103] Cote P, Cassidy JD, Carroll L. The Saskatchewan Health and Back Pain Survey: the prevalence of neck pain and related disability in Saskatchewan adults. Spine 1998;23: 1689–98.

[104] Andersson HI, Ejlertsson G, Leden I, et al. Chronic pain in a geographically defined general population: studies of differences in age, gender, social class, and pain localization. Clin J Pain 1993;9:174–82.

[105] Bovim G, Schrader H, Sand T. Neck pain in the general population. Spine 1994;19:1307–9.

[106] International Headache Society Classification Committee. Classification and diagnostic criteria for headache disorders, cranial neuralgias and facial pain. Cephalagia 1998;8(Suppl 7):9–96.

[107] Bogduk N. The neck and headaches. Neurol Clin 2004;22:151–71.

[108] Kerr FWL. Structural relation of the trigeminal spinal tract to upper cervical roots and the solitary nucleus in cat. Exp Neurol 1961;4:134–48.

[109] Bogduk N. The anatomical basis for cervicogenic headache. J Manipulative Physiol Ther 1992;15:67–70.

[110] Bogduk N. Anatomy and physiology of headache. Biomed Pharmacother 1995;49:435–45.

[111] Bogduk N. Cervical causes of headache and dizziness. In: Grieve G, editor. Modern manual therapy. Edinburgh (UK): Churchill Livingstone. 2nd edition. 1994. p. 317–31.

[112] Michler RP, Bovim G, Sjaastad O. Disorders in the lower cervical spine. A cause of unilateral headache? A case report. Headache 1991;31:550–1.

[113] Bogduk N. The clinical anatomy of the cervical dorsal rami. Spine 1982;7(4):319–29.

[114] Bogduk N. The anatomy of occipital neuralgia. Clin Exp Neural 1980;17:167–84.

[115] Hildebrandt J, Jansen J. Vascular compression of the C2 and C3 roots—yet another cause of chronic intermittent hemicrania? Cephalalgia 1984;4:168–70.

[116] Rosenberg W, Swearingen B, Poletti C. Contralateral trigeminal dysaesthesias associated with second cervical nerve compression: a case report. Cephalalgia 1990;10:259–62.

[117] Sjaastad O, Saunte C, Hovdahl H, et al. "Cervicogenic" headache. An hypothesis. Cephalalgia 1983;3:249–56.

[118] Biondi DM. Cervicogenic headache: a review of diagnostic and treatment strategies. J Am Osteopath Assoc 2005;105(4):16S–22S.

[119] Nilson AN. The prevalence of cervicogenic headache in a random population sample of 20–59 year olds. Spine 1995;20:1884–8.

[120] Pfaffenrath V, Kuabe H. Diagnostics of cervical spine headache. Funct Neurol 1990;5: 157–64.

[121] Balla J, Lansek R. Headache arising from disorders of the cervical spine. In: Hopkins A, editor. Headache: problems in diagnosis and management. London: Saunders; 1988. p. 241–67.

[122] Vernon H, Steiman I, Hagino C. Cervicogenic dysfunction in muscle contraction headache and migraine: a descriptive study. J Manipulative Physiol Ther 1992;15:418–29.

[123] Yi X, Cook AJ, Hamill-Ruth RJ, et al. Cervicogenic headache in patients with presumed migraine: missed diagnosis or misdiagnosis? J Pain 2005;6(10):700–3.

[124] Blau JN, MacGregor EA. Migraine and the neck. Headache 1994;34:88–90.

[125] Bartch T, Goadsby PJ. The trigeminocervical complex migraine: current concepts and synthesis. Curr Pain Headache Rep 2003;7:371–6.
[126] DeNarinis M, Accornero N. Recurrent neck pain as a variant of migraine: description of four cases. J Neurol Neurosurg Psychiatry 1997;62:669–70.
[127] Marcus D, Scharff L, Mercer MA, et al. Musculoskeletal abnormalities in chronic headache; a controlled comparison of headache diagnostic groups. Headache 1999;39:21–7.
[128] Shevel E, Spierings E. Cervical muscles in the pathogenesis of migraine headache. J Headache Pain 2004;5(1):12–4.
[129] Lance J. Mechanism and management of headache. 5th edition. Oxford (UK): Butterworth-Heinemann; 1993.
[130] Brown J. A systemic approach to the dizzy patient. Neurol Clin 1990;8:209–24.
[131] Fisher CM. Vertigo in cerebrovascular disease. Arch Otolaryngol 1967;85:529–34.
[132] Hoffman RM, Einstadter D, Kroenke K. Evaluating dizziness. Am J Med 1999;107:468–78.
[133] Reker V. Cervical nystagmus caused by proprioceptors of the neck. Laryngolica Rhinol Otol Stuttgart 1983;62:312–4.
[134] Cohen L. Role of eye and neck proprioceptive mechanisms in body orientation and motor coordination. J Neurophysiol 1961;24:1–11.
[135] Abrahams VC. The physiology of neck muscles; their role in head movement and maintenance of posture. Can J Physiol Pharmacol 1977;55(3):332–8.
[136] Manzoni D, Pompeiano O, Stampacchia G. Tonic cervical influences on posture and reflex movements. Arch Ital Biol 1979;117(2):81–110.
[137] Cope S, Ryan GMS. Cervical and otolith vertigo. J Laryngol Otol 1959;73:113–20.
[138] Gray LP. Extra labyrinthine vertigo due to cervical muscle lesions. J Laryngol Otol 1956;70(6):352–61.
[139] Weeks VD, Travell J. Postural vertigo due to trigger areas in the sternocleidomastoid muscle. J Pediatr 1955;47(3):315–27.
[140] De Jong PTVM, De Jong JMBV, Cohen B, et al. Ataxia and nystagmus induced by injection of local anesthetics in the neck. Ann Neurol 1977;1:240–6.
[141] Hinoki M. Vertigo due to whiplash injury: a neurotological approach. Acto Otolaryngol (Stockh) Suppl 1985;419:9–29.
[142] Norre ME. Neurophysiology of vertigo with special reference to cervical vertigo. A review. Acta Belg Med Phys 1986;9:183–94.
[143] Phillipszoon A. Neck torsion nystagmus. Pract Otorhinolaryngol (Basel) 1963;25:339–44.
[144] Rubinstein B. Tinnitus and craniomandibular disorders: is there a link? Swed Dent J Suppl 1993;95:1–46.
[145] Young ED, Nelken I, Conley RA. Somatosensory effects on neurons in dorsal cochlear nucleus. J Neurophysiol 1995;73:743–65.
[146] Levine RA. Somatic (craniocervical) tinnitus and the dorsal cochlear nucleus hypothesis. Am J Otolaryngol 1999;20:351–62.
[147] Abel MD, Levine RA. Muscle contractions and auditory perception in tinnitus patients and nonclinical patients. J Craniomandibular Pract 2004;22(3):181–91.
[148] Paparella MM, Jung TTK. Odontalgia. In: Paparella MM, Shumrik DA, Gluckman JL, editors. Otolaryngology. Philadelphia: Saunders; 1991. p. 1237–42.
[149] Kuttila S, Kuttila M, Le Bell Y, et al. Characteristics of subjects with secondary otalgia. J Orofac Pain 2004;18(3):226–34.
[150] Kuttila S, Kuttila M, Le Bell Y, et al. Aural symptoms and signs of temporomandibular disorder in association with treatment need and visits to a physician. Laryngoscope 1999;109:1669–73.
[151] Olsen J, editor. Classification and diagnostic criteria for headache disorders, cranial neuralgias and facial pain. 1st ed. Copenhagen (Denmark): The International Headache Society; 1990.
[152] Spitzer WO, Skovron ML, Salmi LR, et al. Scientific monograph of the Quebec Task Force on Whiplash-Associated Disorders: redefining "whiplash" and its management. Spine 1995;20(8 Suppl):1S–73S.

[153] Jordan A, Manniche C, Mosdal C. The Copenhagen Neck Functional Disability Scale: a study of reliability and validity. J Manipulative Physiol Ther 1998;21(8):520–7.

[154] Feise RJ, Micheal MJ. Functional Rating Index: a new valid and reliable instrument to measure the magnitude of clinical change in spinal conditions. Spine 2001;26(1):78–87.

[155] Manchikanti LS, Peter SS, Vijay S, et al. Evidence-based practice guidelines for interventional techniques in the management of chronic spinal pain. Pain Phys 2003;6:3–81.

[156] Abenhaim L, Rossignol M, Valat J-P, et al. International Paris Task Force on Back Pain. Spine 2000;25(4 Suppl):1S–31S.

[157] Persson LCG, Carlsson C-A, Carlsson JY. Long-lasting cervical radicular pain managed with surgery, physiotherapy, or a cervical collar. Spine 1997;22:751–8.

[158] Bednarik J, et al. The value of somatosensory- and motor-evoked potentials in predicting and monitoring the effect of therapy in spondylotic cervical myelopathy. Prospective randomized study. Spine 1999;24(15):1593–8.

[159] Kadanka Z. Approaches to spondylotic cervical myelopathy: conservative versus surgical results in a 3-year follow-up study. Spine 2002;27(20):2205–10.

[160] Raphael KG, Klausner JJ, Nayak S, et al. Complementary and alternative therapy use by patients with myofascial temporomandibular disorders. J Orofac Pain 2003;17:36–41.

[161] Gross AR, Hoving JL, Haines TA, et al. Cervical overview group manipulation and mobilisation for mechanical neck disorders. Cochrane Database Syst Rev 2004;(1):CD004249.

[162] Aker PD, Gross AR, Goldsmith CH, et al. Conservative management of mechanical neck pain: systematic overview and meta-analysis. Br Med J 1996;313(7068):1291–6.

[163] Hurwitz EL, Aker PD, Adams AH, et al. Manipulation and mobilization of the cervical spine: a systematic review of literature. Spine 1996;21:1746–60.

[164] Jordan A, Bendix T, Nielsen H, et al. Intensive training, physiotherapy, or manipulation for patients with chronic neck pain: a prospective single-blinded randomized clinical trial. Spine 1998;23:311–9.

[165] Nelson BW, Carpenter DM, Dreisinger TE, et al. Can spinal surgery be prevented by aggressive strengthening exercises? A prospective study of cervical and lumbar patients. Arch Phys Med Rehabil 1999;80:20–5.

[166] Rodriquez AA, Bilkey WJ, Agre JC. Therapeutic exercise in chronic neck and back pain. Arch Phys Med Rehabil 1992;73:870–5.

[167] Swezey RL, Swezey AM, Warner K. Efficacy of home cervical traction therapy. Am J Phys Med Rehabil 1999;78(1):30–2.

[168] Jull GA, Trott P, Potter H, et al. A randomized, controlled trial of exercise and manipulative therapy for cervicogenic headache. Spine 2002;27(17):1835–43.

[169] Farrell JP, Jensen GM. Manual therapy: a critical assessment of role in the profession of physical therapy. Phys Ther 1992;12(2):11–20.

[170] Goldstein M. The research status of spinal manipulative therapy 1975. US Department Of Health, Education, and Welfare Publication No. (NIH) 76–998, NINCDS Monograph No. 15.

[171] Korr IM. The neurobiologic mechanisms in manipulative therapy. New York: Plenum Press; 1978.

[172] O'Leary S, Falla D, Jull G. Recent advances in therapeutic exercise for the neck: implications for patients with head and neck pain. Aust Endod J 2003;29(3):138–42.

[173] Kay TM, Gross A, Santaguida PL, et al. Cervical Overview Group. Exercises for mechanical neck disorders. Cochrane Database Syst Rev 2005;(3):CD004250.

[174] Al-Obaidi S, et al. The role of anticipation and fear of pain in the persistence of avoidance behavior in patients with chronic low back pain. Spine 2000;25(9):1126–31.

[175] Wrubel J, et al. Social competence from the perspective of stress and coping. In: Wine J, Smye M, editors. Social competence. New York: Guilford Press; 1981. p. 61–99.

[176] Pincus T. A systematic review of psychological factors as predictors of chronicity/disability in prospective cohorts of low back pain. Spine 2002;27(5):E109–20.

[177] Waddell G, Newton M, Henderson I, et al. A fear-avoidance beliefs questionnaire (FABQ), the role of fear-avoidance belief in chronic low back pain and disability. Pain 1993;52: 157–68.
[178] Wong A, et al. The traction angle and cervical intervertebral separation. Spine 1992;17(2): 136–8.
[179] Joghataei MT, Arab AM, Khaksar H. The effect of cervical traction combined with conventional therapy on grip strength on patients with cervical radiculopathy. Clin Rehabil 2004; 18(8):879–87.

THE DENTAL
CLINICS
OF NORTH AMERICA

Dent Clin N Am 51 (2007) 195–208

Temporomandibular Joint Surgery for Internal Derangement

M. Franklin Dolwick, DMD, PhD

*Division of Oral and Maxillofacial Surgery, University of Florida College of Dentistry,
PO Box 100416, Gainesville, FL 32610-0416, USA*

Surgery of the temporomandibular joint (TMJ) plays a small, but important, role in the management of patients who have temporomandibular disorders (TMDs). The literature has shown that about 5% of the patients who undergo treatment for TMDs require surgical intervention [1]. There is a spectrum of surgical procedures for the treatment of TMDs that ranges from simple arthrocentesis and lavage to more complex open joint surgical procedures. Although each surgical procedure has its enthusiastic supporters, the specific criteria for which cases are most appropriate are lacking. Unfortunately, the literature is based more on observation than on scientifically controlled studies. The success of surgery seems to be based on experience of the surgeon and appropriate case selection. It also is important to recognize that surgical treatment rarely is performed alone; generally, it is supported by nonsurgical treatment before and after surgery. In other words, surgical success is dependent on a total treatment plan that involves nonsurgical and surgical treatment. Surgery performed alone rarely has long-term success.

Each surgical procedure should have strict criteria for which cases are most appropriate. Recognizing that scientifically proven criteria are lacking, this article discusses the criteria for each procedure, ranging from arthrocentesis to complex open joint surgery. The discussion includes indications, brief descriptions of techniques, outcomes, and complications for each procedure.

Temporomandibular joint arthrocentesis

TMJ arthrocentesis is the simplest and least invasive procedure that is performed in the TMJ [2]. Technically, arthrocentesis is not a surgical

---

E-mail address: fdolwick@dental.ufl.edu

doi:10.1016/j.cden.2006.10.003
dental.theclinics.com

procedure; however, because it usually is discussed with surgical procedures, it is included in this article. Arthrocentesis consists of TMJ lavage, placement of medications into the joint, and examination under anesthesia. It usually is performed as an office-based procedure under local anesthesia assisted with conscious intravenous sedation, although it can be performed with local anesthesia alone (Fig. 1).

The technique involves the insertion of two 18-gauge needles into the superior joint space of the TMJ under local anesthesia. Through one needle, 100 to 300 mL of Ringer's lactate solution is injected into the superior joint space; the second needle acts as an outflow portal, which allows lavage of the joint cavity. Lysis of adhesions is achieved by intermittent distention of the joint space by momentarily blocking the outflow needle and injecting under pressure during the lavage. Steroids or sodium hyaluronate may be injected at the end of the lavage to alleviate intracapsular inflammation. Immediately upon completion of the lavage, the needles are removed and the TMJ is examined to determine freedom of movement. After recovery from the sedation, the patient is discharged. The patient is placed on a non-chew soft diet for a few days. Range of motion exercises are started immediately and continued for several days. Analgesics are prescribed as necessary for pain control.

Multiple studies have reported 70% to 90% success rates for arthrocentesis for the management of patients who have painful limited mouth opening [3–7]. Arthrocentesis does seem to reduce pain and improve opening in most patients. Although its primary indication is for painful limited mouth opening, it also may be useful for other conditions that involve

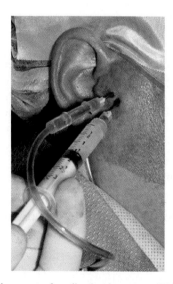

Fig. 1. Arthrocentesis: placement of medication into upper TM joint space after lavage.

inflammation in the joint. The benefit of injecting medications into the joint is unclear, and yet to be proven. There have been no significant complications reported with arthrocentesis. Patients may experience temporary swelling and soreness over the joint area and a slight posterior open bite malocclusion for 12 to 24 hours after the procedure.

Arthrocentesis has become popular and may be the most common procedure that is performed in the TMJ. The advantages of arthrocentesis are that it is a simple, cost-effective, minimally invasive procedure with little morbidity that can be performed in the office.

Indications for temporomandibular joint surgery

Indications for surgery of the TMJ may be divided into relative and absolute [8]. Absolute indications are reserved for those in which surgery has an undisputed role, such as tumors, growth anomalies, and ankylosis of the TMJ.

Because there are no objective criteria for performing TMJ surgery for the more common pain and dysfunction disorders, the decision to perform surgery should be made only after thorough evaluation of the patient. Patient selection seems to be the best determinant of surgical success. The general indications for TMJ surgery for the most common disorder—internal derangement and osteoarthrosis—are significant TMJ pain and dysfunction that are refractory to nonsurgical treatment and there is imaging evidence of disease.

Although the indications for surgery may seem to be clear, they are not specific. The first criterion, significant TMJ pain and dysfunction, may be the most important. What distinguishes the surgical candidate from patients who are not surgical candidates is localization of the pain and dysfunction to the TMJ. The more localized the pain and dysfunction to the TMJ, the better is the prognosis for a successful surgical outcome. Conversely, the more diffuse the pain and dysfunction, the less likely it is that surgical intervention will be successful. Surgical candidates should have localized continuous TMJ pain that is moderate to severe and becomes worse during jaw functions, such as chewing or talking. The pain usually is at its lowest intensity in the morning and worsens as the day progresses. Dysfunction may include painful clicking, crepitus, or locking of the TMJ. Usually, but not always, limited mouth opening is preceded by a period of painful clicking and intermittent locking.

The second criterion, refractory to nonsurgical treatment, also is nonspecific. Although nonsurgical treatment is not specified, most clinicians understand what it implies. Nonsurgical therapy should include some combination of patient education, medications, physical therapy, an occlusal appliance, and possibly, counseling. Most patients respond successfully to this treatment; therefore, surgical consideration is reserved only for patients who fail to respond successfully. The problem is that not all patients who fail nonsurgical treatment are surgical candidates. Surgical treatment is limited to those who have pain and dysfunction that arises from within the TMJ. Patients who have pain and dysfunction that arise from the masticatory muscles or other non-TMJ sources are not surgical candidates and they will be made worse by surgical intervention.

The third criterion, imaging evidence of disease, seems to be the most objective; however, imaging findings should not be interpreted in isolation. The correlation of imaging findings of disk derangement and osteoarthrosis with pain are poor [9,10]. Therefore, imaging evidence should be used to confirm and support the clinical findings. The decision for surgical intervention should be made based on the clinical findings in conjunction with the impact of the pain and dysfunction on the well-being of the patient and the prognosis if no treatment is provided.

Surgical interventions include arthroscopy, condylotomy, and open joint procedures, such as disk repositioning and diskectomy. Randomized clinical trials that compare these procedures do not exist, so the surgical procedure selected is based mostly on the surgeon's experience. Each procedure does have specific benefits as well as risks. Therefore, the procedure that has the highest potential for success with the lowest risks and most cost-effectiveness should be chosen for the patient's specific problem. Based on the author's experience, TMJ arthrocentesis and arthroscopy should be used for painful, limited opening; condylotomy should be used for TMJ pain with little or no restriction of opening; and open TMJ surgery should be reserved for advanced cases of TMJ internal derangement and osteoarthrosis.

Temporomandibular joint arthroscopy

TMJ arthroscopy is a minimally invasive procedure that generally is performed under general anesthesia in the operating room. It is an equipment-dependent procedure that requires considerable manual dexterity on the part of the surgeon. TMJ arthroscopy plays a major role in the surgical management of TMJ internal derangement and osteoarthrosis.

TMJ arthroscopy involves the placement of an arthroscopic telescope (1.8–2.6 mm in diameter) into the upper joint space (UJS) of the TMJ. A camera is attached to the arthroscope to project the image onto a television monitor. The surgeon must conceptualize a three-dimensional space on a two-dimensional image. A second access instrument is placed approximately 10 to 15 mm in front of the arthroscope. The purposes of this instrument are to provide an outflow portal for irrigation and access for instrumentation of the joint space. The UJS is examined systematically starting from the posterior aspect and continuing to the anterior aspect. The examination is started posteriorly by identifying the posterior attachment tissue. The synovial lining is inspected for the presence of inflammation, such as increased capillary hyperemia. The junction of the posterior band of the disk and posterior attachment tissues can be identified (Fig. 2). Movement of the joint allows for the identification of clicking or restriction in movement of the disk. As the arthroscope is moved through the UJS, the articular cartilage is inspected for the presence of degenerative changes (eg, softness, fibrillation, tears). The joint space also is inspected for the presence of adhesions, loose bodies, or other pathology. The integrity of the disk also is determined as the arthroscope is moved throughout the UJS. Perforations of the disk or posterior attachment tissues can be identified. Although the lower joint space (LJS) usually is not examined, the presence of a perforation in the disk or posterior attachment may allow limited examination of the LJS and condyle. Although sophisticated operative techniques, which range from ablation of adhesions with lasers to plication of the disk, have been developed, most surgeons limit the use of arthroscopy to lysis of adhesions and lavage of the UJS. Lysis of adhesions is accomplished most often by sweeping the arthroscope or the irrigation cannula through the adhesion and breaking it. After completion of the examination, the joint space is irrigated thoroughly to remove debris and small blood clots. Usually, the patient is discharged the same day after recovering from the anesthesia. The patient is placed on a nonchew soft diet for a few days. Range of motion exercises are started immediately and continued for several days. Analgesics are prescribed as necessary for pain control.

Multiple studies report an 80% to 90% success rate with arthroscopic lysis and lavage for the management of patients who have painful limited mouth opening [11–16]. Most patients have decreased pain and improved mouth opening. Murakami and colleagues [17,18] showed in studies with 5- and 10-year follow-up that arthroscopic lysis and lavage are successful for all stages of internal derangement, and that results are comparable to those obtained with open surgery procedures. Data from surgical

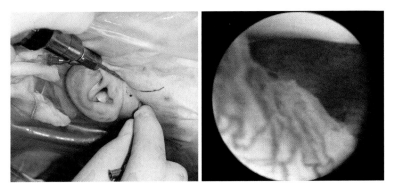

Fig. 2. Placement of arthroscope at the fossa point with view of inflamed posterior attachment and medial capsule.

arthroscopic techniques, such as disk repositioning, are difficult to interpret, and it is unclear that the outcomes are better than those obtained with simple lysis and lavage [19,20].

The advantages of TMJ arthroscopy are that it is minimally invasive and causes less surgical trauma to the joint. Surgical complications are rare and mostly are limited to reversible effects. Patient recovery is rapid and healing time is shorter than with open surgical procedures. The disadvantages include the surgical limitations and the necessity for sophisticated equipment.

Modified condylotomy

The modified TMJ condylotomy is the only TMJ surgical procedure that does not invade the joint structures. It is a modification of the transoral vertical ramus osteotomy that is used in orthognathic surgery. Although some investigators recommend modified condylotomy as the surgical treatment of choice for all stages of TMJ internal derangement, it seems to be most successful when used to treat painful TMJ internal derangement without reduced mouth opening [21]. The objective of the procedure is to surgically reposition the condyle anteriorly and inferiorly beneath the displaced disk effectively by increasing the joint space between the condyle and the fossa.

The modified condylotomy is performed under general anesthesia usually as an outpatient procedure; however, it may require an overnight stay in the hospital. An incision is made intraorally along the anterior border of the mandibular ramus. After exposure of the lateral aspect of the mandibular ramus, a vertical cut is made posteriorly to the lingula from the sigmoid notch to the mandibular angle. After mobilization of the condylar segment the medial pterygoid muscle is stripped from the segment. The mandible is immobilized using maxillomandibular fixation (MMF). Although the surgery is simple, there is a period of postoperative rehabilitation that involves 2 to 3 weeks of MMF followed by training elastics so that the occlusion is maintained (Fig. 3).

Hall and colleagues [21] reported a study on 400 patients over a 9-year period that found good pain relief in about 90% of the patients who were treated with modified condylotomies. In follow-up studies, Hall and colleagues [22] reported a 94% success rate in patients with disk displacement with reduction; 72% of these patients had a normal disk position when evaluated with follow-up MRIs. There was only a 4% complication rate, which consisted primarily of minor occlusal discrepancies. In a group of patients with disk displacement without reduction, the success rate for modified condylotomy was slightly less (88%) [23]. The most significant potential complication of the modified condylotomy is excessive condylar sag that results in malocclusion. Despite the simplicity of the procedure and its high success rate, it has not become widely used. The reasons for this are unclear,

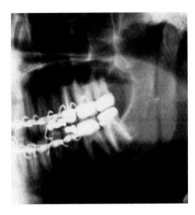

Fig. 3. Modified condylotomy with vertical ramus osteotomy from sigmoid notch to mandibular angle.

but most likely are related to the necessity for MMF and the fear of excessive condylar sag that results in an unstable condylar position with malocclusion.

Open joint surgery (arthrotomy)

Although the use of open joint surgery has decreased significantly, it still has a small, but important, role in the surgical management of TMJ internal derangement. Although other surgical procedures provide a limited range of options, open TMJ surgery provides the surgeon with an unlimited scope of procedures that range from simple debridement of the joint to the removal of the disk. Disk repositioning procedures are performed less commonly today compared with the 1980s and 1990s, because most patients who have disks that can be preserved are treated successfully with simpler procedures. Advanced cases of internal derangement that have degenerative disks and severe arthritic changes may require diskectomy. Arthroplasty in the form of bone contouring of the articular eminence or condyle is sometimes necessary, particularly with disk repositioning procedures.

Open joint surgery is indicated for patients who have TMJ internal derangement and osteoarthrosis that failed to respond to simpler surgical procedures or failed previous open surgery. In the cases of previous surgery, the surgeon must be hesitant to perform repeated surgery because the success rate for repeated surgery is low; in fact after two surgeries, it may approach zero. The surgeon must be certain that the source of the pain or dysfunction is within the joint. Severe mechanical interference, such as loud, hard clicking or intermittent locking associated with loud, hard clicking, is an indication to perform open surgery without performing simpler procedures; experience indicates that simpler procedures are rarely successful in these cases.

Open joint surgery is performed under general anesthesia in the hospital, and usually requires a 1- to 2-day stay. The most common surgical approach is by way of a preauricular incision made in front of the ear. An incision that incorporates the tragus of the ear is used often because it is more cosmetic. Exposure of the capsule is performed carefully to protect the temporal branches of the facial nerve. After exposure of the capsule, the UJS is entered. After entering the UJS it is inspected for the presence of adhesions. The contour and integrity of the fossa and eminence are evaluated, and lastly the disk is visualized. Evaluation of the disk includes its color, position, mobility, shape, and integrity.

Disk repositioning

If the disk is intact and can be repositioned without tension, disk repositioning can be performed by removing excess tissue from the posterior attachment tissues, repositioning the disk, and stabilizing it with sutures. Bone recontouring of the glenoid fossa or articular eminence generally is performed, especially in cases of gross mechanical interference or advanced degenerative joint disease. The goal of disk repositioning surgery is the elimination of mechanical interferences to smooth joint function. After completion of the intra-articular procedures, the UJS is irrigated and the soft tissues are closed.

Immediately after the surgery the patient may experience swelling in front of the ear and a slight change in occlusion and limited mouth opening that usually resolve in about 2 weeks. All patients experience some numbness in front of the ear that resolves in about 6 weeks. Patients normally have moderate discomfort that lasts 1 to 2 weeks. Exercises to improve range of motion are started immediately after the surgery. Continuation of postoperative conservative treatments is important to assure a successful outcome. A soft nonchew diet is recommended for 6 weeks after the surgery.

The literature indicates that disk repositioning surgery is successful in 80% to 95% of cases; however, experience indicates that this success rate may be overstated [24–30]. It has been found that although disk repositioning surgery significantly reduced pain and dysfunction in 51 subjects who were evaluated up to 6 years postoperatively, improvement in disk position was not maintained over the follow-up period for most patients [31]. Despite these findings, the preservation of a healthy, freely mobile disk is justified.

Facial nerve injury is the most significant complication that is associated with open surgery. Although total facial nerve paralysis is possible, it is rare. Inability to raise the eyebrow is the most commonly observed finding. This occurs in about 5% of cases and usually resolves within 3 months. It is permanent in less than 1% of cases. Other complications are limited opening and minor occlusal changes.

Diskectomy

A diseased or deformed disk that interferes with smooth function of the joint and cannot be repositioned should be removed. Only that portion of the disk that is diseased and deformed needs to be removed. The synovial tissues should be preserved as much as possible. Only minimal bone recontouring should be performed after removal of the disk, because exposure of bone marrow may result in heterotopic bone formation. To minimize the risk for heterotopic bone formation, the placement of an interpositional fat graft into the joint space is recommended. After completion of the intra-articular procedures, the joint space is irrigated and the soft tissues are closed (Fig. 4).

The postoperative findings are the same after diskectomy as described for disk repositioning. The postoperative recommendations also are the same, except that a soft, nonchew diet is recommended for 6 months.

Diskectomy of the TMJ has the longest follow-up studies of any procedure for management of TMJ internal derangement. Four studies with at least 30 years of follow-up report excellent reduction in pain and improvement in function in most patients [32–35]. Postoperative imaging studies of patients who underwent diskectomy generally show significant changes in condylar morphology [33]. These changes are believed to be adaptive changes, not degenerative changes. Despite the excellent long-term success that is associated with TMJ diskectomy, surgeons seem to be reluctant to perform this procedure.

The complications that are associated with diskectomy are similar to those that are associated with disk repositioning. The growth of heterotopic bone is more common after diskectomy than after other TMJ surgical procedures. This can be a significant complication that can result in complete ankylosis of the joint. The frequency of occurrence of heterotopic bone formation is unclear.

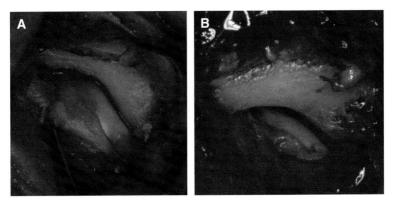

Fig. 4. (*A*) Exposed upper TMJ space showing lateral tubercle of articular eminence and displaced articular disc. (*B*) Exposed upper TMJ space showing recontoured articular eminence and a surgically repositioned articular disc.

Temporomandibular joint replacement

A complete discussion of total TMJ replacement is beyond the scope of this article. Therefore, the discussion is limited to alloplastic total joint replacement in adult patients who have advanced degenerative joint disease, ankylosis, or complications of previously preformed open surgery. The use of alloplastic materials to reconstruct or replace the diseased tissues of the TMJ caused disastrous results in the 1980s and 1990s. The use of Proplast-Teflon and silastic implants caused significant foreign body reactions with severe destruction of the TMJ structures [36–39]. This experience has led some surgeons to reject the use of alloplastic TMJ prostheses in favor of autologous tissues, such as costochondral grafts for TMJ reconstruction [40]. Although there are advantages to using autologous tissues, recently developed alloplastic TMJ prostheses provide safe and predictably successful reconstruction of the TMJ (Fig. 5) [41,42].

The use of TMJ Concepts (TMJ Concepts, Ventura, California) Patient-Fitted Prosthesis and the W. Lorenz TMJ implant (Walter Lorenz Surgical Inc., Jacksonville, Florida) Stock Prosthesis are discussed. The TMJ Concepts Patient-Fitted Prosthesis is a custom-made implant that has been used for more than 10 years [41]. The prosthesis consists of a glenoid fossa implant that has an articular surface made of high molecular weight polyethylene that is attached to a pure titanium mesh. The body of the condylar prosthesis is made of medical-grade titanium alloy with a cobalt chromium molybdenum condylar head. The process for making the prosthesis requires that a head CT be obtained, from which an acrylic model of the patient's skull is made. The planned surgery is performed on the model. The prosthesis is designed on the model and is sent to the surgeon for approval. After approval, the patient's prosthesis is made using computer aided design/computer aided manufacturing (CAD CAM) technology.

The Lorenz TMJ Prosthesis is a stock prosthesis. The prosthesis consists of a glenoid fossa implant that is made of high molecular weight

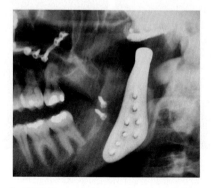

Fig. 5. TMJ Concepts patient-fitted TMJ prosthesis.

polyethylene and a condylar component that is made of cobalt chromium molybdenum alloy. There are three sizes of implants. The fossa implants come in small, medium, and large. The articular surface is the same on all three implants; only the flange varies in size. The condyles come in three lengths: 45 mm, 50 mm, and 55 mm.

The surgical placement is essentially the same for both implants. The surgery requires preauricular and retromandibular incisions for access to the TMJ and mandibular ramus. A gap arthroplasty is performed by removing the diseased condyle or ankylosed bone. Generally, a coronoidectomy also is performed. After the teeth are placed into MMF, the implants are fitted in the patient and secured using titanium screws. The Lorenz implants are more difficult to place than are the patient-fitted implants, because the bony structures must be reshaped to fit the implants. The MMF is released, the occlusion is verified, and the range of motion is determined. If these are acceptable, the wounds are irrigated, a fat graft is placed around the condyle, and the soft tissues are closed.

The surgical outcomes for both prostheses have been excellent. The criteria that are used to determine success in complex patients who have chronic TMJ pain are relative, and, as such, precise success rates are difficult to determine. Successful outcome generally means that the patient has reduced pain levels, increased range of motion, improved function, and an absence of surgical complications. Using these criteria, the success rates are high for both prostheses. Patients who have had multiple TMJ surgical procedures and who suffer from chronic pain generally experience about a 50% pain reduction and gain 10 to 15 mm of mandibular opening. It should be emphasized that total TMJ replacement is not necessarily a solution to the management of chronic pain. The TMJ prosthesis can be used to predictably restore occlusion and increase range of motion, but pain relief is variable. Conversely, both TMJ prostheses predictably provide pain-free restoration of occlusion and range of motion for patients who have TMJ reconstruction for ankylosis, tumors, or other conditions in which pain is not a component.

The most significant complication following TMJ reconstruction with alloplastic implants is facial nerve injury. Although uncommon, it does occur more frequently than following routine open joint surgical procedures, especially in patients who have had multiple TMJ surgeries. The formation of heterotopic bone is a common complication that occurs in as many as 20% of cases. Other complications, such as infection, foreign body and allergic reactions, malocclusion, and implant failure, can occur but are rare. Complications that require implant removal are unusual.

Unquestionably, TMJ Concepts Patient-Fitted Prosthesis provides the best TMJ reconstruction. The surgery is easier to perform and the implants fit more accurately than do the Lorenz stock prostheses; however, there is a need for both types of implants. Patient-fitted implants require 1 to 3 months to manufacture, so immediate TMJ reconstruction is not possible.

They also are more expensive than are stock prostheses. There also are several situations in which two surgeries are necessary to use patient-fitted prosthesis. These are (1) patients who have large malocclusions that require significant reposition of the mandible to correct; (2) patients who have extensive bony ankylosis that requires large amounts of bone removal; (3) combinations of 2 and 3; and (4) patients who have foreign bodies, such as a previously placed alloplastic TMJ prosthesis, that must be removed before an accurate CT can be obtained. When two surgeries are required it can be problematic to maintain the occlusion and function after the first surgery during the time that the prosthesis is being made. Additionally, two surgeries are inconvenient for the patient; they cause longer healing times, expose the patient to greater risks for complications, and are more expensive. Stock joints can provide adequate reconstruction with a single operation in these situations. Conversely, there are situations in which a stock prosthesis cannot be used. These occur in patients who have extensive bone loss at the lateral aspect of the fossa and articular eminence or the mandibular ramus that result in inadequate bone for placement of a stock prosthesis. There is great flexibility in the design of patient-fitted prostheses, which allows them to be adapted to a variety of complex clinical situations.

In conclusion, patient-fitted and stock TMJ prostheses are available that provide safe and predictably successful reconstruction of the TMJ in adult patients. Both types of prostheses are necessary to meet the needs of the variety of TMJ conditions that require TMJ replacement.

Summary

TMJ surgery has a small, but important, role in the treatment of patients who have TMJ pain and dysfunction conditions. Patient selection is the most important consideration in determining a successful outcome. The most important diagnostic finding is that the pain and dysfunction arises from within the TMJ. The more localized the pain and dysfunction is to the joint, the better is the prognosis for surgical intervention. Conversely, the more diffuse the signs and symptoms, the less successful is the surgery. When surgery is unsuccessful, it usually is because of a failure to recognize and manage factors, such as parafunction.

Several surgical procedures have been shown to be successful. The simplest procedure that has the best prognosis with the least morbidity should be selected for each patient's specific problem. Unfortunately, there have not been any randomized controlled studies on surgery; therefore, the decision to operate and the choice of procedure are based on clinical experience.

Several alloplastic total joint prostheses are approved by the US Food and Drug Administration and have been shown to be safe and successful. These devices have greatly improved the management of complicated cases that involve TMJ degeneration, ankylosis, and tumors.

References

[1] McNeill C. Temporomandibular disorders: guidelines for classification, assessment and management. 2nd edition. Chicago: Quintessence Books; 1993.

[2] Nitzan DW, Dolwick MF, Martinez A. Temporomandibular joint arthrocentesis: a simplified treatment for severe, limited mouth opening. J Oral Maxillofac Surg 1991;49: 11163–7.

[3] Dimitroulis G, Dolwick MF, Martinez A. Temporomandibular joint arthrocentesis and lavage for the treatment of closed lock: a follow-up study. Br J Oral Maxillofac Surg 1995;33: 23–6.

[4] Hosaka H, Murakami K, Goto K, et al. Outcome of arthrocentesis for temporomandibular joint with closed lock at 3 years follow-up. Oral Surg Oral Med Oral Pathol Oral Radiol Endod 1996;82:501–4.

[5] Nitzan DW, Samson B, Beher H. Long-term outcome of arthrocentesis for sudden-onset, persistent, severe closed lock of the temporomandibular joint. J Oral Maxillofac Surg 1997;55:151–7.

[6] Alpaslan GH, Alpaslan C. Efficacy of temporomandibular joint arthrocentesis with and without injection of sodium hyaluronate in treatment of internal derangement. J Oral Maxillofac Surg 2001;59:613–8.

[7] Alpaslan C, Dolwick MF, Heft NW. Five-year retrospective evaluation of temporomandibular joint arthrocentesis. Int J Oral Maxillofac Surg 2003;32:263–7.

[8] Dimitroulis G. The role of surgery in the management of the temporomandibular joint: a critical review of the literature Part 2. Int J Oral Maxillofac Surg 2005;34:231–7.

[9] Kircos LT, Ortendahahl DA, Mark AS, et al. Magnetic resonance imaging of the TMJ disc in asymptomatic volunteers. J Oral Maxillofac Surg 1987;45:397–401.

[10] Kozeniauskas JJ, Ralph WJ. Bilateral arthrographic evaluation of unilateral temporomandibular joint pain and dysfunction. J Prosth Dent 1988;60:98–105.

[11] McCain J. Arthroscopy of the human temporomandibular joint. J Oral Maxillofac Surg 1988;46:648–55.

[12] Moses JJ, Poker I. TMJ arthroscopic surgery: an analysis of 237 patients. J Oral Maxillofac Surg 1989;47:790–4.

[13] Holmlund A, Gynther G, Axelsson S. Efficiency of arthroscopic lysis and lavage in patients with chronic locking of the temporomandibular joint. Int J Oral Maxillofac Surg 1994;23: 262–5.

[14] Kurita K, Goss AN, Ogi N. Correlation between pre-operative mouth-opening and surgical outcome after arthroscopic lavage in patients with disk displacement without reduction. J Oral Maxillofac Surg 1998;56:1394–7.

[15] Sorel B, Piecuch JF. Long-term evaluation following temporomandibular joint artgroscopy with lysis and lavage. Int J Oral Maxillofac Surg 2000;29:259–63.

[16] Dimitroulis G. A review of 56 cases of chronic closed lock treated with temporomandibular joint arthroscopy. J Oral Maxillofac Surg 2002;60:519–24.

[17] Murakami KI, Tsuboi Y, Bessho K, et al. Outcome of arthroscopic surgery to the temporomandibular joint correlates with stage of internal derangement: five-year follow-up study. Br J Oral Maxillofac Surg 1998;36:30–4.

[18] Murakami KI, Segami N, Okamoto M, et al. Outcome of arthroscopic surgery for internal derangement of the temporomandibular joint: long term results covering 10 years. J Craniomaxillofac Surg 2000;5:264–71.

[19] McCain JP, De La Rua H. Principles and practice of operative arthroscopy of the human temporomandibular joint. Oral Maxillofac Clin North Am 1989;1:135–52.

[20] McCain JP, Podrasky AE, Zabiegalski NA. Arthroscopic disc repositioning and suturing: a preliminary report. J Oral Maxillofac Surg 1992;50:568–73.

[21] Hall HD, Nickerson JW, McKenna SL. Modified condylotomy for treatment of the painful joint with reducing disc. J Oral Maxillofac Surg 1993;51:133–42.

[22] Hall HD, Navarro EZ, Gibbs SL. One and three-year prospective outcome study of modified condylotomy for treatment of reducing disc displacement. J Oral Maxillofac Surg 2000;58(1):7–17.

[23] Hall HD, Navarro EZ, Gibbs SL. Prospective study of modified condylotomy for treatment of non-reducing disc displacement. Oral Surg 2000;89:147.

[24] McCarthy WL, Farrar WB. Surgery for internal derangement of the temporomandibular joint. J Prosth Dent 1979;42:191–6.

[25] Marciani RD, Zeigler RC. Temporomandibular joint surgery: a review of 51 operations. Oral Surg Oral Med Oral Pathol 1983;56:472–6.

[26] Hall MB. Meniscoplasty of the displaced temporomandibular meniscus without violating the inferior joint space. J Oral Maxillofac Surg 1984;42:788–92.

[27] Dolwick MF, Sanders B. TMJ internal derangement and arthrosis—surgical atlas. St. Louis (MO): CV Mosby Co.; 1985.

[28] Piper MA. Microscopic disc preservation surgery of the temporomandibular joint. Oral Maxillofac Clin North Am 1989;1:279–302.

[29] Dolwick MF, Nitzan DW. [TMJ disc surgery: 8-year follow-up evaluation]. Fortschr Kiefer Gesichtschir 1990;35:162–7 [in German].

[30] Dolwick MF, Nitzan DW. The role of disc repositioning surgery for internal derangement of the temporomandibular joint. Oral Maxillofac Clin North Am 1994;6:271–5.

[31] Montgomery MT, Gordon SM, VanSickels JE, et al. Changes in signs and symptoms following temporomandibular joint disc repositioning surgery. J Oral Maxillofac Surg 1992;50:320.

[32] Silver CML. Long-term results of meniscectomy of the temporomandibular joint. J Craniomandib Pract 1984;3:46–9.

[33] Eriksson L, Westesson P-L. Long–term evaluation of meniscectomy of the temporomandibular joint. J Oral Maxillofac Surg 1985;43:263–6.

[34] Tolvanem M, Oikarinen VJ, Wolf J. A 30 year follow-up study of temporomandibular joint menisctomies: a report of 5 patients. Br J Oral Maxillofac Surg 1988;26:311–3.

[35] Takaku S, Toyoda T. Long-term evaluation of diskectomy of the temporomandibular joint. J Oral Maxillofac Surg 1994;52:722–6.

[36] Dolwick MF, Aufdemorte TB. Silicone induced foreign body reaction and lymphadenopathy after temporomandibular joint arthroplasty. Oral Surg Oral Med Oral Pathol 1985;59: 449–52.

[37] Heffez L, Mafee MF, Rosenberg H, et al. CT evaluation of temporomandibular disc replacement with a Teflon laminate. J Oral Maxillofac Surg 1987;45:657–60.

[38] Westesson P-L, Ericksson L, Lindstrom C. Destructive lesions of the mandibular condyle following discectomy with temporary silastic implants. Oral Surg Oral Med Oral Pathol 1987;63:143–50.

[39] Kaplan PA, Tu HK, Williams SM. Erosive arthritis of the temporomandibular joint caused by teflon-proplast implants: plain film features. AJR Am J Roentgenol 1988;151:337–40.

[40] MacIntosh RB. The use of autogenous tissues for temporomandibular joint reconstruction. J Oral Maxillofac Surg 2000;58:63–9.

[41] Mercuri LG. The use of alloplastic prostheses for temporomandibular joint reconstruction. J Oral Maxillofac Surg 2000;58:70–5.

[42] Quinn PD. Alloplastic reconstruction of the temporomandibular joint. J Oral Maxillofac Surg 2000;7:1.

Dent Clin N Am 51 (2007) 209–224

THE DENTAL
CLINICS
OF NORTH AMERICA

Neuropathic Orofacial Pain: Proposed Mechanisms, Diagnosis, and Treatment Considerations

Christopher J. Spencer, DDS,
Henry A. Gremillion, DDS*

*Department of Orthodontics, Parker E. Mahan Facial Pain Center, University of Florida
College of Dentistry, P.O. Box 100437, Gainesville, FL 32610-0437, USA*

Today's health care professional is faced with the stark reality that the most common reason patients seek medical or dental care in the United States is due to pain or dysfunction. Recent studies reveal that the head and neck region is the most common site of the human body to be involved in a chronic pain condition [1]. The orofacial region is plagued by a number of acute, chronic, and recurrent painful maladies. A population-based survey of 45,711 households revealed that 22% of the United States population experienced orofacial pain on more than one occasion in a 6-month period [2]. Pain involving the teeth and the periodontium is the most common presenting concern in dental practice. Non-odontogenic pain conditions also occur frequently. Recent scientific investigation has provided an explosion of knowledge regarding pain mechanisms and pathways and an enhanced understanding of the complexities of the many ramifications of the total pain experience. Therefore, it is mandatory for the dental professional to develop the necessary clinical and scientific expertise on which he/she may base diagnostic and management approaches. Optimum management can be achieved only by determining an accurate and complete diagnosis and identifying all of the factors associated with the underlying pathosis on a case-specific basis. A thorough understanding of the epidemiologic and etiologic aspects of dental, musculoskeletal, neurovascular, and neuropathic orofacial pain conditions is essential to the practice of evidence-based dentistry/medicine.

* Corresponding author.
E-mail address: hgremillion@dental.ufl.edu (H.A. Gremillion).

0011-8532/07/$ - see front matter © 2007 Elsevier Inc. All rights reserved.
doi:10.1016/j.cden.2006.09.006

Pain has been characterized as nociceptive, neuropathic, and mixed. Nociceptive pain is defined as pain transmitted by normal physiologic pathways via peripheral nerves to the central nervous system in response to potentially tissue-damaging stimuli [3]. Examples include frank dental pain, myofascial pain, and degenerative joint disease. It is typically described as diffuse aching, stiffness, or tenderness. Neuropathic pain refers to pain initiated or caused by a primary lesion or dysfunction in the nervous system [3]. Conditions representative of neuropathic pain are postherpetic neuralgia, trigeminal neuralgia, trauma-induced neuropathy, atypical odontalgia /non-odontogenic toothache, idiopathic oral burning, and complex regional pain syndrome. Neuropathic pain conditions are frequently associated with qualities with which the patient is not familiar. This may make it difficult for the patient to communicate their pain experience. Typical descriptors used by patients include stabbing, burning, electric-like, or sharp, with numbness or tingling projected to a cutaneous area [4,5]. Aching pain does not preclude the possibility of a neuropathic basis for the patient's pain [6]. Mixed pain is caused by a combination of primary injury or secondary effects. It is described by a myriad of terms that may be diagnostically confusing to the practitioner. Each of these types of pain is associated with variable mechanisms that must be targeted to optimize treatment outcomes.

Neuropathic orofacial pain

Neuropathic orofacial pain is relatively common. It is diagnosed in approximately 25 to 30% of patients presenting in a tertiary care University-based Facial Pain Center (H.A. Gremillion, unpublished data, 2006). It is associated with significant interpatient variability regarding presentation and response to treatment. Current scientific evidence supports a complex pathophysiology.

Chronic neuropathic pain may result from nerve injury or damage. In the vast majority of cases, chronic neuropathic pain cannot be satisfactorily treated with conventional analgesics and is generally resistant to opioids [7]. It is characterized by spontaneous pain that is often unprovoked. Box 1 lists relevant clinical features that are associated with neuropathic orofacial pain.

Pathophysiology

The pathophysiology of neuropathic orofacial pain has not been fully elucidated, but a number of mechanisms have been suggested. Change in excitability of primary nociceptive afferents may be the single most important factor in generation and maintenance of acute chemogenic pain or chronic neuropathic pain in humans [8].

Box 1. Clinical features associated with neuropathic orofacial pain

- Precipitating factors, such as trauma or disease, can typically be identified.
- There may be a delay in onset after initial injury/insult (days to months).
- Typical patient complaints of pain may include burning, paroxysmal lancinating, or sharp episodes.
- Additional complaints may be related to paresthesia or dysesthesia. Paresthesia is expressed as abnormal, not necessarily unpleasant, sensations such as heaviness, tingling, or numbness. Dysesthesia is regarded as abnormal or unpleasant sensations such as burning, stinging, or stabbing.
- The area in which pain is experienced may exhibit sensory deficit.
- Physical examination may reveal allodynia, hyperalgesia, or sympathetic hyperfunction. Allodynia is defined as pain resulting from a stimulus that does not normally cause pain. Hyperalgesia is an increased or exaggerated response to painful stimuli.
- Local pathophysiology is associated with an abnormal nerve healing (eg, sprouting, neuroma formation).

Deafferentation is defined as a continuous pain after complete or partial damage to a nerve. It may occur after facial trauma, dental extraction, placement of dental implants, endodontic therapy (surgical and nonsurgical), crown preparation, periodontal therapy, and bleaching of teeth. It may develop after the most perfect procedure if there is a predisposition or if peripheral or central neural sensitization occurs.

Deafferentation pain is associated with the following clinical characteristics: pain in the structure before amputation, persistent pain after the injured tissue has healed, discrete trigger areas in the affected region, and pain that is refractory to usually effective treatments. The estimated incidence of deafferentation pain postendodontic treatment has been reported to be 3 to 6% [9,10]. Pulpal extirpation is followed by a degenerative process of primary trigeminal axons and neurons in the spinal trigeminal nucleus, specifically in subnucleus caudalis. This finding suggests that a central mechanism plays a role in the ongoing pain condition [11,12].

Demyelination is a degenerative process that is associated with a loss of integrity of the myelin sheath that normally protects nerve fibers. This may result in an aberration in nerve impulse generation and conduction. Demyelination can occur peripherally or centrally. Multiple sclerosis is the most well known example of a central demyelinating disease. When the disease affects the trigeminal ganglion, it can present as trigeminal neuralgia. The peripheral nervous system neurons can undergo pathologic damage from numerous sources, such as vascular compression, radiation, inflammation, trauma, infection, and exposure to neurotoxins [13]. This damage occurs in two primary ways: demyelination and axotomy (deafferentation with severance of the axon). It has long been known that these two phenomena can produce numbness and paresthesia. More recently it has been shown that these pathologic entities can cause ectopic discharge or impulse generation from the sites along the axon where the damage has occurred, rather than just at the sensory nerve ending [13]. Demyelination can have a disastrous impact on the individual's quality of life because spontaneous nociceptive impulses can create severe and unpredictable pain. These same impulses can cause central sensitization, which can lead to a peripheral allodynia and hyperalgesia.

New information reveals that the root of this peripheral problem is not at the synaptic cleft between neurons but rather occurs as a result of membrane hyperexcitability along the axon [13]. Under normal conditions, the sensory nerve endings, and an adjacent region of the axon, bring about the transduction of a stimulus (electrogenesis) to initiate a train of electrical impulses (repetitive firing of the neuron) that are propagated and carried by the axon. Beyond the initial receptors, axons normally have few regions where repetitive firing can originate, with the exception of the nodes of Ranvier [14]. Single impulses (a quick sharp electrical feeling) can originate anywhere, such as can occur with a needle trauma to the lingual or inferior alveolar nerve during a local anesthetic injection.

With demyelination or axotomy, areas of involvement along an axon can become ectopic sites of repetitive firing that occur spontaneously or secondary to a stimulus. This process involves an abnormal "pacemaking" ability whereby the neuronal membrane demonstrates a depolarizing resonance (a fluctuating depolarizing cycle) just below the firing threshold. When combined with a depolarization after potential, it exceeds the threshold and causes repetitive firing [15]. This pacemaking ability can also create spontaneous activity in adjacent uninjured neurons including C-fibers (small-diameter, unmyelinated nociceptive fibers) [16]. C-fiber damage is generally associated with burning neuropathic pain.

Studies have recently demonstrated that membrane remodeling, particularly involving Na^+ channels, is responsible for the ectopic repetitive firing [17,18]. There are three primary ways in which sodium channels affect a change in membrane hyperexcitability and repetitive firing in damaged axons. First, there is a change in the rate of protein synthesis of various Na^+ channels as a result of neuronal injury. More Na^+ channels mean more sensitivity. For example, $Na_v1.3$ channels have been found to potentially influence the pacemaking activity previously mentioned. The elevated rate of synthesis of these proteins occurs concurrently with axonal ectopic firing and the initiation of allodynia [19]. Second, there is an intracellular regulation of the Na^+ channels that allows the channels to remain open longer and create more hypersensitivity and even spontaneous firing of damaged neurons [20]. The third way involves the interruption of axonal transport. If an axon is transected [21], exposed to certain toxins, or undergoes demyelination [22,23], then the axonal transport system responsible for moving Na^+ channel proteins from the cell nucleus to the axon sensory nerve endings is disrupted. This results in accumulation of transport vesicles at the damaged region. Furthermore, once damage occurs, neuromas (aberrant nerve regeneration) may form. Transport vesicles and Na^+ channel proteins build up in the multiple sprouting endings of the neuroma endbulb because they can no longer go to their original destination. Apparently, the Na^+ channels are then inserted into the cellular membrane where the integrity of the myelin sheath has been compromised or in the neuroma causing an abnormal, elevated concentration of these channels. The membrane hypersensitivity is directly dependent upon the concentration of Na^+ channels [14]. The concentration of Na^+ channels and hypersensitivity of the neuronal membrane after nerve injury is increased, resulting in spontaneous or easily stimulated repetitive firing of nociceptive neurons, causing the neuropathic pain.

An understanding of the mechanisms of neuropathic pain can provide the clinician/scientist with a basic rationale for treatment. Because the pathogenesis of neuropathic pain has not been determined, the practitioner must be aware of the various classes of pharmacotherapeutic agents that have been suggested to provide relief in selected cases. Pharmacotherapy for neuropathic pain encompasses a variety of agents with analgesic potential. A systematic approach to drug trials and ongoing assessment by a responsible, informed practitioner is key to successful control of neuropathic pain. Diverse agents in numerous classes may be used effectively in the heterogenous population with pain of neuropathic nature. Adjuvant analgesics are drugs that have primary indications other than pain but may be analgesic in specific circumstances. Some of the medications that have been suggested to be effective are included in Box 2.

Because the synaptic cleft is not predictably involved in the etiology of neuropathic pain, it is not surprising that drugs that inhibit synaptic transmission are many times ineffective; however, these drugs should remain a consideration. Examples of drugs that act at the synaptic cleft include clonidine or benzodiazepines. Rather, the membrane-stabilizing drugs, such as the anticonvulsant drugs (eg, carbamazepine, lamotrigine, oxcarbazepine, and phenytoin), are more predictably effective because they suppress the hyperexcitability of the axonal membrane [24]. Tricyclic antidepressants, such as amitriptyline, may be effective at low dosages because they also work as membrane stabilizers in addition to their trans-synaptic effects [25].

Local anesthesia has been used as diagnostic aid in the evaluation of the patient who has orofacial pain. Devor [13] has suggested that a positive

---

Box 2. Adjuvant analgesic drugs that may be used in the treatment of neuropathic orofacial pain

Antidepressants
Tricyclic antidepressants
- Amitriptyline
- Nortriptyline
- Imipramine

Serotonin–norepinephrine selective reuptake inhibitors
- Venlafaxine
- Duloxetine

Anticonvulsants/antiepileptic drugs
- Carbamazepine
- Oxcarbazepine
- Phenytoin
- Gabapentin
- Pre-gabalin
- Lamotrigine
- Topiramate
- Tiagabine
- Levetiracetam
- Clonazepam
- Valproic acid
- Zonisamide

Local anesthetics
Muscle relaxants
- Lioresal
- Tizanidine

---

response to local anesthetic provides validation of the axonal membrane etiology for neuropathic pain. Local anesthetics have a membrane-stabilizing effect and provide an additional treatment consideration for neuropathic pain. One study demonstrates the effectiveness of lidocaine for the suppression of nerve growth factor and the resultant sympathetic neurite sprouting in the dorsal root ganglion and in peripheral nerves [26]. This could suppress pain connections in the dorsal root ganglion and the hypersensitivity peripherally. Systemic lidocaine also was demonstrated to have a selective depression of C-fiber activity in the spinal cord, which could affect transmission of certain neuropathic pain types [27]. In summary, lidocaine can be applied topically with other medication in transdermal preparations, injected locally, or administered systemically for therapeutic benefit and not just for short-term pain relief [28,29].

Trigeminal neuralgia

Trigeminal neuralgia (TN) is a neuropathic orofacial pain originating in one or more branches of the Vth cranial nerve sensory distribution. TN can be idiopathic or secondary to demyelinating diseases (eg, multiple sclerosis) or the result of trauma. The pathology involves the structures of the neurons rather than the peripheral structures innervated by them.

One study reported the results for visits to neurology practice and found that the three main neuropathic pain-related diagnoses were postherpetic neuralgia, TN, and diabetic neuropathy [30]. In this study, 7.95% of the patient referrals were found to be for neuropathic pain; TN was one of the main diagnoses. The incidence of trigeminal neuralgia has been reported to be 2 to 27 individuals per 100,000 of the general population [31,32]. The larger number reported was generated from actual patient visits in the United Kingdom from a review of over 6 million visits to primary care physicians and not purely referrals to neurology-based practices. If this last report is accurate, then TN may be markedly under diagnosed.

Women are reported to experience TN with a greater frequency then are men. The onset of idiopathic TN occurs typically after 50 years of age and rarely occurs before the age of 30. Dentistry plays an important role in recognizing TN in its early stages because this condition can mimic dental pain, prompting dental approaches before a definitive diagnosis is made.

TN occurs primarily in the maxillary or mandibular divisions of the trigeminal nerve distribution unilaterally and may involve one or both divisions. It is rarely expressed in the ophthalmic division. Individuals who suffer from TN report a sharp, shooting, or lancinating pain that lasts from a few seconds to 2 minutes. These paroxysms may occur at intervals or nearly continuously. The patient may enter a refractory period that can last for minutes to hours where the pain cannot be triggered. TN can go into a period of remission, may never return, or may be re-expressed in an even more refractory state. This pain often is associated with a trigger zone that, when stimulated, triggers the lightening bolt–like pain with a light touch or a light breeze on the face. Other commonly reported triggers are chewing, talking, swallowing, brushing the teeth, combing the hair, putting on make-up, or washing one's face. Some individuals have multiple trigger zones, whereas others have spontaneous pain with no identified trigger zones. The most common trigger zones are lateral to the ala of the nose (nasolabial fold area) in the maxillary distribution or near the commissure of the lip in the mandibular distribution. Trigger zones can include intraoral sites including teeth, mucosa, and the tongue. One study reported that 64.5% of patients presented with an intraoral trigger zone [33]. TN can refer pain to the teeth. This can make the diagnosis difficult because dental pulpal pain often mimics neuropathic pain. Failure to address the proper diagnostic entity results in well intentioned, but misdirected, care and perpetuation or exacerbation of the pain. The same study reported that 31 of 48 patients

underwent dental procedures for their facial pain before TN was diagnosed
[33]. Along with this lightening bolt–like pain, 15 to 20% of patients who
have TN also exhibit sensory loss in the affected trigeminal division, which
is rarely reported [34]. This can lead to confusion in diagnosis and prompt
multiple tests to rule out other entities discussed later in this article.

Pre-trigeminal neuralgia

The diagnosis if TN may take months or more to confirm because the
condition may be initially expressed as pre-trigeminal neuralgia (PTN). At
this stage, the condition may present with a dull aching pain (a toothache
or sinus-like pain) with a sporadic sharp, lancinating component. The
pain is of spontaneous onset but with no specific trigger zone. Pain may
be triggered by routine activity such as chewing, drinking hot or cold liq-
uids, tooth brushing, yawning, or talking. The duration of PTN-related
pain may be minutes to hours or in some cases constant, in comparison
to a duration of seconds to minutes characteristic for classic TN. The
pain is likely to decrease with the use of diagnostic anesthesia. In PTN,
the differential diagnosis must include neoplasm, atypical odontalgia, odontogenic pain, lower-half headache, sinusitis, myofascial pain, temporomandibular joint dysfunction, and osseous pathology due to the overlap of
symptoms. PTN typically progresses to classic TN.

The mechanisms associated with TN and PTN have been debated for
many years. There must exist a malfunction at the peripheral or central neuronal components of the trigeminal system. One theory suggests a demyelination of the root of the trigeminal nerve by vascular compression in the area
[34]. Intracranially, an artery may rub against the trigeminal axons, causing
a hyperexcitability in the primary afferent neurons and a decreased efficacy
of the inhibitory controls. One author suggests that this creates an increased
spontaneous firing of the wide dynamic neurons in the subnucleus caudalis
(nociceptive neurons) and hypersensitivity (lowering of the threshold) of the
low-threshold mechanoreceptors in the subnucleus oralis [35]. Another theory proposes nerve entrapment at the foremen rotundum or foramen ovale
and suggests that this phenomenon may explain the right-sided (3:2) predi-
lection of TN [36]. The result is that low-threshold mechanoreceptors fire
spontaneously or when stimulated by what would normally be a nonpainful
stimulus, such as light touch. The action potential is carried by A_{beta} fibers
(large-diameter, heavily myelinated fibers that carry nonpainful sensations
and proprioception) that trigger a paroxysmal firing of the A_{delta} fibers
(lightly myelinated nociceptive fibers), causing the electrical-like pain that
is characteristic of TN.

Treatment of TN can be divided into two primary modalities: pharmacotherapy and surgical. Pharmacotherapy generally involves using the membrane-stabilizing anticonvulsant class of medications. Carbamazepine is
the gold standard, but multiple adverse effects frequently prohibit its use.

Other anticonvulsants, including oxcarbazepine, lamotrigine, gabapentin, and pregabalin, may be efficacious. Other adjuvant medications in the antispasmodic, muscle relaxants, antidepressants, and local anesthetic drug classifications can be used in combination with the primary medication.

TN can also be treated by neurosurgery. Surgical approaches may be necessary if pharmacotherapy becomes ineffective or is medications are not tolerated. In some cases, surgical intervention should be the first line of treatment. One effective surgical treatment is microvascular decompression, or the Janetta procedure. Entry is made into the cranium behind the mastoid process, and a synthetic material is placed between the trigeminal rootlets and the vascular structures found to be compressing the nerve. Studies report that a 90 to 96% incidence of vascular compression is identified in patients undergoing the microvascular decompression procedure [37]. One study reported 80% complete pain relief over a 20-year period [38].

Other surgical options involve ablation of the neurons in the trigeminal ganglion responsible for the patient's pain. This can be accomplished several ways. An instrument is inserted through the cheek and fluoroscopically directed through the foremen ovale into the trigeminal ganglion. Once the instrument is in place, the patient is awakened to confirm which specific area is responsible for the pain. The patient is reanesthetized, and the rootlets in the area are ablated. Three techniques are used for this type of procedure: radiofrequency thermocoagulation, glycerol, and balloon (mechanical) compression. These procedures have been reported to provide 90% relief [39–41] that is often immediate. Potential adverse effects include anesthesia, paresthesia, hemorrhage, infection, or anesthesia dolorosa (ongoing pain in the anesthetized area). Gamma knife radiosurgery is a relatively new approach that uses stereotactic surgery of the trigeminal ganglion targeting the offending afferent neurons with columnated gamma rays. This technique is fast and minimally invasive; however, it demonstrates a slow onset of pain relief, sometimes requiring months to provide full benefit.

As compared with idiopathic TN, traumatic secondary TN has a known cause: trauma to one or more of the divisions of the trigeminal nerve. This trauma can be associated with a surgical procedure that violates the myelin sheath of the nerve or any other overt trauma that causes nerve injury. The prevalence has been noted to be mild in 32% and "disturbing" in 3% of cases after orthognathic surgery [42]. The incidence of inferior alveolar nerve damage after 3rd molar removal was reported to be 5.5% at 24 hours, 3.9% at 7 to 10 days, and 0.9% after 1 year [43].

There have been case reports of neuropathic pain and secondary TN after the placement of implants, endodontic instruments, endodontic filling cements, or hydroxyapatite into the mandibular canal resulting in damage to the inferior alveolar nerve. Local anesthetic injections have been known to damage the lingual nerve or the inferior alveolar nerve. Clinical presentation involves patients often reporting numbness, tingling, or sharp, lancinating, or burning pain. In the affected peripheral region of pain, the skin, mucosa, or gingiva may exhibit a total sensory loss (anesthesia) or a partial sensory loss (paresthesia) to sharp and dull testing. MRI T2-weighted imaging can aid in the diagnosis of peripheral nerve damage. A hyperintense signal from gadolinium-enhanced axonal edema makes peripheral damage visible [44].

Neural damage can cause pain, but how this occurs is yet to be determined. One study demonstrated the importance of C-fiber involvement in stimulus-induced and spontaneous types of neuropathic pain conditions [44]. An increase of neuropeptides (pain modulatory substances), such as Substance P, calcitonin gene-related peptide, and vasoactive intestinal polypeptide, have been shown to be expressed as a result of injuries to the lingual or inferior alveolar nerves. These same neuropeptides can invoke changes at the injury site by increasing the "rate of discharge" of the neuron and at the trigeminal ganglion involving sodium channels and certain enzymes [8].

Treatment usually involves surgical repair of damaged nerves. Microsurgeries can be attempted to the lingual or inferior alveolar nerves. If the damage is extensive, neural grafts may be necessary. Time is of the essence. Once damage has been confirmed, surgical intervention needs to be accomplished within a few months for optimal treatment outcomes. Finally, pharmacotherapy involving the antiepileptic drugs may be needed as adjunctive treatment (see Box 2). In some injury sites involving neuroma formation, corticosteroid injection can reduce some of the mechanically induced hyperactivity of that branch of the trigeminal nerve [45].

Atypical odontalgia/non-odontogenic toothache

Atypical odontalgia/non-odontogenic toothache is a condition that is associated with constant pain in a tooth with no obvious source of local pathology. The typical age of occurrence ranges from 25 to 65 years, with a mean age of 48 years. Molars are affected at 58%, premolars at 26%, and incisors at 10%. The maxilla was found to be involved two times more often than the mandible. The pain was typically reported to be moderate in intensity, with a rating of 46/100 on the VAS scale [46].

Clinically, atypical odontalgia presents as a continuous pain in a particular tooth that is unchanging for at least for 3 months. Radiograph reveals no pathology. Diagnostic anesthetic response is equivocal and may result in resolution of the pain for the duration of anesthetic effect in one instance but not another [46]. The tooth exhibits hyperesthesia demonstrated by a positive response to percussion, sensitivity to cold, or pain associated with chewing. Along with the clinical presentation, there are associated features, such as depression, oral dysesthesias, and excessive concern with oral hygiene [47]. No studies have supported psychopathology as the primary or sole etiology in this condition.

There is no defined mechanism for this disorder. Theories have suggested vascular mechanisms, sympathetic dysregulation, psychologic mechanisms, or a neural pathology. This poses a problem because the patient perceives pain in a tooth and can be frustrated with the lack of resolution that dental approaches provide. A diagnosis of exclusion must be made before successful treatment can be rendered or, in the case of non-odontogenic toothache, no dental treatment at all. Tricyclic antidepressants and benzodiazepines have been used with equivocal results.

Post-herpetic neuralgia

Post-herpetic neuralgia (PHN) is a neuropathic pain that persists after the outbreak of the herpes zoster virus (HZV). The varicella virus is responsible for the primary infection and is the cause of chicken pox, which is seen mostly in young children [48–50]. The rash associated with HZV presents shortly after hyperesthesia or dysesthesia is expressed, usually involving the scalp, face, and trunk. It is estimated that 95% of the American population will have been exposed to the HZV by adulthood, with approximately four million cases reported each year [51].

After active infection, during the latency stage, the varicella virus goes through a morphologic transformation referred to as the varicella-zoster virus (VZV) [49]. In this form, the virus migrates to the ganglion of the peripheral nervous system. The most prevalent location for the VZV is the dorsal root ganglion of the thoracic spine, where the virus is located in 55% of cases. In 15% of cases, the virus is found in the ganglion associated with the cranial nerves. Of the cranial nerves, the trigeminal (CN V) and facial nerves (CN VII) are most frequently involved [48,49]. The cervical distribution of the spinal nerves is involved in 12% of the cases. Of most interest to the dentist is VZV expressed in the cranial and cervical distributions. Once the virus reaches the ganglion, it may remain dormant indefinitely. The virus may be activated by some "trigger," which in most instances is unknown. Once reactivated, the condition is referred to as "shingles." Suspected triggers are stress (physical or emotional), colds, spinal cord injury, steroid use, a compromised immune system, use of immunosuppressants, and cancer [49,52]. The clinical course of shingles is similar to chicken pox. In contrast to chicken pox, the herpes zoster virus cannot be contracted from exposure to the rash [53]. Shingles may present without vesicle formation (Zoster Sine Herpete), making diagnosis problematic. Shingles is a severe and debilitating condition that affects over 500,000 people per year in the United States [51]. It has been reported that there are over 9000 hospitalizations per year, many with viral pneumonia, related to the zoster virus [51]. Disseminated shingles can result in blindness and deafness [51].

In the trigeminal system, the virus may be expressed in any of the three divisions alone or in combination [48]. The ophthalmic branch is most commonly involved. Cervical nerve involvement usually follows the C-3 and C-4 distribution. Although zoster can involve more than one nerve distribution, it generally is expressed unilaterally [48]. Complications of a zoster infection include myelitis, meningoencephalitis, systemic toxicity, bacterial sepsis, viral pneumonia, and postherpetic neuralgia.

Reactivation of the dormant virus

When triggered, the herpes zoster virus invades the nerves and ganglion of the peripheral nervous system. If the immune system becomes sufficiently impaired, an intense necrotizing reaction causing nerve injury associated with glutamate receptor-mediated excitotoxicity ensues [54]. This central and peripheral nerve damage is the primary cause of the pain experienced in PHN. PHN may present in the exact area as the pain and rash of the shingles or may encompass larger or smaller zones. Descriptors of the pain include deep, aching, burning, stabbing, itching, electrical, unbearable, and fire under the skin [55]. Many individuals who experience PHN report that stimuli such as light touch, wind, or temperature change causes severe pain [56]. About 87% of patients who have PHN experience allodynia, hyperesthesia, dysesthesia, or anesthesia [56]. Such debilitating pain may cause poor sleep and result in a compromise in activities of daily living. Social isolation due to the severe pain is likely a major reason for the common finding of depression and anxiety in those who suffer with PHN.

The incidence of PHN increases with age [50,55]. On average, one in five people who have shingles develop PHN. The older one is when an outbreak of shingles occurs, the greater the likelihood of developing PHN [48]. At the age of 55, approximately one in four individuals develops PHN. At age 60, the incidence increases to two in four; at age 70 or older, three in four are afflicted. There is also some indication that patients who have diabetes have an increased risk of PHN [51].

There is no cure for PHN. Therefore, the major focus should be on prevention. This fact led the FDA to approve a vaccine for VZV in 1995. The effectiveness of the vaccine preventing chicken pox is between 70 and 90%. However, the vaccine is of limited quantity due to the lack of a suitable animal model [57]. Because of the large number of previously HZV-infected cases, there exists a high probability of the development of shingles and subsequently PHN. This fact mandates that other approaches to management of the pain associated with PHN be identified.

There are a number of modalities available to address PHN pain, including oral pharmacotherapy, nerve blocks, topical medications, electrical stimulation, and complementary alternative treatments (eg, acupuncture and nutrition). Pharmacotherapy is hallmarked by the use of opioids, antivirals, antidepressants, and anticonvulsants. Famciclovir, valacyclovir, and acyclovir are the most common antivirals that are used during the viral replication phase and in immunocompromised individuals [50,51,58]. The tricyclic antidepressants that have been shown to be of most benefit are amitriptyline and nortriptyline in small doses [59]. Gabapentin, an anticonvulsant, has recently been approved by the FDA to treat PHN [51,60]. Peripheral and sympathetic anesthetic nerve blocks have provided relief for PHN pain. Topical medications come in many forms. The lidocaine patch [61,62] is approved by the FDA for PHN pain. Capsaicin cream (made from the seeds of hot peppers) has also been used in the management of pain associated with PHN. Complementary alternative treatments (eg, acupuncture) have been of limited efficacy in the control of PHN pain. Nutritional supplements (eg, L-lysine, vitamin C, vitamin E, vitamin B complex, zinc, calcium and magnesium) can be used to support nerve health and provide protection from free radicals. Herbals, such as green tea, are used to provide antiviral, antioxidant, and anti-inflammatory support. Licorice has limited benefit as a topical agent [53].

Summary

Based upon current understanding of neuropathic orofacial pain, successful management is dependent upon recognizing several basic principles.

1. Neuropathic orofacial pain represents a number of subcategories of conditions that are associated with a primary lesion or dysfunction in the nervous system.
2. Neuropathic pain conditions are many times overlaid with psychosocial issues.
3. The primary means of management of most neuropathic orofacial pain conditions is through rational pharmacotherapy.
4. Limit the use of invasive and irreversible approaches to cases where there is a high probability that the procedure will eliminate or significantly reduce the complaint.
5. Do not escalate physical treatments without comprehensive re-evaluation, which should include psychological and behavioral aspects.
5. Ongoing pain can become a disease in and of itself.
6. Complete and accurate diagnosis on a case-specific basis provides for the development of the most efficacious individualized approach to care.
7. Many cases of neuropathic orofacial pain are best managed by a multidisciplinary team involving dentists, neurologists, neurosurgeons, clinical and health psychologists, and other health care disciplines.
8. The health care professional must be aware of the existence of comorbid conditions and address them appropriately to optimize treatment outcomes.

References

[1] Donaldson D, Kroening R. Recognition and treatment of patients with chronic orofacial pain. J Am Dent Assoc 1979;99:961–6.
[2] Lipton JA, Ship JA, Larach-Robinson D. Estimated prevalence and distribution of reported orofacial pain in the United States. J Am Dent Assoc 1993;124:115–21.

[3] Merskey H, Bogduk N. Classification of chronic pain: descriptions of chronic pain syndromes and definitions of pain terms. 2nd edition. Seattle (WA): IASP Press; 1994.

[4] Rowbotham M, Harden N, Stacey B, et al, for the Gabapentin Postherpetic Neuralgia Study Group. Gabapentin for the treatment of postherpetic neuralgia: a randomized controlled trial. JAMA 1998;280:1837–42.

[5] Rice ASC, Maton S, , for the Postherpetic Neuralgia Study Group. Gabapentin in postherpetic neuralgia: a randomized, double blind study. Pain 2001;94:215–24.

[6] Osterberg A, Boivie J, Holmgren H, et al. The clinical characteristics and sensory abnormalities of patients with central pain caused by multiple sclerosis. In: Gebhart GF, Hammond DL, Jensen TS, editors. Proceedings of the 7th World Congress on Pain, Progress in Pain Research and Management, vol. 2. Seattle (WA): IASP Press; 1994. p. 789–96.

[7] Hansson P. Neurogenic pain. Pain Clin Updates 1994;II:1–4.

[8] Koltzenburg M, Torebjork HE, Wahren LK. Nociceptor modulated central sensitization causes mechanical hyperalgesia in acute chemogenic and chronic neuropathic pain. Brain 1994;117:579–91.

[9] Marbach JJ, Hulbrock J, Hohn C, et al. Incidence of phantom tooth pain: an atypical facial neuralgia. Oral Surg Oral Med Oral Pathol 1982;53:190–3.

[10] Campbell RL, Parks KW, Dodds RN. Chronic facial pain associated with endodontic therapy. Oral Surg Oral Med Oral Pathol 1990;69:287–90.

[11] Westrum LE, Canfield RC, Black RG. Transganglionic degeneration in the spinal trigeminal nucleus following removal of tooth pulps in adult cats. Brain Res 1976;101:137–40.

[12] Keller O, Kalina M, Juec E, et al. Projection of tooth pulp afferents to the brainstem and to the cortex in the cat. Neurosci Lett 1981;25:233–7.

[13] Devor M. Sodium channels and mechanisms of neuropathic pain. J Pain 2006;7(Suppl 1): s3–12.

[14] Priestley T. Voltage-gated sodium channels and pain. Curr Drug Targets CNS Neurol Disord 2004;3:441–56.

[15] Liu C-N, Michaelis M, Amir R, Devor M. Spinal nerve injury enhances subthreshold membrane potential oscillations in DRG neurons: relation to neuropathic pain. J Neurophysiol 2000;84:205–15.

[16] Wu G, Ringkamp M, Murinson BB, et al. Degeneration of myelinated efferent fibers induces spontaneous activity in uninjured C-fiber afferents. J Neurosci 2002;22:7746–53.

[17] Wood JN, Abrahamsen B, Baker MD, et al. Ion channel activities implicated in pathological pain. Novartis Found Symp 2004;261:32–40 [discussion: 40–54].

[18] Takahashi N, Nikuchi S, Dai Y, et al. Expression of auxiliary beta subunits of sodium channels in primary afferent neurons and effect of nerve injury. Neuroscience 2003;121:441–50.

[19] Chung JM, Dib-Hajj SD, Lawson SN. Sodium channel sub-types and neuropathic pain. In: Dostrovsky JO, Carr DB, Koltzenburg M, editors. Proceedings of the 10th World Congress of Pain, Progress in Pain Research and Management, vol. 24. Seattle (WA): IASP Press; 2003. p. 99–114.

[20] Chahine M, Ziane R, Vijayvaragavan K, et al. Regulation of Na v channels in sensory neurons. Trends Pharmacol Sci 2005;26:496–502.

[21] Kretschmer T, Happel LT, England JD, et al. Accumulation of PN1 an PN3 sodium channels in painful human neuroma-evidence from immunocytochemistry. Acta Neurochir (Wien) 2002;144:803–10.

[22] Craner MJ, Lo AC, Black JA, et al. Abnormal sodium channel distribution in optic nerve axons in a model of inflammatory demyelination. Brain 2003;126:1552–61.

[23] Dugandzija-Novakovic S, Koszowski AG, Levinson RS, et al. Clustering of Na^+ channels and node of Ranvier formation in remyelinating axons. J Neurosci 1995;15:492–503.

[24] Stacey BR. Management of peripheral neuropathic pain. Am J Phys Med Rehabil 2005; 84(Suppl):S4–16.

[25] McQuay M, Moore A. An evidence-based resource for pain relief. Oxford: Oxford University Press; 1998.

[26] Takatori M, Kuroda Y, Hirose M. Local anesthetics suppress nerve growth factor-mediated neurite outgrowth by inhibition of tyrosine kinase activity of TrkA. Anesth Analg 2006;102: 462–7.

[27] Woolf CJ, Wiesenfeld-Hallin Z. The systemic administration of local anaesthetics produces a selective depression of C-afferent fibre evoked activity in the spinal cord. Pain 1985;23: 361–74.

[28] Sawynok J. Topical analgesics in neuropathic pain. Curr Pharm Des 2005;11:2995–3004.

[29] Dressler RL. Systemic lidocaine or mexiletine for neuropathic pain. American Family Physician Cochrane for Clinicians 2006;74:4–5.

[30] Carneado-Ruiz J, Morera-Guitart J, Alfaro-Saez A, et al. Neuropathic pain as the reason for visiting neurology: an analysis of its frequency. Rev Neurol 2005;41:643–8 [comment: 641–2].

[31] Brewis M, Poskanzer DC, Rolland C, et al. Neurological disease in an English city. Acta Neurol Scand 1966;42(Suppl 24):1–89.

[32] Hall GC, Carroll D, Parry D, et al. Epidemiology and treatment of neuropathic pain: the UK primary care perspective. Pain 2006;122:156–62.

[33] Sicuteri F, Nicolodi M, Fusco BM, et al. Idiopathic headache as a possible risk factor for phantom tooth pain. Headache 1991;31:577–81.

[34] Rozen TD. Trigeminal neuralgia and glossopharyneal neuralgia. Neurol Clin N Am 2004;22: 185–206.

[35] Fromm GH. Pathophysiology of trigeminal neuralgia. In: Fromm GH, Sessle BJ, editors. Trigeminal neuralgia: current concepts regarding pathogenesis and treatment. Boston: Butterworth-Heinemann; 1991. p. 105–30.

[36] Neto HS, Camilli JA, Marques MJ. Trigeminal neuralgia caused by maxillary and mandibular nerve entrapment: greater incidence of right sided facial symptoms is due to the foremen rotundum and foremen ovale being narrower on the right side of the cranium. Med Hypotheses 2005;65:1179–82.

[37] Hamlyn PJ, King TT. Neurovascular compression in trigeminal neuralgia: a clinical and anatomical study. J Neurosurg 1992;76:948–54.

[38] Barker GG, Janetta PJ, Bissonette DJ, et al. The long term outcome of microvascular decompression for trigeminal neuralgia. N Engl J Med 1996;334:1077–83.

[39] Lopez BC, Hamlyn PJ, Zakrzewska JM. Systematic review of ablative neurosurgical techniques for the treatment of trigeminal neuralgia. Neurosurg 2004;54(4):973–82.

[40] Onofrio BM. Radiofrequency percutaneous gasserian ganglion lesions: results in 140 patients with trigeminal pain. J Neurosurg 1975;42:132–9.

[41] Arias MJ. Percutaneous retrogasserian glycerol rhizotomies for trigeminal neuralgia: a prospective study of 100 cases. Neurosurgery 2000;65:32–6.

[42] Panula K, Finne K, Oikarinen K. Incidence of complications and problems related to orthognathic surgery: a review of 655 patients. J Oral Maxillofac Surg 2001;59:1128–36.

[43] Carmichael FA, McGowan DA. Incidence of nerve damage following third molar removal: a West of Scotland Oral Surgery Research Group study. Br J Oral Maxillofac Surg 1992;30: 78–82.

[44] Koltzenburg M, Bendszus M. Imaging of peripheral nerve lesions. Curr Opin Neurol 2004; 17:621–6.

[45] Robinson PP, Boissonade FM, Loescher AR, et al. Peripheral mechanisms for the initiation of pain following trigeminal nerve injury. J Orofac Pain 2004;18:287–92.

[46] Graff-Radford SB, Solberg WK. Atypical odontalgia. Craniomandibular Disord 1992;6: 260–5.

[47] Graff-Radford SB, Solberg WK. Is atypical odontalgia a psychological problem? Oral Surg Oral Med Oral Pathol 1993;75:579–82.

[48] Jensen JL, Barr RJ. Lesions of the facial skin. In: Wood NK, Goaz PW, editors. Differential diagnosis of oral and maxillofacial lesions. 5th edition. St. Louis (MO): Mosby; 1997. p. 557–8.

[49] Kennedy PG. Varicella-Zoster virus latency in human ganglia. Rev Med Virol 2002;12: 327–34.

[50] Stankus SJ, Diugopolski M, Packer D. Management of herpes zoster (shingles) and post-herpetic neuralgia. Am Fam Phys 2000;61:2437–48.

[51] Gnann JW, Whitley RJ. Herpes zoster. N Engl J Med 2002;347(5):340–6.

[52] Sumpf MP, Laidlaw Z, Jansen VA. Herpes viruses hedge their bets. Proc Natl Acad Sci 2002; 99(23):15234–7.

[53] Madison LK. Shingles update: common questions in caring for a patient with shingles. Orthop Nurs 2000;19(1):59–62.

[54] Dugan LL, Choi DW. Excitotoxicity, free radicals and cell membrane changes. Ann Neurol 1994;(suppl):517–21.

[55] Goh CL, Khoo L. A retrospective study of the clinical presentation and outcome of herpes zoster in a tertiary dermatology referral clinic. Int J Dermatol 1997;36:667–72.

[56] Rowbotham MC, Fields HL. The relationship of pain, allodynia, and thermal sensation in post-herpetic neuralgia. Brain 1996;119:347–54.

[57] Fleetwood-Walker SM, Quinn JP, Wallace C, et al. Behavior changes in the rat following infection with varicella-zoster virus. J Gen Virol 2002;80:2433–6.

[58] Bowsher D. Post-herpetic neuralgia in older patients, incidence, and optimal treatment. Drugs Aging 1994;5:411–8.

[59] Bryson HM, Wilde MI. Amitriptyline: a review of it's pharmacological properties and therapeutic use in chronic pain states. Drugs Aging 1996;8:459–76.

[60] Scheinfeld N. The role of gabapentin in treating diseases with cutaneous manifestations and pain. Int J Dermatol 2003;42:491–5.

[61] Ahmad M, Goucke CR. Management strategies for the treatment of neuropathic pain in the elderly. Drugs Aging 2002;19:929–45.

[62] Campbell BJ, Rowbotham M, Davies PS, et al. Systemic absorption of topical lidocaine in normal volunteers, patients with post-herpetic neuralgia, and patients with acute herpes zoster. J Pharm Sci 2002;9:1343–50.

Dent Clin N Am 51 (2007) 225–243

THE DENTAL
CLINICS
OF NORTH AMERICA

ELSEVIER
SAUNDERS

Four Oral Motor Disorders: Bruxism, Dystonia, Dyskinesia and Drug-Induced Dystonic Extrapyramidal Reactions

Glenn T. Clark, DDS, MS*,
Saravanan Ram, BDS, MDS

*Department of Diagnostic Sciences, Orofacial Pain and Oral Medicine Center,
University of Southern California School of Dentistry, 925 West 34th Street,
Room B-14, Los Angeles, CA 90089-0641, USA*

Four oral movement disorders

The literature is replete with articles that discuss motor disorders, such as Parkinson's disease, Bell's palsy, essential tremor, poststroke paralysis, dystonia, and dyskinesia. The focus of this article is on those motor disorders that are known to affect the masticatory system and its adjacent muscles. The term "orofacial motor disorder" (OMD) encompasses a spectrum of movement aberrations, both hyperactive and hypoactive, which involves the muscles of the orofacial complex and are innervated by cranial nerves V, VII, and XII. OMDs generally present as localized problems that affect only the masticatory system, but they are driven by alterations in central nervous system (CNS) functioning. Dentists must be able to recognize and become involved with management of these problems, because such behaviors cause pain and dysfunction of the jaw and interfere with needed dental care on patients [1–3].

The most common OMDs are sleep bruxism and sustained habitual forceful clenching (day or night). In addition to bruxism, this article reviews three other vexing oral motor disorders: focal orofacial dystonia, oromandibular dyskinesia, and medication-induced extrapyramidal syndrome (EPS)–dystonic reactions. Table 1 provides a brief definition, the main clinical features, and management approaches that are used for these four OMDs. When severe, these motor disorders may cause strong headaches,

---

* Corresponding author.
  E-mail address: gtc@usc.edu (G.T. Clark).

0011-8532/07/$ - see front matter © 2007 Elsevier Inc. All rights reserved.
doi:10.1016/j.cden.2006.09.002
                                    dental.theclinics.com

Table 1
Oral motor disorders: dystonia, dyskinesia, bruxism and dystonic extrapyramidal reactions

Oral motor disorders	Definition	Clinical features	Management
Bruxism (ICD-9 #306.8)	Sleep bruxism can be defined as nonfunctional jaw movement that includes clenching, grinding, clicking, and gnashing of teeth during sleep.	Dental attrition Tooth pain TMJ dysfunction Headaches	Pharmacologic treatment data not convincing. Most cases treated with an occlusal appliance, severe cases treated with botulinum toxin injections.
Oromandibular dystonia (ICD-9 #333.6)	Involuntary, repetitive, sustained muscle contraction that results in an abnormal posturing of a structure. Depending on the muscle involved, it may produce a twisting motion of involved structure.	Involuntary jaw opening. Lateral movements of the jaw. Protrusion of the tongue. Present during the day. Disappears during deep sleep. Dystonic spasms increase in intensity during stress, emotional upset, or fatigue.	Pharmacologic treatment. Chemodenervation with botulinum toxin injections. Select use of neurosurgical treatment.
Orofacial dyskinesia (ICD9 #333.82)	The presence of excessive, repetitive, stereotypic oral movements.	Facial grimacing. Repetitive tongue protrusion. Puckering, smacking and licking of the lips. Side-to-side motion of the jaw.	Withdrawal of neuroleptic medications or other offending agent. Pharmacologic treatment.
Drug induced dystonic-type extrapyramidal reactions (ICD-9 #333.9)	Medications and illegal drugs produce a motor response that is classified better as an unspecified extrapyramidal syndrome reaction.	3 presentations: Dystonia Akathisia Parkinsonism	Withdraw offending drug. Pharmacologic trials.

damage the temporomandibular joint (TMJ), or create such motor control difficulty that patients are unable to eat and may start to lose weight. These motor disorders can affect the tongue musculature to such a degree that it compromises the patient's ability to speak clearly. The social embarrassment that patients must endure affects their daily living; many patients refuse or strongly avoid leaving their homes. Fortunately, there are various medications, including botulinum toxin injections, and surgical interventions that reduce the severity of the OMDs.

Bruxism

The prevalence of chronic bruxism is unknown, because no large, probability-based, random sample study has been performed using polysomnography (which is needed to measure bruxism). Based on a combination of attrition assessment and reports by parents, spouses, or roommates, it is estimated that 5% to 21% of the population has substantial sleep bruxism [4,5]. Many bruxers do not have substantial attrition and many do not make tooth-grinding sounds during sleep, so sleep partner or parental reports are not always accurate. The pathophysiology of bruxism is unknown. The most cogent theory describes bruxism as a neuromotor dysregulation disorder. This theory proposes that bruxism occurs because of the failure to inhibit jaw motor activity during a sleep state arousal. There are numerous clear-cut neuromotor diseases that exhibit bruxism as a feature of the disease (eg, cerebral palsy). The disorder of periodic limb movements is similar to an OMD, except that it occurs in the leg muscles [6]. There are many articles that describe the clinical presentation and consequences of bruxism; most agree that the single most effective way to protect the teeth from progressive attrition, fracture, or clenching-induced pulpitis is to fabricate an occlusal appliance and have the patient use it at night [7]. The problem with an occlusal-covering appliance is that it does little or nothing to stop the bruxism in the long term. Most alter the behavior for a few weeks when first used, but this only offers a brief respite from some headaches and bruxism-induced TMJ derangement or arthritis problems. In cases in which the disorder is severe and the damaging consequences are well beyond the teeth, one option is to inject the masseter or temporalis about every 3 to 6 months to minimize the power of the bruxism activity. The literature supports this concept; one of the first reports was by Van Zandijcke and Marchau [8] in 1990 who provided a brief note on the treatment of a brain-injured patient who exhibited severe bruxism with botulinum toxin type-A injections (100 U total into the masseter and temporalis). Seven years later, Ivanhoe and colleagues [9] described the successful treatment of a brain-injured patient who had severe bruxism with botulinum toxin type-A. In this case, the patient was injected with a total of 50 U to each of four muscles (right and left masseter and temporalis) for a total of 200 U. Of course, the successful treatment of a single case of brain injury–induced bruxism does not make a compelling story for its routine use in managing bruxism. The story was extended by a more recent report [10]. The investigators reported on the long-term treatment of 18 cases of severe bruxism with botulinum toxin type-A. These patients all had severe bruxism, which had been causing symptoms for an average of 14.8 ± 10.0 years and all had no success with previous medical or dental treatment. Similar to previous reports, the masseter muscle was injected with a mean dose of 61.7 ± 11.1 U per side. The efficacy of these injections was rated by the subjects as a 3.4 on a scale from 0 to 4 (with 4 being equal to total cessation of the behavior). The investigators described one subject who experienced dysphagia as a side effect of the injections. Finally, another investigator described a young child (age 7) who had severe brain injury–induced bruxism that was treated successfully with botulinum toxin [11]. The primary management method for strong bruxism and clenching is still a full-arch occlusal appliance, which does not stop the behavior but limits its dental damage [12]. Fortunately, the most severe cases of bruxism and clenching now have several motor suppressive medications; in extreme cases, botulinum toxin injections can be added to occlusal appliance treatment.

Oromandibular dystonia

Oromandibular dystonia is one form of a focal dystonia that affects the orofacial region and involves the jaw openers (lateral pterygoids and anterior digastrics), tongue muscles, facial muscles (especially orbicularis oris and buccinator), and platysma. When this occurs in association with blethrospasm (focal dystonia of the orbiculares oculi muscles), it is called Meige's syndrome [13]. Dystonia is considered present when repeated, often asynchronous spasms of muscles are present. Most dystonias are idiopathic and the focal form of dystonia occurs 10 times more often than does the generalized systemic form [14]. The prevalence of all forms of idiopathic dystonia ranges between 3 and 30 per 100,000 [15]. Focal dystonias can be primary or secondary; the secondary form of dystonias occurs as a result of a trauma (peripheral or central), brainstem lesion, systemic disease (eg, multiple sclerosis, Parkinson's disease), vascular disease (eg, basal ganglia infarct), or drug use [16]. Most dystonias are primary or "idiopathic" and demonstrate no specific CNS disease. Of course, various pathophysiologic mechanisms have been proposed to explain dystonia (eg, basal ganglia dysfunction, hyperexcitability of interneurons involved in motor signaling [15], reduced inhibition of spinal cord and brainstem signals coming from supraspinal input and dysfunction of neurochemical systems involving dopamine, serotonin, and noradrenaline [14]). All dystonias are involuntary but tend to be more intermittent than dyskinesias (see later discussion) and are compromised of short, but sustained, muscle contractions that produce twisting and repetitive movements or abnormal postures [17,18].

One interesting aspect of the involuntary motor disorders is that patients can control or suppress the movement partially with the use of tactile stimulation (eg, touching the chin in the case of orofacial dystonia or holding an object in their mouth). This suppressive effect has been called "geste antagonistique" [19]. These tactile maneuvers may lead physicians to the erroneous diagnosis of malingering or hysteria. Other examples of sensory tricks include placing a hand on the side of the face, the chin, or the back of the head, or touching these areas with one or more fingers, which, at times, will reduce the neck contractions that are associated with cervical dystonia. With some dystonias, patients have discovered that placing an object in the mouth (eg, toothpick, piece of gum) may reduce dystonic behaviors of the jaw, mouth, and lower face (oromandibular dystonia). Finally, most of the focal and segmental dystonias only occur during waking periods and disappear entirely during sleep.

For treatment, there are several medications that can be used to suppress hyperkinetic muscles (see later discussion). After medications, the other primary method for treating dystonia is chemodenervation using botulinum toxin. In 1989, Blitzer and colleagues [20] first described the injection of botulinum toxin for oromandibular dystonia. They described injecting many of the orofacial muscles in oromandibular dystonia and claimed that masseter and temporalis injections helped with suppressing the overall oromandibular dystonia. These early reports did not specifically look at tongue movement changes nor were tongue botulinum toxin injection performed. In 1991, Blitzer and colleagues [21] described the first use of botulinum toxin in patients who had lingual dystonia, but cautioned clinicians that dysphagia was a problem in some of their cases; unfortunately, doses and injections sites were not described carefully. In 1997, Charles and colleagues [22] reported on nine patients who had repetitive tongue protrusion that resulted from oromandibular dystonia or Meige's syndrome. They were treated with botulinum toxin injections into the genioglossus muscle at four sites by way of a submandibular approach. Six of these patients were helped, and the average dose injected was 34 U, which produced a 3- to 4-month effect. Clearly, there is a need to explore when, where, and to what degree botulinum toxin may become useful in the management of the patient who has galloping tongue or tongue-based severe dyskinesia. There are many variations of oromandibular dystonia, but one common one is involuntary jaw-opening dystonia. One complication of jaw-opening dystonia is that the TMJ can become locked physically in the wide-open position, so that even after the dystonic contraction stops, the jaw will not close easily. In 1997, Moore and Wood [23] described the treatment of recurrent, involuntary TMJ dislocation using botulinum toxin A. The injected target was the lateral pterygoid muscle, and they injected each lateral pterygoid using electromyographic guidance. The investigators described that the effect lasted for 10 months. The lateral pterygoid is the muscle that is most responsible for opening; it is a difficult injection, which has a high potential for misplacement of the solution into other adjacent muscles.

Dyskinesia

Risk factors for the development of tardive dyskinesia are older age, female sex, and the presence of affective disorders [24]. For spontaneous dyskinesias, the prevalence rate is 1.5% to 38% in elderly individuals, depending on age and definition. Elderly women are twice as likely to develop the disorder [25]. When this disorder is associated with a drug use, the medications that are implicated most commonly are the neuroleptic medications that are now in widespread use as a component of behavioral therapy. The prevalence of drug-induced dyskinesia (tardive form) is approximately 15% to 30% in patients who receive long-term treatment with neuroleptic medications [26]. These medications chronically block dopamine receptors in the basal ganglia. The result would be a chemically-induced denervation supersensitivity of the dopamine receptors which leads to excessive movement; however, other neurotransmitter abnormalities in γ-aminobutyric acid (GABA)ergic and cholinergic pathways have been suggested. There are isolated reports in the literature that implicate dental treatment as a factor in the onset of spontaneous orofacial dyskinesia. Orofacial dyskinesia occurs as involuntary, repetitive, stereotypical movement of the lips, tongue, and sometimes the jaw during the day [27,28]. Sometimes the dyskinesia is induced by medication (tardive) or it can occur spontaneously. The spontaneous form of dyskinesia often affects the elderly. Typically, the tardive form of dyskinesia occurs in mentally ill patients who have a long-term exposure to medications that are used to treat the mental illness [29]. By definition, tardive dyskinesia requires at least 3 months of total cumulative drug exposure, which can be continuous or discontinuous. Moreover, the dyskinesia must persist more than 3 months after cessation of the medications in question. Most dopamine receptor antagonists cause oral tardive dyskinesia to one degree or another. The typical antipsychotics—and in recent years, even the atypical antipsychotics—including clozapine, olanzapine, and risperidone were reported to cause tardive dystonia and tardive dyskinesia. No adequate epidemiologic data exist regarding whether any particular psychiatric diagnosis constitutes a risk factor for the development of tardive reactions to medications; however, the duration of exposure to antipsychotics that is required to cause tardive reaction is from months to years. Exposure to antipsychotics need not be long, and a minimum safe period is not apparent. This duration of neuroleptic exposure seems to be shorter for women. A longer duration of exposure to neuroleptics does not correlate with the severity of the reaction. Treatment of orofacial dyskinesia is largely with medications (see later discussion).

Drug-induced dystonic-type extrapyramidal reactions

There are patients who have developed a medication-induced oral motor hyperactivity that does not fit into the dyskinesia category [30]. These medications and illegal drugs produce a motor response that is classified better as an unspecified extrapyramidal syndrome (EPS) reaction. EPS responses typically have three presentations: dystonia, akathisia, and parkinsonism. Dystonic reactions consist of involuntary, tonic contractions of skeletal muscles [31–33]. Akathisia reactions occur as a subjective experience of motor restlessness [34,35]. Patients may complain of an inability to sit or stand still, or a compulsion to pace or cross and uncross their legs. Parkinsonian reactions manifest themselves as tremor, rigidity, and akinesia, which shows as a slowness in initiating motor tasks and fatigue when performing activities that require repetitive movements (bradykinesia). When a medication or drug induces a dystonic EPS reaction, it typically involves the muscles of the head, face, and jaw that produce spasm, grimacing, tics, or trismus. Most of the literature has focused on the more severe acute dystonic EPS reactions that occur with use of antipsychotic medications. In addition to the antipsychotics, several antiemetics with dopamine receptor–blocking properties have been associated with tardive dystonia. These include prochlorperazine, promethazine, and metoclopramide. Of course, other less severe reactions do occur that vary in intensity and even wax and wane over time. The most commonly reported offending agents that are not neuroleptics are the selective serotonin reuptake inhibitors (SSRIs) and the stimulant medications and illegal drugs.

Serotonergic agents that cause extrapyramidal reactions

SSRIs (eg, fluoxetine, fluvoxamine, paroxetine, sertraline, citalopram, escitalopram) are used for depression and a variety of other mental illnesses. Unfortunately, these drugs are reported to produce the side effect of increased clenching and bruxism [36–39]. Actually the term "SSRI-induced bruxism" may not be accurate in that the actual motor behavior does not present as brief, strong, sleep state–related contractions as seen in bruxism, but more of an increased sustained nonspecific activation of the jaw and tongue musculature. Patients generally describe an elevated headache and tightness in their jaw, tongue, and facial structures. The best information available about the effect of SSRI class medications on oromandibular structures comes from a study in 1999, which examined the acute effects of paroxetine on genioglossus activity in obstructive sleep apnea [40]. It found that paroxetine, 40 mg, produced a clear augmentation of peak inspiratory genioglossus activity during non-rapid eye movement (NREM) sleep. Of course, the recent widespread use of SSRIs is based on a perception that these drugs have a lower side effect profile than do other categories of antidepressant medications (eg, tricyclics and monoamine oxidase inhibitors). Unfortunately, only case-based literature exists at this time; further polysomnographic studies on the motor effects of SSRIs are necessary to define prevalence and risk factors and to establish a causal relationship between SSRI use and oral motor disorders.

Stimulant drugs and other medications that cause extrapyramidal reactions

Illegal drugs, such as methamphetamine cocaine and 3,4-methylenedioxymethamphetamine (Ecstasy), and legal prescription stimulants, such as methylphenidate, phentermine, pemoline, dextroamphetamine, amphetamines, and diethylproprion, have been reported to induce bruxism and dystonic extrapyramidal reactions [41–45]. All stimulant drugs have the potential to cause extrapyramidal reactions and they are being used in greater numbers to treat obesity or as stimulants for children who have attention deficit hyperactivity disorder or narcolepsy and even for severe depression [46].

Differential diagnosis of orofacial motor disorder

The most important aspect of any clinician's skill is the ability to provide a differential diagnosis. With the exception of bruxism, all of the other motor disorders require a neurologic consultation to achieve a definitive diagnosis. This includes Bell's palsy, essential tremor, the focal and multifocal dystonias, the dyskinesias, the motor and vocal tics, and hemifacial spasm. Although the dentist will not be doing this examination, it is necessary to identify whether a patient has had a correct assessment before participating in the management of the patient. A proper initial diagnostic work-up for a movement disorder involves a full clinical examination, including a thorough neurologic examination. This is necessary to rule out the possibility that the motor dysfunction may be due to a central degenerative, demyelinating, or sclerotic lesion of the nervous system. Depending on the exact nature of the motor disorder, the examining physician may add a thorough medication and illegal drug history to the work-up. Standard, enhanced, and angiographic-type MRI will be taken of the brain and spinal cord to rule in or out a neurologic infarct or tumor or compression of these tissue; an electromyographic assessment may be ordered to identify specifically which muscles are involved and to assess the patient for a motor nerve or sensory nerve conduction deficit or a peripheral-origin myopathic disease or motor neuron abnormality; and for the most severe forms of bruxism and some myoclonic-type bruxism problems, it will be necessary to conduct a nocturnal polysomnogram, which includes an electroencephalogram. For the dystonias that affect a specific motor system (eg, blepharospasm or torticollis), it is necessary to assess that system thoroughly to ensure that no local infection or neoplastic or arthritic disease is present, to name only a few of the considerations. For disorders that involve the masticatory muscles, the tongue, or the perioral muscles, it is necessary for the dentist to conduct a careful examination to rule out local pathologic entities.

Treatment of orofacial motor disorders

If the dentist chooses to become involved in medicating patients who have OMDs, it is essential to be familiar with the pharmacodynamic and pharmacokinetic effects of medications that are prescribed as well as risk/benefit considerations. For dystonia and dyskinesia that have undergone a confirming medical differential diagnosis, it is preferable for the dentist to work in conjunction with a neurologist or psychiatrist who specializes in movement disorder, because pharmacologic management can be exceedingly complex and frustrating. This frustration is that although the medications described below can work effectively, more often only a small effect is seen and side effects can be substantial. Only a dentist who is well versed in pharmacologic approaches should attempt drug management, albeit this also should be done with continuing medical interaction. As far as surgical approaches for movement disorder, these are reserved for the most severe cases (see later discussion on interventional approaches).

There is no impressive data in the literature that suggest that a medication (other than botulinum toxin injections) can suppress bruxism reliably for more than a few days. Behavioral approaches should be addressed by the appropriate health care provider; they offer some help to patients who are having an acute stress problem that is influencing bruxism and clenching behavior, but again, data on true suppression of bruxism with a straight behavioral approach is lacking. Most of the time, the best treatment for bruxism is to fabricate an occlusal guard and try to protect the teeth from further attrition. Botulinum toxin injections are helpful for the more severe motor disorders, including bruxism.

General medical treatment strategy

For most OMDs, there is no well-defined treatment protocol except to rule out CNS disease and local pathology and to try one or more of the medications that may be helpful in these cases. If the disorder is severe enough and focal enough to consider, and the medications are not adequate, botulinum toxin injections can be considered. For patients who cannot be helped with the above, it is reasonable to consider neurosurgical therapy or implanted medication pumps that can deliver intrathecal medications. The use of motor blocking injections (botulinum toxin) can be considered. This method has proven to be most helpful for the focal dystonias and dyskinesias. In these disorders, injection of botulinum toxin is used successfully to block the transmission from the motor nerve to the motor end plate on the muscle for a period of 2 to 3 months (until the nerve sprouts and reconnects to the muscle). In the specific case of bruxism, some of the damage that is done by this behavior can be mitigated with the use of an intraoral appliance. For hemifacial spasm of spontaneous origin, intracranial surgical decompression surgery is used occasionally to remove the source of the irritation on the nerve.

Overview of interventional approaches

Surgical microvascular decompression

This approach can be used for hemifacial spasm if the clinician has determined that there is a compressive lesion of the facial nerve [47]. The involved blood vessel is lifted off from the facial nerve and often a sponge is placed between the vessel and the nerve bundle.

Myectomy

If a specific muscle is involved (focal dystonia) or predominates on the OMD presentation, severing it may offer a solution when the patient has been refractory to other, more conservative approaches and cannot function. Blepharospasm may respond to cutting of the orbicularis oculi muscle [48].

Pallidotomy

The globus pallidus is a functional entity within the basal ganglia in the brain. This procedure involves creating a surgical lesion (localized damage) in this area of the brain that is involved with motion control; this can be of value for certain dystonias and torticollis [49]. This is one surgical approach that is used for managing Parkinson's disease.

Deep brain stimulation

Deep brain stimulation uses an implanted electrode to deliver continuous high-frequency electrical stimulation to the thalamus, globus pallidus, or any part of the brain that is involved with the control of movement [50]. In spite of these methods, the prognosis for curing a specific OMD is poor; however, some of them can be managed successfully with a combination of education, medications, and selective injections of botulinum toxin.

Treatment of drug-induced dyskinesia and dystonic extrapyramidal reactions

The general rule is that the offending medication is withdrawn and it is hoped that the dyskinesia or dystonic reaction goes away [51]. Fortunately, acute dystonic reactions secondary to neuroleptic drugs are infrequent and disappear upon discontinuation of the medication; however, this may take days to months, depending upon the drug, its dose, and the patient. The same is true for less severe dystonic EPS reactions that are associated with SSRIs and stimulant drugs.

If the suspected medication cannot be stopped or if the motor hyperactivity is severe, the following methods are used to treat the motor hyperactivity: diphenhydramine, 50 mg, or benztropine, 2 mg intravenously (IV) or intramuscularly (IM) [52–54]. The preferred route of administration is IV, but if this is not feasible, IM drug administration can be used. Finally, amantadine, 200 to 400 mg/d by mouth [55], and diazepam, 5 mg IV [56], have been shown to be effective for recurrent neuroleptic-induced dystonic reactions. Some patients who have SSRI-induced dystonic EPS have relief when the dosage of SSRI or the other stimulant drug is reduced (eg, fluoxetine changed from 20 mg/d to 10 mg/d). Other patients respond to the addition of buspirone in dosages of 5 to 15 mg/d [57,58]. Other patients developed bruxism within the first few weeks of SSRI therapy; however, they were treated successfully with buspirone, 10 mg two to three times daily. Buspirone seems to be an effective treatment based on a few case reports. This drug may have an additional benefit of relieving anxiety if it is present. It is usually tolerated well and carries a low risk for significant side effects. Finally, switching to antidepressants that have not been associated with bruxism, such as mirtazapine or nefazodone, is an option.

Treatment of spontaneous dyskinesias and dystonias

With any new-onset movement disorders without obvious cause, a motor suppressive medication trial is logical. The commonly used medications are presented in Table 2. If the disorder is severe enough and focal enough to consider, and the medications are not adequate, botulinum toxin injections should be considered. Finally, for patients who cannot be helped with the above methods, and the scientific evidence to support alternative approaches is reasonable, consider neurosurgical therapy or implanted medication pumps that can deliver intrathecal medications. Regarding the prognosis of motor suppressive medications, a recent meta-analysis of the literature made several conclusions that should be shared with patients before starting treatment [59]. First, this review suggested that botulinum toxin has obvious benefit for the treatment of focal dystonias, such as cervical dystonia and blepharospasm. Second, trihexyphenidyl in high dosages is effective for the treatment of segmental and generalized dystonia in younger patients. Third, all other methods of pharmacologic intervention for generalized or focal dystonia, including botulinum toxin injections, have not been confirmed as being highly effective according to accepted evidence-based criteria.

Motor suppressive medications

There are multiple motor suppressive medications used in motor disorder management.

Anticholinergic therapy

The anticholinergic drugs, such as trihexyphenidyl hydrochloride, biperiden, or benztropine are the first line of motor suppressive medications used for dystonia, although they are only partially effective when compared with botulinum toxin injections [60,61]. It is critical to start at a low dose and increase the dose very slowly to try to minimize the adverse effects (dry mouth, blurred vision, urinary retention, confusion, memory loss).

Gamma-aminobutyric acid receptor agonist therapy

Baclofen is a GABA-ergic agent that is used in spasm [62]. The starting dosage is 10 mg at bedtime. The dosage should be increased by 10 mg

Table 2
Medications used for management of hyperkinetic motor disorders

Drug	Group	Starting dose	Usual dose	Indications	Receptor action
Trihexyphenidyl HCl (Artane)	Cholinergic antagonists	1 mg/d	6–15mg/d	Idiopathic parkinson's, extrapyramidal reactions, primary dystonias	Antagonizes acetylcholine receptors
Benztropine (Cogentin)	Cholinergic antagonists	1 mg bid	6 mg/d	Parkinsonism, extrapyramidal reactions, acute-onset secondary dystonias	Antagonizes acetylcholine and histamine receptors
Biperiden (Akineton)	Cholinergic antagonists	2 mg tid	16 mg/d	Parkinsonism, extrapyramidal disorders	Antagonizes acetylcholine receptors
Baclofen (Lioresal)	GABA agonist/ antispasmodic	10 mg/d	30–80 mg/d	Spasticity	Mechanism unclear, but most likely a GABA effect
Clonazepam (Klonipin)	GABA agonist/ tricyclic antidepressant	0.25 mg/d	1–4 mg/d	Seizures, absence anxiety, panic disorder, periodic leg movements, neuralgia	Binds to benzodiazepine receptors and enhances GABA effect
Tiagabine (Gabitril)	Anticonvulsant	4 mg/d	8–32 mg/d	Partial seizures	GABA reuptake inhibitor
Buspirone (Buspar)	Anxiolytic/hypnotic	7.5 mg bid	20–30 mg/d	Anxiety	Nonbenzodiazepine, but mechanism unclear

Amantadine (Symmetrel)	Antiviral/ antiparkinsonian	100 mg bid	100–300 mg/d	Influenza A, extrapyramidal reactions, parkinsonism	Mechanism unclear
Carbi/levodopa (Sinemet)	Antiparkinsonian	25–100 mg tid	200–2000 mg/d	Parkinson's associated tremor	Inhibits peripheral dopamine decarboxylation, dopamine precursor
Diphenhydramine (Benadryl)	Antihistamine	25 mg tid	400 mg/d	Dystonic reactions	Antagonizes central and peripheral H1 receptors (nonselective)
Clonidine (Catapres)	α-2 adrenergic agonist	0.1 mg bid	0.3 mg bid	Shown helpful for tardive dyskinesia	Stimulates α-2 adrenergic receptor
Botulinum toxin type A (Botox)	Neuromuscular blocker	20–50 U per large jaw closer muscle	Max: 200 units every 3 months	Focal dystonia	Blocks release of acetylcholine from motor end plate

Abbreviations: bid, twice a day; Max, maximum; tid, three times a day.

each week to a maximum of 30 mg three or four times daily. The best data for baclofen is not for oral medications, but for intrathecal injections of baclofen that are delivered with an implantable pump [63,64]. The main side effects include drowsiness, confusion, dizziness, and weakness. Finally, a recent report suggests that tiagabine, a GABA reuptake inhibitor that is used as an adjunctive anticonvulsant treatment for partial seizures, can be helpful in bruxism reduction [65]. The dosages of tiagabine that are used to suppress nocturnal bruxism at bedtime (4–8 mg) are lower than those that are used to treat seizures.

Benzodiazepine therapy

Benzodiazepines can be effective for suppression of focal, segmental, and generalized dystonia [66]. They bind to a specific benzodiazepine receptor on GABA receptor complex, which increases GABA affinity for its receptor. No study has found a significant difference between the various benzodiazepines and clonazepam, which has been widely used in movement disorders. The starting dose for clonazepam is 0.25 mg at bedtime and gradually increasing the dosage to a maximum of 1 mg four times daily. The main side effects include drowsiness, confusion, trouble concentrating, and dizziness.

Dopamine therapy

A specific subset of dystonias that have an onset in childhood was shown to respond remarkably well to low-dosage L-dopa, such as carbi/levodopa. These dystonias are referred to as dopa-responsive dystonias (DRD), and have been shown in recent years to encompass adult parkinsonism, adult-onset parkinsonism, adult-onset oromandibular dystonia, spontaneously remitting dystonia, developmental delay and spasticity mimicking cerebral palsy, and limb dystonia that is not only diurnal but related clearly to exercise [67,68].

Miscellaneous drugs for movement disorder therapy

There are several miscellaneous drugs that have been reported to suppress motor disorders. One medication that is used to suppress motor activity is buspirone, which is a nonbenzodiazepine anxiolytic drug [60,69]. Another drug whose mechanism is unclear is amantadine, which is used to suppress extrapyramidal reactions [70]. Other drugs that suppress motor activity are diphenhydramine [71] and clonidine [72].

Skeletal muscle relaxants

There are numerous drugs that are approved by the US Food and Drug Administration and used for relief of local regional musculoskeletal pain and spasm, including carisoprodol, chlorzoxazone, cyclobenzaprine hydrochloride, metaxalone, methocarbamol, and orphenadrine citrate [73].

Generally, these medications are used only for acute clinical proven spasm and are not recommended for long-term use. This is because the evidence is weak that these muscle relaxants are beneficial for individuals who have chronic muscle pain that affects the neck and lower back [74,75]. As far as chronic involuntary oral motor disorders are concerned, these drugs are ineffective and do not play a role in their management.

Botulinum toxin

In 2003, a thorough review of botulinum toxin for oral motor disorders was published; it described the potential uses and current evidence basis for using this medication in the orofacial region [76]. The toxin that is used in botulinum toxin injections is produced by the anaerobic bacterium *Clostridium botulinum*. This injectable drug is able to block motor nerve conduction, and once injected, it suppresses muscle activity for a time period that ranges from 8 weeks to 16 weeks for botulinum toxin type-A. Any clinician who has used this medication will testify to its powerful and dramatic effect in some cases. Unfortunately, this treatment is only palliative. Botulinum acts by interfering with vesicular exocytosis, which blocks the release of neurotransmitters that are contained within these vesicles. The blockage occurs when the toxin enters the nerve and cleaves proteins that are needed for the docking and release of the vesicle contents into the synaptic cleft [77]. Acetylcholine is believed to be the main neurotransmitter that is blocked by the BoNT/A. BoNT/A is manufactured by Allergan, Inc. (Irvine, California), as Botox [78]. This agent is supplied in vials in a lyophilized form, at a dose of 100 U per vial. The typical expiration date is 24 months when stored at -5 to $-20°$C. Another serotype, BoNT/B, is marketed by Solstice Neurosciences, Inc. (San Diego, California) as Myobloc®. Another BoNT/A formulation, Dysport, is marketed outside of the United States by Ipsen Ltd. in Europe. All of these preparations—Botox, Myobloc, and Dysport⁻differ in formulation and potency; hence, their units are not interchangeable. Side effects can be divided into site-of-injection side effects and medication-related side effects. With regard to site-of-injection side effects, the needles that are used for most injections are small (27–30-gauge needles); if the skin is cleaned properly, then the chances of local hematoma, infection, or persistent pain in the injection site is extremely low. Medication-related side effects generally are few, transitory, and tolerated well by patients. The most common medication-related side effect is adjacent muscle weakness (eg, an inadvertent weakening of the muscles of facial expression or swallowing when this is not desired). For patients who have had injections into the lateral pterygoid or palatal muscles, slurred speech with palatal weakness also is a distinct possibility. In general, these "inadvertent weakness" complications that are due to local diffusion of the drug can and do occur. Moreover, this complication is technique and dose-dependent [79–81]. A second side effect with botulinum toxin injections of the masticatory muscle is an alteration in the character of the saliva of patients who have not had direct salivary gland injections. Although this is an uncommon problem, some patients report that their saliva is diminished and thicker (ie, ropy saliva); it is more likely with higher doses and for injections around the parotid or submandibular gland. Obviously, this effect is desired at times if there is a substantial sialorrhea problem.

In most cases, the above complications are less problematic than are the untreated original motor disorder and generally do not stop the patient from seeking additional injections. If the injections are being used primarily to treat pain secondary to contraction, these complications might be more bothersome. Fortunately, persistent, more significant complications are distinctly rare. For example, systemic complications are uncommon and although several studies have reported a flulike syndrome, particularly after the first injection, such symptoms also have been reported following placebo injection. Finally, some patients develop antibodies to the toxin. It is unclear exactly what factors predispose to development of antibodies, but some studies suggest that the risk is increased by higher-dose and more frequent injections. For this reason, injections are not done more often than once every 12 weeks.

References

[1] Clark GT, Koyano K, Browne PA. Oral motor disorders in humans. J Calif Dent Assoc 1993;21(1):19–30.
[2] Kato T, Thie NM, Montplaisir JY, et al. Bruxism and orofacial movements during sleep. Dent Clin North Am 2001;45(4):657–84.
[3] Winocur E, Gavish A, Volfin G, et al. Oral motor parafunctions among heavy drug addicts and their effects on signs and symptoms of temporomandibular disorders. J Orofac Pain 2001;15(1):56–63.
[4] Reding GR, Rubright WC, Zimmerman SO. Incidence of bruxism. J Dent Res 1966;45(4): 1198–204.
[5] Glaros AG. Incidence of diurnal and nocturnal bruxism. J Prosthet Dent 1981;45(5):545–9.
[6] Wetter TC, Pollmacher T. Restless legs and periodic leg movements in sleep syndromes. J Neurol 1997;244(4)(Suppl 1):S37–45.
[7] van der Zaag J, Lobbezoo F, Wicks DJ, et al. Controlled assessment of the efficacy of occlusal stabilization splints on sleep bruxism. J Orofac Pain 2005;19(2):151–8.
[8] Van Zandijcke M, Marchau MM. Treatment of bruxism with botulinum toxin injections. J Neurol Neurosurg Psychiatry 1990;53(6):530.
[9] Ivanhoe CB, Lai JM, Francisco GE. Bruxism after brain injury: successful treatment with botulinum toxin-A. Arch Phys Med Rehabil 1997;78(11):1272–3.
[10] Tan EK, Jankovic J. Treating severe bruxism with botulinum toxin. J Am Dent Assoc 2000; 131(2):211–6.
[11] Pidcock FS, Wise JM, Christensen JR. Treatment of severe post-traumatic bruxism with botulinum toxin-A: case report. J Oral Maxillofac Surg 2002;60(1):115–7.
[12] Clark GT, Minakuchi H. The role of oral appliances in the management of TMDs. In: Laskin D, Green C, Hylander W, editors. Temporomandibular disorders: an evidenced approach to diagnosis and treatment. Chicago: Quintessence Publishing Co, Inc; 2006. p. 1–15.
[13] Tolosa E, Marti MJ. Blepharospasm-oromandibular dystonia syndrome (Meige's syndrome): clinical aspects. Adv Neurol 1988;49:73–84.

[14] Richter A, Loscher W. Pathology of idiopathic dystonia: findings from genetic animal models. Prog Neurobiol 1998;54(6):633–77.

[15] Cardoso F, Jankovic J. Dystonia and dyskinesia. Psychiatric Clin North Am 1997;20(4):821–38.

[16] Korczyn AD, Inzelberg R. Dystonia. Curr Opin Neurol Neurosurg 1993;6(3):350–7.

[17] Defazio G, Abbruzzese G, Livrea P, et al. Epidemiology of primary dystonia. Lancet Neurol 2004;3(11):673–8.

[18] Le KD, Nilsen B, Dietrichs E. Prevalence of primary focal and segmental dystonia in Oslo. Neurology 2003;61(9):1294–6.

[19] Gomez-Wong E, Marti MJ, Cossu G, et al. The 'geste antagonistique' induces transient modulation of the blink reflex in human patients with blepharospasm. Neurosci Lett 1998; 251(2):125–8.

[20] Blitzer A, Brin MF, Greene PE, et al. Botulinum toxin injection for the treatment of oromandibular dystonia. Ann Otol Rhinol Laryngol 1989;98(2):93–7.

[21] Blitzer A, Brin MF, Fahn S. Botulinum toxin injections for lingual dystonia. Laryngoscope 1991;101(7)(Pt 1):799.

[22] Charles PD, Davis TL, Shannon KM, et al. Tongue protrusion dystonia: treatment with botulinum toxin. South Med J 1997;90(5):522–5.

[23] Moore AP, Wood GD. Medical treatment of recurrent temporomandibular joint dislocation using botulinum toxin A. Br Dent J 1997;183(11–12):415–7.

[24] Tanner CM, Goldman SM. Epidemiology of movement disorders. Curr Opin Neurol 1994; 7(4):340–5.

[25] Jankovic J. Cranial-cervical dyskinesias: an overview. Adv Neurol 1988;49:1–13.

[26] Brasic JR. Clinical assessment of tics. Psychol Rep 2001;89(1):48–50.

[27] Blanchet PJ, Abdillahi O, Beauvais C, et al. Prevalence of spontaneous oral dyskinesia in the elderly: a reappraisal. Mov Disord 2004;19(8):892–6.

[28] Klawans HL, Tanner CM, Goetz CG. Epidemiology and pathophysiology of tardive dyskinesias. Adv Neurol 1988;49:185–97.

[29] Casey DE. Pathophysiology of antipsychotic drug-induced movement disorders. J Clin Psychiatry 2004;65(Suppl 9):25–8.

[30] Fernandez HH, Friedman JH. Classification and treatment of tardive syndromes. Neurologist 2003;9(1):16–27.

[31] Chouinard G. New nomenclature for drug-induced movement disorders including tardive dyskinesia. J Clin Psychiatry 2004;65(Suppl 9):9–15.

[32] Trosch RM. Neuroleptic-induced movement disorders: deconstructing extrapyramidal symptoms. J Am Geriatr Soc 2004;52(12 Suppl):S266–71.

[33] Tarsy D, Baldessarini RJ, Tarazi FI. Effects of newer antipsychotics on extrapyramidal function. CNS Drugs 2002;16(1):23–45.

[34] Tarsy D. Neuroleptic-induced extrapyramidal reactions: classification, description, and diagnosis. Clin Neuropharmacol 1983;6:9–26.

[35] Van Putten T, May PRA, Marder SR. Akathisia with haloperidol and thiothixene. Arch Gen Psychiatry 1984;41:1036–9.

[36] Ellison JM, Stanziani P. SSRI-associated nocturnal bruxism in four patients. J Clin Psychiatry 1993;54(11):432–4.

[37] Romanelli F, Adler DA, Bungay KM. Possible paroxetine-induced bruxism. Ann Pharmacother 1996;30(11):1246–8.

[38] Gerber PE, Lynd LD. Selective serotonin-reuptake inhibitor-induced movement disorders. Ann Pharmacother 1998;32(6):692–8.

[39] Lobbezoo F, van Denderen RJ, Verheij JG, et al. Reports of SSRI-associated bruxism in the family physician's office. J Orofac Pain 2001;15(4):340–6.

[40] Berry RB, Yamaura EM, Gill K, et al. Acute effects of paroxetine on genioglossus activity in obstructive sleep apnea. Sleep 1999;22(8):1087–92.

[41] Peroutka SJ, Newman H, Harris H. Subjective effects of 3,4-methylenedioxymeth-amphetamine in recreational users. Neuropsychopharmacology 1988;1(4):273–7.

[42] Vollenweider FX, Gamma A, Liechti M, et al. Psychological and cardiovascular effects and short-term sequelae of MDMA ("ecstasy") in MDMA-naive healthy volunteers. Neuropsychopharmacology 1998;19(4):241–51.
[43] Fazzi M, Vescovi P, Savi A, et al. [The effects of drugs on the oral cavity]. Minerva Stomatol 1999;48(10):485–92 [in Italian].
[44] See SJ, Tan EK. Severe amphetamine-induced bruxism: treatment with botulinum toxin. Acta Neurol Scand 2003;107(2):161–3.
[45] Winocur E, Gavish A, Voikovitch M, et al. Drugs and bruxism: a critical review. J Orofac Pain 2003;17(2):99–111.
[46] Malki GA, Zawawi KH, Melis M, et al. Prevalence of bruxism in children receiving treatment for attention deficit hyperactivity disorder: a pilot study. J Clin Pediatr Dent 2004;29(1):63–7.
[47] Yuan Y, Wang Y, Zhang SX, et al. Microvascular decompression in patients with hemifacial spasm: report of 1200 cases. Chin Med J (Engl) 2005;118(10):833–6.
[48] Bates AK, Halliday BL, Bailey CS, et al. Surgical management of essential blepharospasm. Br J Ophthalmol 1991;75(8):487–90.
[49] Eltahawy HA, Saint-Cyr J, Giladi N, et al. Primary dystonia is more responsive than secondary dystonia to pallidal interventions: outcome after pallidotomy or pallidal deep brain stimulation. Neurosurgery 2004;54(3):613–9.
[50] Bertrand C, Molina-Negro P, Martinez SN. Combined stereotactic and peripheral surgical approach for spasmodic torticollis. Appl Neurophysiol 1978;41(1–4):122–33.
[51] Scott BL. Evaluation and treatment of dystonia. South Med J 2000;93(8):746–51.
[52] Raja M. Managing antipsychotic-induced acute and tardive dystonia. Drug Saf 1998;19(1):57–72.
[53] Gelenberg AJ. Treating extrapyramidal reactions: some current issues. J Clin Psychiatry 1987;Sep(Suppl 48):24–7.
[54] Donlon PT, Stenson RL. Neuroleptic induced extrapyramidal symptoms. Dis Nerv Sys 1976;37:629–35.
[55] Borison RL. Amantadine in the management of extrapyramidal side effects. Clin Neuropharmacol 1983;6(Suppl 1):S57–63.
[56] Gagrat D, Hamilton J, Belmaker RH. Intravenous diazepam in the treatment of neuroleptic-induced acute dystonia and akathisia. Am J Psychiatry 1978;135:1232–3.
[57] Pavlovic ZM. Buspirone to improve compliance in venlafaxine-induced movement disorder. Int J Neuropsychopharmacol 2004;20:1–2.
[58] Bostwick JM, Jaffee MS. Buspirone as an antidote to SSRI-induced bruxism in 4 cases. J Clin Psychiatry 1999;60(12):857–60.
[59] Balash Y, Giladi N. Efficacy of pharmacological treatment of dystonia: evidence-based review including meta-analysis of the effect of botulinum toxin and other cure options. Eur J Neurol 2004;11(6):361–70.
[60] Bhidayasiri R. Dystonia: genetics and treatment update. Neurologist 2006;12(2):74–85.
[61] Costa J, Espirito-Santo C, Borges A, et al. Botulinum toxin type A versus anticholinergics for cervical dystonia. Cochrane Database Syst Rev 2005;25(1):CD004312.
[62] Gracies JM, Nance P, Elovic E, et al. Traditional pharmacological treatments for spasticity. Part II: General and regional treatments. Muscle Nerve Suppl 1997;6:S92–120.
[63] Rawicki B. Treatment of cerebral origin spasticity with continuous intrathecal baclofen delivered via an implantable pump: long-term follow-up review of 18 patients. J Neurosurg 1999;91(5):733–6.
[64] Ford B, Greene PE, Louis ED, et al. Intrathecal baclofen in the treatment of dystonia. Adv Neurol 1998;78:199–210.
[65] Kast RE. Tiagabine may reduce bruxism and associated temporomandibular joint pain. Anesth Prog 2005;52(3):102–4.
[66] Davis TL, Charles PD, Burns RS. Clonazepam-sensitive intermittent dystonic tremor. South Med J 1995;88(10):1069–71.

[67] Bressman SB. Dystonia update. Clin Neuropharmacol 2000;23(5):239–51.
[68] Nygaard TG, Marsden CD, Fahn S. Dopa-responsive dystonia: long-term treatment response and prognosis. Neurology 1991;41:174–81.
[69] Bonifati V, Fabrizio E, Cipriani R, et al. Buspirone in levodopa-induced dyskinesias. Clin Neuropharmacol 1994;17(1):73–82.
[70] Konig P, Chwatal K, Havelec L, et al. Amantadine versus biperiden: a double-blind study of treatment efficacy in neuroleptic extrapyramidal movement disorders. Neuropsychobiology 1996;33(2):80–4.
[71] van't Groenewout JL, Stone MR, Vo VN, et al. Evidence for the involvement of histamine in the antidystonic effects of diphenhydramine. Exp Neurol 1995;134(2):253–60.
[72] Wagner ML, Walters AS, Coleman RG, et al. Randomized, double-blind, placebo-controlled study of clonidine in restless legs syndrome. Sleep 1996;19(1):52–8.
[73] Arulmozhi DK, Veeranjaneyulu A, Bodhankar SL. Migraine: current concepts and emerging therapies. Vascul Pharmacol 2005;43(3):176–87.
[74] Pettengill CA, Reisner-Keller L. The use of tricyclic antidepressants for the control of chronic orofacial pain. Cranio 1997;15(1):53–6.
[75] Saarto T, Wiffen PJ. Antidepressants for neuropathic pain. Cochrane Database Syst Rev 2005;20(3):CD005454.
[76] Clark GT. The management of oromandibular motor disorders and facial spasms with injections of botulinum toxin. Phys Med Rehabil Clin N Am 2003;14(4):727–48.
[77] Meunier FA, Schiavo G, Molgo J. Botulinum neurotoxins: from paralysis to recovery of functional neuromuscular transmission. J Physiol (Paris) 2002;96(1–2):105–13.
[78] Anderson ER. Non-cosmetic uses of botulinum neurotoxin: scientific and clinical update. Am J Health Syst Pharm 2004;61(Suppl 6):S3–4.
[79] Eleopra R, Tugnoli V, Caniatti L, et al. Botulinum toxin treatment in the facial muscles of humans: evidence of an action in untreated near muscles by peripheral local diffusion. Neurology 1996;46(4):1158–60.
[80] Wohlfarth K, Schubert M, Rothe B, et al. Remote F-wave changes after local botulinum toxin application. Clin Neurophysiol 2001;112(4):636–40.
[81] Klein AW. Contraindications and complications with the use of botulinum toxin. Clin Dermatol 2004;22(1):66–75.

ELSEVIER
SAUNDERS

THE DENTAL
CLINICS
OF NORTH AMERICA

Dent Clin N Am 51 (2007) 245–261

A Critical Review of the Use of Botulinum Toxin in Orofacial Pain Disorders

Glenn T. Clark, DDS, MS[a],*, Alan Stiles, DMD[b],
Larry Z. Lockerman, DDS[c], Sheldon G. Gross, DDS[d]

[a]*Department of Diagnostic Sciences, Orofacial Pain and Oral Medicine Center,
University of Southern California, 925 West 34th Street, Los Angeles, CA 90089, USA*
[b]*Oral and Maxillofacial Surgery Department, Thomas Jefferson University,
909 Walnut Street, Third Floor, Philadelphia, PA 19107, USA*
[c]*Temporomandibular Joint/Headache Center, University of Massachusetts Memorial Medical
Center, University of Massachusetts Medical School, 119 Belmont Street,
Worcester, MA 01605, USA*
[d]*University of Connecticut Health Center, Farmington, CT 06030, USA*

This paper is divided into two parts; the first part provides a background on botulinum neurotoxin (BoNT) for medical uses as well as a description of how to use it. The second part provides a critical review of the evidence regarding the use of BoNT for pain in the orofacial region. This review was based on published literature gathered from Medline databases. Specifically, the authors looked for papers that were randomized, double-blind, placebo-controlled trials (RBCTs) that were published in peer-reviewed journals. Where these were not widely available, they describe the case report and open-label clinical trials–based evidence.

Regarding the medical use of BoNT, as soon as it became evident that victims of food poisoning experienced motor paralysis as a part of their disease and that the bacterium *Clostridium botulinum* was responsible, the idea that a toxin that is produced by this bacteria might have medical uses was not far behind. It was in the 1920s that BoNT was purified first [1]. It was not a single toxin that was produced by this anaerobic bacterium; seven serologically distinct forms were discovered (BoNT/A, B, C, D, E, F, G) [2]. From that point to the point at which the United States Food and Drug Association (FDA) approved BoNT/A was 60 plus years [3]. Toxin A was

* Corresponding author.
E-mail address: gtc@usc.edu (G.T. Clark).

0011-8532/07/$ - see front matter © 2007 Elsevier Inc. All rights reserved.
doi:10.1016/j.cden.2006.09.003

dental.theclinics.com

found to be the most potent and longest lasting of these seven toxins, and it has since proven to be a valuable treatment for focal muscle hyperactivity disorders (eg, focal dystonias). BoNT/A was approved for use by the FDA for the temporary treatment of two eye muscle disorders (blepharospasm and strabismus), and for cervical dystonia 1 year later [4]. The injections clearly reduce the severity of motor contraction–induced abnormal head position and accompanying neck pain. Also in 2000, the FDA approved BoNT/B for the treatment of cervical dystonia in patients who developed BoNT/A resistance. Since then, BoNT/A has been approved for the treatment of primary axillary hyperhidrosis (excessive sweating) and for the reduction of deep glabellar lines in the face. Table 1 contains the FDA-approved use specifications for BoNT/A and BoNT/B. BoNT/A is supplied in vials in a lyophilized form, at a dose of 100 units (U) per vial. The typical expiration date is 24 months when stored at -5 to $-20°C$. Another serotype, BoNT/B, is marketed by Solstice Neurosciences, Inc. (San Diego, California) as Myobloc. Another BoNT/A formulation, Dysport, is marketed outside of the United States by Ipsen Ltd. in Europe. All of these preparations—Botox, Myobloc, and Dysport—differ in formulation and potency; hence, their units are not interchangeable.

Off-label botulinum neurotoxin use

In addition to the above on-label uses, BoNT/A is used off-label in the orofacial region to help treat primary and secondary masticatory and facial muscle spasm, severe bruxism, facial tics, orofacial dyskinesias, dystonias, and even idiopathic hypertrophy of the masticatory muscles. A recent review of the literature describes the muscle hyperactivity–related indications for BoNT/A in the orofacial muscles [5]. With the exception of hypertrophy, the common link for these conditions is that they are involuntary motor hyperactivity disorders; although their treatment with BoNT is off-label, they are similar in pathophysiology to the condition for which BoNT is approved by the FDA. Even more "off-label" is the suggested use of BoNT for pain disorders without a clear-cut motor hyperactivity basis. These pain disorders include conditions, such as chronic migraine headache, chronic daily headache (CDH), chronic myofascial pain, focal sustained neuropathic pain, and, more recently, episodic trigeminal neuralgia.

Using a drug off-label sometimes generates interest by the medical, legal, and federal regulatory communities. Off-label drug use is not illegal, and the FDA recognizes that the off-label use of drugs often is appropriate and, in time, may represent the standard of practice for a specific condition. The purpose of establishing an approved or labeled use of a drug by the FDA is to protect patients from unsafe or ineffective drugs; however, it is the prerogative of practitioners to use their professional judgment in providing the best treatment possible for their patients. Off-label use of a medication is not

Table 1
US Food and Drug Administration–approved (on-label) uses of botulinum neurotoxin

Disease or condition	FDA approval	Age limitation	Dosing recommendations (initially always use lower dose)[a]
Blepharospasm, strabismus association with dystonia, including benign essential blepharospasm or VII nerve disorders.	12/29/1989	Adults (>12 y)	Botox: dose is 1.25–2.5 U (0.05 mL to 0.1 mL at each site) injected into the medial and lateral pretarsal orbicularis oculi of the upper lid and into the lateral pretarsal orbicularis oculi of the lower lid.
Cervical dystonia in adults to decrease the severity of abnormal head position and neck pain associated with cervical dystonia.	12/21/2000	Adults (>16 y)	Botox: dose for cervical dystonia is between 198–300 U IM, divide dose among affected muscles; use < 100 U into SCM muscle to decrease dysphagia risk; duration 3 months. Myobloc: dose for cervical dystonia is between 2500–5000 U IM divided among affected muscles.
Cosmetic use for moderate to severe glabellar lines associated with corrugator or procerus muscle activity.	4/12/2002	Adults (≤65 y)	Botox Cosmetic: dose is 0.1 ml IM times 5 sites. This solution is injected into each corrrugator muscle and into the centrally located procerus muscle.
Primary axillary hyperhidrosis: Botox is indicated for the treatment of severe primary axillary hyperhidrosis that is inadequately managed with topical agents.	7/12/2004	Adults (>18 y)	Botox: dose for primary axillary hyperhidrosis is 50 U intradermal/axilla; divide dose into 10–15 injections of 3–4 U per injection positioned 1–2 cm apart.

Pediatric dose: safety and effectiveness in children younger than the age of 12 have not been established for blepharospasm or strabismus and younger than the age of 16 for cervical dystonia or 18 for hyperhidrosis.

Geriatric use: clinical studies of Botox did not include sufficient numbers of subjects aged 65 and older to determine whether they respond differently from younger subjects. Other reported clinical experience has not identified differences in responses between the elderly and younger patients. There were too few patients older than the age of 75 to enable any comparisons. In general, dose selection for an elderly patient should be cautious, usually starting at the low end of the dosing range, reflecting the greater frequency of decreased hepatic, renal, or cardiac function, and of concomitant disease or other drug therapy.

Abbreviations: IM, intramuscularly; SCM, sternocleidomastoid.

[a] Renal and hepatic dosing: not defined.

a license to use any product off-label without regard for the published scientific evidence of efficacy. The practitioner who elects to use a drug "off-label" bears some inherent liability risk. Legal rulings have suggested that off-label drug use in itself is not sufficient evidence of negligence; however, the practitioner should do so only when one believes that the off-label use is outweighed by the potential benefit to the patient. In such situations, the risks and benefits should be explained to the patient, and a consent form (Fig. 1) should be signed by the patient. The clinician also should be familiar with a reasonable body of scientific evidence that supports the application of the drug (in this case BoNT/A) specifically for the disorder under treatment. It also is important that the patient be informed that the expected therapeutic benefit may only extend weeks to months, and that the treatment will need to be repeated to have an ongoing effect.

BOTULINUM TOXIN Consent Form

I, _____, request that Dr. _____ DDS, perform BOTULINUM TOXIN injection into the necessary muscles (or sites) to treat my symptoms (or my musculoskeletal and/or neuropathic symptoms) as needed.

- I understand that this use of Botulinum Toxin is considered off-label by the Federal Drug Administration.

- I understand that Botulinum toxin injection treatments have a temporary effect and serial treatments may be required to maintain results, or attain further improvement.

- I understand that Botulinum toxin injection treatments contain human-derived albumin and carries a theoretical risk of virus transmission. I understand that there have been no proven cases of disease transmission through Botulinum toxin injections.

- I understand the possible side effects and complications. to the treated areas and adjacent skin to include redness, swelling, mild pain, bruising, numbness, infection, flu-like symptoms, temporary muscle aching, as well as paralysis of nearby muscle (which can cause droopy eyelids, double vision, of neck weakness.)

- I understand that the following complications, although uncommon, can occur and have been reported in the medical literature: anaphylaxis, erythema multiforme, dysphagia, dyspnea, respiratory compromise, syncope, acute closed angle glaucoma, focal facial paralysis, arrhythmias, myocardial infarction, dysphonia, ptosis, headache, neck pain, ocular dryness, punctuate keratitis, cough, flu symptoms, rhinitis, dizziness, muscle weakness, local numbness, xerostomia, injection site pain, speech disturbance, visual disturbance and skin rash.

- I acknowledge that I am not pregnant, nursing, and if of childbearing age, I am using adequate contraception.

- I acknowledge that I do not have a known allergy to albumin

- I acknowledge that I am not taking a blood thinner (other than baby aspirin).

- I understand that Botulinum toxin injections should not be used with any neuromuscular disorders like Myasthenia gravis or amyotrophic lateral sclerosis (ALS), a motor neuropathy, atrophy at the planned site or preexisting ptosis. It should not be used in patients with a cardiovascular disease.

- I understand that Botulinum toxin injections may not be effective if used with certain medications including: D-Penicillamine used for rheumatoid arthritis; Antimalarials such as chloroquine, chloroquine phosphate, hydroxychloroquine; Aminoglycosides, Antibiotics such as clindamycin, streptomycin, gentamycin, kanamycin; and Immunosuppressant such as cyclosporine; and magnesium sulfate, quinidine, succinylcholine and non-polarizing neuromuscular blockers.

- I understand the above and have had the risks, benefits, and alternatives explained to me. I give my informed consent for Botulinum toxin injections today as well as for the future treatments as needed.

Patient Signature: _____ Date: _____

Witness Signature: _____ Date: _____

Dentist Signature: _____ Date: _____

Fig. 1. Botulinum toxin consent form.

Mechanism of action

BoNT inhibits the exocytosis of acetylcholine (ACh) on cholinergic nerve endings of motor nerves [6]. Autonomic nerves also are affected by the inhibition of ACh release at the neural junction in glands and smooth muscle [7]. BoNT achieves this effect by its endopeptidase activity against SNARE proteins, which are 25-kd synaptosomal-associated proteins that are required for the docking of the ACh vesicle to the presynaptic membrane. It was suggested that when BoNT was used for the treatment of neuromuscular disorders—particularly focal dystonias and spastic conditions—patients reported a marked analgesic benefit [8]. Initially, this benefit was believed to be due to the direct muscle relaxation effect of BoNT; however, various observations have suggested that BoNT may exert an independent action on peripheral nociceptors by blocking exocytosis of such neurotransmitters as substance P, glutamate, and calcitonin gene–related peptide (CGRP). In addition, because BoNT does not cross the blood–brain barrier, and because it is inactivated during its retrograde axonal transport, the effect is believed to be in the first-order sensory nerve and not more centrally [9]. The actual experimental evidence that examines this analgesic claim is presented below.

Training and injection procedures

Training in the use of BoNT/A usually is accomplished by way of short training programs or preceptorships in the office of an experienced caregiver. As with any injected medication, it is imperative that clinicians undergo training that includes knowledge of anatomy, injection techniques, handling of the materials, side effects, and appropriate dosing, because different dosages are used in the different areas of the mouth, face, and neck for different medical conditions. Although the skills to inject BoNT into a muscle are learned easily, some training in this arena is suggested. Essentially, BoNT is injected in the same manner as are local anesthetics, and a 23- to 30-gauge needle is placed into the target muscle. Targeting is confirmed by palpation in larger muscles. When a muscle is difficult to palpate, such as the anterior digastric or lateral pterygoid muscles, confirmation of correct needle position before injection can be confirmed by use of a Teflon-coated monopolar injection needle that also has the ability to record the electromyographic (EMG) signals from the muscle. This technique requires specific training in the use of an EMG machine. The authors wish to emphasize that EMG guidance is not a requirement for injecting most orofacial muscles, because they can be injected safely by using palpation confirmation of location. Depending on the equipment used, the recording is displayed on a screen or turned into the sound pattern. The graphic display or sound increases in amplitude, frequency, or volume when the muscle contracts. To be sure that the practitioner is in the correct muscle, the patient may be asked to make a specific movement or effort to activate the target muscle. One can reduce the risk for BoNT dispersion into unwanted adjacent sites by using superficial injections, having the patient keep activity to minimum, and not massaging the area for 4 hours; this allows the toxin to penetrate mainly the target nerves. Ultrasound, fluoroscopy, or CT also may be used, but is needed rarely for the orofacial muscles.

Injection preparation, dosing, and effect duration

BoNT/A is kept frozen (2–4°C) in a vial until it is ready to use. The drug is put into solution, following manufacturer's guidelines, by adding normal saline (preservative-free 0.9% saline solution). Once prepared it should be used within 4 hours. The preferred syringe is a calibrated 1.0-mL tuberculin syringe, and the needle selected for injection usually is between 26 and 30 gauge. Skin preparation involves alcohol wipes and dry sterile gauze sponges. Aspiration before injection is recommended. Usually, dosing is established by the diagnosis and reason for use of the toxin, size of the muscle, and medical conditions or medications. Until studies narrow down all specifics, the final dilution and dosage used is left to the clinical experience and discretion of the practitioner. The number of injection sites usually is determined by the size of the muscle. Theoretically, it may be appropriate to inject more sites with smaller doses, and using more injection sites should facilitate a wider distribution of BoNT/A to nerve terminals; however, too many injection sites may cause local injection site pain. The proper targeting of muscles is a crucial factor in achieving efficacy and reducing adverse effects from BoNT/A injections. The therapeutic effects of BoNT/A first appear in 1 to 3 days, peak in 1 to 4 weeks, and decline after 3 to 4 months.

Adverse events and side effects

BoNT is classified as a Category C drug by the FDA, because its reported use in pregnant and lactating women is scant. Approximately 1% of patients who receive BoNT/A injections may experience severe, debilitating headaches that may persist at high intensity for 2 to 4 weeks before fading gradually [10]. Care in choosing the injection site and dose used may limit undesirable muscle weakness. A small group of patients eventually may develop antibodies; this problem generally occurs when patients receive higher doses, especially at more frequent intervals. Therefore, the FDA-approval label recommends injecting no more frequently than once every 3 months and using the lowest effective dose to minimize antibody formation.

Cautions and contraindications

When using BoNT/A, caution must be used when injecting individuals who have peripheral motor neuropathic diseases or neuromuscular junctional disorders. Moreover, drugs that interfere with neuromuscular transmission, such as aminoglycosides, magnesium sulfate, anticholinesterases, succinylcholine chloride, polymyxins, quinidine, and curare-like nondepolarizing blockers, can potentiate the effect of BoNT/A. BoNT/A treatment is contraindicated in the presence of infection, especially at the injection site and in individuals who have known hypersensitivity to any ingredient in the formulation. Formation of neutralizing antibodies to BoNT/A may reduce its effectiveness by inactivating the biologic activity of the toxin and the rate of formation of these neutralizing antibodies in patients who receive BoNT/A treatment; its long-term effects have not been studied well. The reformulated BoNT/A has a lower protein content that may decrease the risk for antibody formation and the development of resistance. Patients who have neuromuscular disorders who receive BoNT/A could have amplified effects of the drug, such as severe dysphagia and respiratory difficulties. Patients who have BoNT/A injections in the cervical region, tongue, or posterior region of the mouth may experience dysphagia. Rare cases of arrhythmia and myocardial infarction have been reported. Some of these patients had pre-existing cardiovascular disease. Caution also should be exercised when injecting patients who have excessive atrophy or weakness in target muscle, ptosis, excessive dermatochalasis, deep dermal scarring, thick sebaceous skin, marked facial asymmetry, and inflammatory skin disorder at the planned injection site. Box 1 contains a preinjection checklist.

Box 1. Preinjection check list

- Appropriate emergency drugs, such as epinephrine, should be available when a toxin is to be injected.
- The practitioner should have an established injection protocol that includes the specific locations and appropriate doses for the condition to be treated.
- All injection sites should have been evaluated properly. If the region to be injected has been surgerized previously, potential anatomic variations should be taken into consideration.
- The practitioner must be aware of all medications and supplements that are taken by the patient to minimize any effect on the potency of the BoNT/A.
- The practitioner should be aware of all medical conditions; vital signs, such as blood pressure, should be noted before injecting.
- It is strongly recommended that a consent form be explained to and signed by the patient (see Fig. 1).

Botulinum neurotoxin and experimental pain in animals

Regarding the evidence for BoNT as a pain control agent, it is appropriate to look first at how BoNT affects experimental pain in animals. Two animal studies examined how the release of pain-inducing neurotransmitters is suppressed in nociceptive afferents and sensory ganglia neurons by BoNT/A treatment [11,12]. In another rat model, the effect of BoNT on pain from nerve fibers in the bladder was examined. This was done by filling the bladder with a 0.3% acetic acid solution in BoNT/A-treated rats. Rats who had received BoNT/A previously showed a significantly decreased CGRP release at day 7 after the injection compared with control (non-BoNT/A) rats [13]. These neurochemistry studies are supported by an animal pain behavior study that examined the effect of BoNT on pain involved a subcutaneous injection of formalin into the paw of a rat [14]. This injection is known to cause the release of glutamate from the primary afferent neuron, which induces increased paw-licking behavior in the rat. The investigators reported that preconditioning the animal by giving it a BoNT injection into the paw before the formalin injection reduced paw licking. They suggested that this was evidence of a direct analgesic response from BoNT. Finally, in another pain behavior study, the antinociceptive effect of BoNT/A was examined using a rat model of carrageenan (1%)- and capsaicin (0.1%)-induced paw pain [15]. Mechanical and thermal responses were recorded. The investigators reported on the use of BoNT/A (5 U/kg) that was applied 6 days or 1 day before peripheral carrageenan or capsaicin injections. When used 6 days before injection, enhanced sensitivity to mechanical and thermal stimuli was reduced significantly or abolished. Based on these data, it was suggested that BoNT inhibits trigeminal hyperexcitability by blocking the antidromic flow of substance P and CGRP. This results in a decrease in peripheral sensitization of nociceptive fibers, which indirectly reduces central sensitization. Another pain inhibitory effect of BoNT/A may be by blocking stimulated CGRP release from sensory ganglia neurons [16].

Botulinum neurotoxin and experimental pain in humans

Two recent RBCTs examined experimental pain and BoNT in humans. These studies show conflicting results. A 2002 study specifically measured cutaneous nociception in 50 healthy adult volunteers who received bilateral subcutaneous forearm injections of 100 units of BoNT/A or placebo [17]. Pain thresholds for heat and cold in the treated skin areas were measured quantitatively. Quantitative sensory testing was performed before and 4 and 8 weeks after BoNT injection. The heat and cold pain thresholds increased by 1.4°C from baseline to week 4 and by 2.7°C by week 8. In comparison, the placebo site showed 1.1°C and 1.2°C changes at weeks 4 and 8, respectively. A similar trend was seen for electrical-induced pain thresholds, but none of these differences was statistically significant. The investigators concluded that no strong direct cutaneous antinociceptive effect for BoNT/A was demonstrated by their study. In contrast, Barwood and colleagues [18], in 2000, studied the analgesic effect of BoNT on 16 young children (mean age, 4.7 years) for management of their spastic cerebral palsy. These investigators reported that, compared with the placebo, BoNT/A injections reduced pain scores by 74% ($P < .003$). They did not measure pain threshold using quantitative sensory testing, and pain measurement in children this young might be problematic.

Previous systematic review of botulinum neurotoxin for pain

The animal, and, to a lesser degree, the human data that were reviewed in the preceding two sections provide the underpinnings for the theory that pain may be reduced by BoNT. It is not known which orofacial chronic pain disorders might be modulated by BoNT. This question was examined in a previous systematic review [19]. The reviewers examined published data on various head and neck pain conditions by performing a thorough search of the medical literature, striving to find RBCTs that evaluated the effect of BoNT on specific conditions. They reported that two RBCTs were found for cervicogenic headache; however, the results were in conflict, and therefore, nonconclusive. They also identified two studies that addressed chronic neck pain, but neither revealed significant efficacy data. Only one small trial was found that involved temporomandibular disorders (TMD) (N = 15 patients), but no conclusive effect was evident. No RBCT was identified for the use of BoNT in cluster headache, chronic paroxysmal hemicrania, or trigeminal neuralgia. Therefore, the investigators were unable to draw any definite conclusions about the effectiveness of BoNT on these conditions.

Myofascial trigger points

Myofascial trigger points are believed to be the result of abnormal motor end-plate activity that produces an excessive continuous release of the neurotransmitter ACh [6]. In theory, using neuromuscular blocking agents, such as BoNT, for myofascial trigger point pain would eliminate the end-plate dysfunction by blocking the release of Ach, and, thereby, reduce pain. An open-label case series on 77 patients that was published in 2003 reported reduced visual analog scale (VAS) pain levels after using BoNT/A for persistent trigger points [20]. In contrast, in 2006 an RBCT parallel clinical study examined the effect of BoNT on pain from muscle trigger points [21]. Although BoNT did not reduce motor end-plate activity, it had no better effect on pain or pain thresholds when compared with isotonic saline. The investigators concluded that BoNT does not have a specific antinociceptive or analgesic effect. In 2006, another double-blind, randomized, controlled crossover BoNT trial was reported on 31 subjects who had neck and shoulder

myofascial pain [22]. The investigators concluded that there was no difference between the effect of small doses of botulinum toxin A and those of
physiologic saline in the treatment of myofascial pain syndrome. Finally,
three other randomly assigned, double- or single-blind studies compared
BoNT/A with a control/comparison treatment. The first of these RBCTs
compared trigger point pain that was treated with BoNT/A versus saline
[23]. The study included 132 patients who had cervical or shoulder myofascial pain with active trigger points; it used VAS pain reports, pressure algo-
metry, and pain medication usage as the outcome measure. The
investigators reported no significant differences between the groups. Another recent randomized, double-blind, cross-over study compared BoNT/A
with bupivacaine and included 18 patients [24]. The investigators compared
the effectiveness of trigger point injections using the two agents in combination with a home-based rehabilitation program. After being injected, the
subjects were followed until their pain returned to at least 75% of their
preinjection pain for two consecutive weeks. After an additional 2-week
wash-out period, the subjects received the other treatment injection. Both
treatments were effective in reducing pain when compared with baseline
($P = .0067$), but there was no significant difference between the injected
agents in the duration or magnitude of pain relief, function, or satisfaction.
A third randomized, single-blind treatment comparison study, which evaluated BoNT/A with dry needling and lidocaine injections into cervical myofascial trigger points, was reported in 2005 [25]. This study involved 29
patients. Pain pressure thresholds and pain scores improved significantly
in all three groups, with a slightly greater response in the groups that received lidocaine and BoNT/A. Overall, these RBCTs suggest that BoNT
is no better or longer lasting than are the other standard trigger point– based
therapies. Overall, the literature suggests that BoNT is not better or longer
lasting than is placebo or other standard trigger point–based therapies.

Temporomandibular pain and dysfunction

The first open-label study for an acceptable size group of patients that
was diagnosed with a temporomandibular disorder occurred in 1999 [26].
This study reported on 15 adult patients who had a nonspecific heterogeneous diagnosis of temporomandibular joint pain and dysfunction. All subjects were given BoNT/A, 150 U, divided among the right and left masseter
and temporalis muscles. The investigators reported that jaw pain (VAS) and
muscle tenderness decreased, with no reported side effects. In 2000, these investigators expanded their data set and reported on a larger case series of 60
patients who had mixed temporomandibular disorders, many of whom
qualified as having chronic tension-type headaches (CTTHs; n = 46).
BoNT/A was used under open-label uncontrolled conditions [27,28]. The investigators reported significant results for all measured outcomes, except for

maximum bite force. In 2001, another open-label study reported on the effect of BoNT/A for chronic facial pain in 41 patients who had the diagnosis of temporomandibular dysfunction [29]. The investigators injected an average of 200 U of BoNT/A on each side into the jaw closing muscles, and followed the patients for an average of 6.7 months. They reported that 80% of patients improved, with a mean pain reduction of 45% (VAS). One patient had reversible speech and swallowing difficulties. A recent report (also an open-label case series) looked specifically at temporomandibular disk function in 26 patients [30]. The investigators used BoNT/A (12.5 U) injected into the lateral pterygoid muscle, although some patients also received injections into the temporalis, medial pterygoid, and masseter muscles when severe tenderness was noted. Except for clicking of the right joint, all outcome measures (pain, opening, left temporomandibular joint clicking, headache) improved.

Open-label case reports do not constitute strong evidence, and all such preliminary reports need to have RBCTs conducted to assess fully the true effect of the therapy being examined. The full story that underlies TMD and BoNT can be better understood by looking at two RBCTs. The first involved 90 patients who had a heterogeneous diagnosis of chronic facial pain, including temporomandibular dysfunction. Sixty subjects received masticatory muscle injections with BoNT/A, whereas 30 subjects received a placebo injection [31]. This study was only single-blinded (ie, the injectors knew what substance was being injected), which increases the risk for inducing bias in the study outcome. Moreover, the technique was not described clearly and it was unknown whether the investigators injected bilaterally in most patients. If they did and they used 70 U per muscle (medial pterygoid, masseter, temporalis), one must assume that they applied nearly 400 U of BoNT/A per patient. Ninety-one percent of the patients who received BoNT/A showed an improved VAS pain score. The mean change was 3.2 points on a 10-point scale, which was significantly different from the change seen with placebo injections (0.4 points). In contrast to the above study is another RBCT on jaw muscle pain in a smaller sample [32]. This second RBCT included 15 women who had chronic moderate to severe jaw muscle pain. The study was double-blind, using a total of 150 U of BoNT/A divided between the right and left temporalis and masseter muscles. Data were collected at baseline and at 8, 16, and 24 weeks after injection. A major difference compared with the previous study was that the subjects were crossed over to the comparison treatment after 16 weeks. Five subjects did not complete the study. For the 10 patients who finished, no statistically significant difference was found in pain variables. The investigators concluded that the results do not support the use of BoNT/A for moderate to severe jaw closing muscle pain. Based on these two studies, it is not clear whether the effect of BoNT/A injections for jaw muscle pain, using doses in the 100- to 150-U range, will be sustained.

Chronic migraine

That patients experienced relief of migraine symptoms as a unexpected side benefit of having BoNT injections for hyperfunctional facial lines was reported in 2000 [33]. Two additional studies have concluded that BoNT/A is an effective and safe prophylactic treatment for headache across a range of patient types [34,35], including migraine of cervical origin [36]. A recent review of the literature summarized the data on BoNT/A for migraine prophylaxis [37]. Based on a combination of open-label data and three RBCTs on episodic migraine, it was concluded that BoNT/A is effective in migraine prophylaxis. Its main effect was to reduce the frequency, severity, and disability that is associated with migraine headaches. The first of these studies, in 2002, examined 123 subjects using a random-assignment, double-blind, vehicle-controlled approach. All subjects had a history of two to eight moderate-to-severe migraine attacks per month, with or without aura [38]. Diaries were kept during a 1-month baseline and for 3 months following the injection period. The group that received BoNT/A, 25 U, showed significantly fewer migraine attacks per month, a reduced maximum severity of migraines, a reduced number of days of acute migraine medication use, and a reduced incidence of migraine-associated vomiting [39]. The second study was less clear-cut and examined 60 patients who had migraines using an RBCT method. Subjects received BoNT/A or placebo injections. There were no significant differences between the groups with respect to reduction of migraine frequency, number of days with migraine, and the number of total single doses to treat a migraine attack. Overall, this study did not report any added efficacy of BoNT/A for the prophylactic treatment of migraine beyond placebo; however, subsequently, it was questioned whether the dose (16 U) was too low. Finally, a third RBCT study looked at a subset of 228 patients on the use of BoNT/A or placebo for the prophylaxis of CDH, presumed to be of migrainous origin, without the confounding factor of concurrent prophylactic medications [40]. The subjects were adults with 16 or more headache days per 30-day period; all had a history of migraine or probable migraine and were not receiving concomitant prophylactic headache medications. One hundred and seventeen subjects received BoNT/A and 111 subjects received placebo injections. The maximum change in the mean frequency of headaches per 30 days was −7.8 with BoNT/A compared with only −4.5 with placebo. This difference was statistically significant; the investigators concluded that BoNT/A was an effective and well-tolerated prophylactic treatment for migraine headaches in patients who had CDHs are were not using other prophylactic medications.

Chronic tension-type headache

In contrast to the open-label studies, in which some benefit was shown [41,42], the RBCTs that examined the use of BoNT/A for patients who have CTTH or CDH suggest little to no benefit. Specifically in 2001, an RBCT that involved 60 subjects concluded "in the important outcome variables, such as pain intensity, number of pain free days and consumption of analgesics, there were no statistical differences between the [BoNT/A] and control group" [43]. In 2004, another RBCT on BoNT/A was performed that involved 40 subjects who had CTTH [44]. The investigators concluded that there was no significant difference between the two treatment groups (BoNT/A or saline) on the patient's assessment of improvement after 12 weeks. Finally, a large, multiple-center RBCT was performed [45]. This study examined 112 patients who had CTTH using BoNT/A or placebo injections; there were no significant differences between the two groups. Again, these investigators concluded that there is no evidence of improvement with the use of botulinum toxin A on CTTH. In 2006, two additional RBCTs reported that "for the primary endpoint, the mean change from baseline in the number of TTH-free days per month, there was no statistically significant difference between placebo and four BoNTA groups" [46], and "the between-group difference of 1.5 headache-free days favored BoNT-A treatment, although the difference between the groups was not statistically significant" [47]. Based on these five RBCTs that examined the use of BoNT/A in CTTH, the authors conclude that the evidence for efficacy of BoNT in CTTHs and CDHs is non-existent or weak at best.

Focal chronic orodental neuropathic pain

Based on the animal studies and pharmacology of the drug, BoNT/A may well be effective as a treatment for focal trigeminal neuropathic pain (eg, atypical toothache, phantom tooth pain, and possibly neuromas) that is caused by nerve injury. Although not proof that oral neuropathic pain will respond, one study examined localized postamputation pain before and after BoNT injections [48]. This open-label case report described four cases of chronic phantom pain of more than 3 years that were treated successfully. The investigators used BoNT/A injected into four muscle trigger points in the amputation stump of each patient. All trigger points were painful to compression before injection, and all patients reported referred sensations in the phantom foot from at least one of the trigger sites. In all cases, the phantom pain was reduced by about 60% to 80%. In the absence of reports of BoNT that is used to treat atypical odontalgia, phantom tooth pain, or trigeminal neuroma pain, it is impossible to formulate an opinion on whether BoNT/A will be helpful in treating these problems.

Trigeminal neuralgia

Several investigators have described the effects of botulinum toxin injections on trigeminal neuralgia. Unfortunately, all of these studies have been open-label, uncontrolled reports. The first was a report on 11 patients who had chronic facial pain that was due to trigeminal neuralgia. The investigators reported that 75% (8 of 11) of patients responded favorably, and claimed that the beneficial effect lasted between 2 and 4 months. In this open-label study, BoNT/A was used at doses that ranged from 25 to 75 U per patient [49]. Three additional case reports followed this initial report. The sample sizes for these three studies ranged from a single patient to 13 patients. All of these reports described substantial pain reduction as a result of BoNT injections, the dose ranged between 10 U and 100 U, and the improvement lasted between 2 and 6 months [50–52]. Although these case reports are interesting, they do not provide enough quality data to make any recommendation about the efficacy of BoNT injections for trigeminal neuralgia.

Trigeminal autonomic cephalalgia

Trigeminal autonomic cephalalgias include cluster headache, shortlasting unilateral neuralgiform headache attacks with conjunctival injection and tearing (SUNCT), and chronic paroxysmal hemicrania. These painful, highly disruptive pain disorders are not prevalent enough in most clinics for a randomized, blinded, clinical trial to be conducted to assess the effect of botulinum toxin. For this reason, no RBCTs can be used to guide us about the efficacy of BoNT for suppressing trigeminal autonomic cephalalgia pain events.

Summary

The animal experimental literature suggests that BoNT can inhibit peripheral pain processes, but BoNT cannot produce remarkable cutaneous anesthesia in the area above an injection site. Although anesthesia is not critical to blocking chronic pain phenomena if it were present, this would strengthen the theory that BoNT might decrease neural input to the trigeminal nuclei, and, thus, potentially reverse chronic neuropathic pains that are manifested in the head, neck, and orofacial regions. When the quality data on this application are analyzed with regard to its use on patients who have orofacial pain, the following conclusion are suggested:

> The studies for resistant myofascial trigger points demonstrate no difference from already accepted lidocaine injections or even placebo injections.
> For temporomandibular pain and dysfunction, the published data are flawed in that a heterogeneous population has been used, and the methodology and number of patients tested also can be called into question. Insufficient evidence is available to make specific treatment recommendations.

For migraine prophylaxis, there is a general consensus among clinicians who treat migraine that BoNTs may have an effective role in the population that has failed other modalities. It is the opinion of the authors that the most evidence exists for migraine prophylaxis, and that in the more refractory cases, BoNT is a viable treatment modality.

For CTTHs, the evidence does not support the use of BoNT injections.

For the trigeminal neuropathic conditions (eg, atypical facial and odontogenic pain and phantom tooth pain, and neuromas), acceptable evidence is lacking.

For the use of BoNT in trigeminal neuralgia, the literature is limited to case reports; few individuals have been treated. BoNT has not been tested in a placebo-controlled, double-blind fashion in trigeminal neuralgia; therefore, it is the opinion of the authors that insufficient evidence exists to be able to come to a definitive recommendation for the use of BoNT for trigeminal neuralgia.

For the autonomic cephalalgias (eg, cluster headache, chronic paroxysmal hemicrania, and SUNCT), the literature is not sufficient; therefore, the authors are unable to come to a definitive recommendation.

References

[1] Schantz EJ. Historical perspective. In: Jankovic J, Hallett M, editors. Therapy with botulinum toxin. New York: Marcel Dekker; 1994. p. xxiii–xxvi.

[2] Coffield JA, Considine RV, Simpson LL. The site and mechanism of action of botulinum toxin. In: Jankovic J, Hallett M, editors. Therapy with botulinum toxin. New York: Marcel Dekker; 1994. p. 3–13.

[3] Anderson ER. Non-cosmetic uses of botulinum neurotoxin: scientific and clinical update. Am J Health Syst Pharm 2004;61(Suppl 6):S3–4.

[4] Use of botulinum toxin-A in pain associated with neuromuscular disorders. Available at: http://www.health.state.mn.us/htac/botox.htm. Accessed October 21, 2006.

[5] Clark GT. The management of oromandibular motor disorders and facial spasms with injections of botulinum toxin. Phys Med Rehabil Clin N Am 2003;14(4):727–48.

[6] Meunier FA, Schiavo G, Molgo J. Botulinum neurotoxins: from paralysis to recovery of functional neuromuscular transmission. J Physiol (Paris) 2002;96(1–2):105–13.

[7] Bhidayasiri R, Truong DD. Expanding use of botulinum toxin. J Neurol Sci 2005;235(1–2): 1–9.

[8] Aoki KR. Evidence for antinociceptive activity of botulinum toxin type A in pain management. Headache 2003;43(Suppl 1):S9–15.

[9] Dressler D, Adib Saberi F. Botulinum toxin: mechanisms of action. Eur Neurol 2005;53(1): 3–9.

[10] Alam M, Arndt KA, Dover JS. Severe, intractable headache after injection with botulinum A exotoxin: Report of 5 cases. J Am Acad Dermatol 2002;46(1):62–5.

[11] Welch MJ, Purkiss JR, Foster KA. Sensitivity of embryonic rat dorsal root ganglia neurons to Clostridium botulinum neurotoxins. Toxicon 2000;38(2):245–58.

[12] Durham PL, Cady R, Cady R. Regulation of calcitonin gene-related peptide secretion from trigeminal nerve cells by botulinum toxin type A: implications for migraine therapy. Headache 2004;44(1):35–43.

[13] Chuang YC, Yoshimura N, Huang CC, et al. Intravesical botulinum toxin a administration produces analgesia against acetic acid induced bladder pain responses in rats. J Urol 2004; 172(4 Pt 1):1529–32.

[14] Cui M, Khanijou S, Rubino J, et al. Subcutaneous administration of botulinum toxin A re-
     duces formalin-induced pain. Pain 2004;107:125–33.
[15] Bach-Rojecky L, Lackovic Z. Antinociceptive effect of botulinum toxin type a in rat model
     of carrageenan and capsaicin induced pain. Croat Med J 2005;46(2):201–8.
[16] Fielder T, Durham PL. Stimulation of CGRP secretion from trigeminal ganglia neurons by
     nitric oxide and repression by botulinum toxin type A. Soc Neurosci Abstr Viewer Itiner
     2003;ABS588.6.
[17] Blersch W, Schulte-Mattler WJ, Przywara S, et al. Botulinum toxin A and the cutaneous no-
     ciception in humans: a prospective, double-blind, placebo-controlled, randomized study.
     J Neurol Sci 2002;205(1):59–63.
[18] Barwood S, Baillieu C, Boyd R, et al. Analgesic effects of botulinum toxin A: a randomized,
     placebo-controlled clinical trial. Dev Med Child Neurol 2000;42(2):116–21.
[19] Sycha T, Kranz G, Auff E, et al. Botulinum toxin in the treatment of rare head and neck pain
     syndromes: a systematic review of the literature. J Neurol 2004;251(Suppl 1):I19–30.
[20] De Andres J, Cerda-Olmedo G, Valia JC, et al. Use of botulinum toxin in the treatment of
     chronic myofascial pain. Clin J Pain 2003;19(4):269–75.
[21] Qerama E, Fuglsang-Frederiksen A, Kasch H, et al. A double-blind, controlled study of bot-
     ulinum toxin A in chronic myofascial pain. Neurology 2006;67(2):241–5.
[22] Ojala T, Arokoski JP, Partanen J. The effect of small doses of botulinum toxin a on neck-
     shoulder myofascial pain syndrome: a double-blind, randomized, and controlled crossover
     trial. Clin J Pain 2006;22(1):90–6.
[23] Ferrante FM, Bearn L, Rothrock R, et al. Evidence against trigger point injection technique
     for the treatment of cervicothoracic myofascial pain with botulinum toxin type A. Anesthe-
     siology 2005;103(2):377–83.
[24] Graboski CL, Shaun Gray D, Burnham RS. Botulinum toxin A versus bupivacaine trigger
     point injections for the treatment of myofascial pain syndrome: a randomised double blind
     crossover study. Pain 2005;118(1–2):170–5.
[25] Kamanli A, Kaya A, Ardicoglu O, et al. Comparison of lidocaine injection, botulinum toxin
     injection, and dry needling to trigger points in myofascial pain syndrome. Rheumatol Int
     2005;25(8):604–11.
[26] Freund B, Schwartz M, Symington JM. The use of botulinum toxin for the treatment of tem-
     poromandibular disorders: preliminary findings. J Oral Maxillofac Surg 1999;57(8):916–20
     [discussion 920–1].
[27] Freund B, Schwartz M, Symington JM. Botulinum toxin: new treatment for temporoman-
     dibular disorders. Br J Oral Maxillofac Surg 2000;38(5):466–71.
[28] Freund BJ, Schwartz M. Relief of tension-type headache symptoms in subjects with tempo-
     romandibular disorders treated with botulinum toxin-A. Headache 2002;42(10):1033–7.
[29] von Lindern JJ. Type A botulinum toxin in the treatment of chronic facial pain associated
     with temporo-mandibular dysfunction. Acta Neurol Belg 2001;101(1):39–41.
[30] Karacalar A, Yilmaz N, Bilgici A, et al. Botulinum toxin for the treatment of temporoman-
     dibular joint disk disfigurement: clinical experience. J Craniofac Surg 2005;16(3):476–81.
[31] von Lindern JJ, Niederhagen B, Berge S, et al. Type A botulinum toxin in the treatment of
     chronic facial pain associated with masticatory hyperactivity. J Oral Maxillofac Surg 2003;
     61(7):774–8.
[32] Nixdorf DR, Heo G, Major PW. Randomized controlled trial of botulinum toxin A for
     chronic myogenous orofacial pain. Pain 2002;99(3):465–73.
[33] Klein AW, Glogau RG. Botulinum toxin: beyond cosmesis. Arch Dermatol 2000;136(4):
     539–41.
[34] Barrientos N, Chana P, De la Cerda A, et al. Efficacy and safety of botulinum toxin in mi-
     graine: 1-year follow-up. J Neurol Sci 2003;214(1–2):91.
[35] Binder WJ, Brin MF, Blitzer A, et al. Botulinum toxin type A (BOTOX) for treatment of
     migraine headaches: an open-label study. Otolaryngol Head Neck Surg 2000;123(6):
     669–76.

[36] Krusz JC. Intradermal botulinum toxin type B for migraine of cervical origin. Am J Pain Manag 2004;14(3):81–4.

[37] Gobel H. Botulinum toxin in migraine prophylaxis. J Neurol 2004;251(Suppl 1):I8–11.

[38] Silberstein S, Mathew N, Saper J, et al. Botulinum toxin type A as a migraine preventive treatment. For the BOTOX Migraine Clinical Research Group. Headache 2000;40(6): 445–50.

[39] Evers S, Vollmer-Haase J, Schwaag S, et al. Botulinum toxin A in the prophylactic treatment of migraine–a randomized, double-blind, placebo-controlled study. Cephalalgia 2004; 24(10):838–43.

[40] Dodick DW, Mauskop A, Elkind AH, et al. BOTOX CDH Study Group. Botulinum toxin type A for the prophylaxis of chronic daily headache: subgroup analysis of patients not receiving other prophylactic medications: a randomized double-blind, placebo-controlled study. Headache 2005;45(4):315–24.

[41] Relja M, Telarovic S. Botulinum toxin in tension-type headache. J Neurol 2004;251(Suppl 1): I12–4.

[42] Blumenfeld A. Botulinum toxin type A as an effective prophylactic treatment in primary headache disorders. Headache 2003;43(8):853–60.

[43] Schmitt WJ, Slowey E, Fravi N, et al. Effect of botulinum toxin A injections in the treatment of chronic tension-type headache: a double-blind, placebo-controlled trial. Headache 2001; 41(7):658–64.

[44] Padberg M, de Bruijn SF, de Haan RJ, et al. Treatment of chronic tension-type headache with botulinum toxin: a double-blind, placebo-controlled clinical trial. Cephalalgia 2004; 24(8):675–80.

[45] Schulte-Mattler WJ, Krack P, BoNTTH Study Group. Treatment of chronic tension-type headache with botulinum toxin A: a randomized, double-blind, placebo-controlled multi-center study. Pain 2004;109(1–2):110–4.

[46] Silberstein SD, Gobel H, Jensen R, et al. Botulinum toxin type A in the prophylactic treatment of chronic tension-type headache: a multicentre, double-blind, randomized, placebo-controlled, parallel-group study. Cephalalgia 2006;26(7):790–800.

[47] Mathew NT, Frishberg BM, Gawel M, et al, BOTOX CDH Study Group. Botulinum toxin type A (BOTOX) for the prophylactic treatment of chronic daily headache: a randomized, double-blind, placebo-controlled trial. Headache 2005;45(4):293–307.

[48] Kern U, Martin C, Scheicher S, et al. [Treatment of phantom pain with botulinum-toxin A. A pilot study.] Schmerz 2003;17(2):117–24 [in German].

[49] Borodic GE, Acquadro MA. The use of botulinum toxin for the treatment of chronic facial pain. J Pain 2002;3:21–7.

[50] Türk U, Ilhan S, Alp R, et al. Botulinum toxin A and intractable trigeminal neuralgia. Clin Neuropharmacol 2005;28:161–2.

[51] Allam N, Brasil-Neto JP, Brown G, et al. Injections of botulinum toxin type a produce pain alleviation in intractable trigeminal neuralgia. Clin J Pain 2005;21(2):182–4.

[52] Piovesan EJ, Teive HG, Kowacs PA, et al. An open study of botulinum-A toxin treatment of trigeminal neuralgia. Neurology 2005;65(8):1306–8.

ELSEVIER
SAUNDERS

THE DENTAL
CLINICS
OF NORTH AMERICA

Dent Clin N Am 51 (2007) 263–274

Complementary and Alternative Medicine for Persistent Facial Pain

Cynthia D. Myers, PhD, LMT[a,b,*]

[a]*Integrative Medicine Program, H. Lee Moffitt Cancer Center & Research Institute,
12902 Magnolia Drive, Tampa, FL 33612, USA*
[b]*Department of Interdisciplinary Oncology, College of Medicine,
University of South Florida, Tampa, FL, USA*

Complementary and alternative medicine (CAM) is described by the National Institutes of Health (NIH) National Center for Complementary and Alternative Medicine (NCCAM) as a group of unconventional medical systems, practices, and products not presently considered part of the conventional biomedical care provided by medical doctors and other conventionally trained health professionals [1]. For most CAM therapies, there are unanswered questions regarding safety, cost-effectiveness, efficacy, and mechanisms of action. Facilitating the scientific evaluation of CAM is a key objective of NCCAM.

NCCAM groups CAM therapies into the following five categories: mind–body interventions, manipulative and body-based therapies, biologically based therapies, energy therapies, and alternative medical systems. Mind–body interventions aim to increase the mind's capacity to enhance bodily function and reduce symptoms. Examples from this category include biofeedback, relaxation, meditation, hypnosis, and yoga and other movement therapies involving a component of mental focus. Spiritual approaches, such as prayer, are categorized as mind–body interventions. Additional mind–body interventions once considered to be outside of conventional medical or dental treatment have achieved integration into multidisciplinary pain treatment and mainstream care on the basis of evidence for their safety and improved treatment outcomes resulting from their inclusion in combined treatments [2]. These include patient education, cognitive-behavioral

* Integrative Medicine Program, MRC-PSY H. Lee Moffitt Cancer Center & Research Institute, 12902 Magnolia Drive Tampa, FL 33612.
E-mail address: myerscd@moffitt.usf.edu

0011-8532/07/$ - see front matter © 2007 Elsevier Inc. All rights reserved.
doi:10.1016/j.cden.2006.09.008   *dental.theclinics.com*

coping skills training, and behavioral modification techniques such as habit reversal.

NCCAM defines manipulative and body-based therapies as physical modalities such as massage therapy, chiropractic adjustments, and osteopathic manipulations. Biologically based therapies include foods, vitamins, minerals, herbal products, and other natural substances used as dietary supplements. Energy therapies are of two types. In the first type, practitioners intend to manipulate biofields theorized to exist within and around the patient. The second type of energy therapy involves the unconventional use of electromagnetic fields for therapeutic purposes.

The final category delineated by NCCAM, the alternative medical systems, is comprised of complete systems of theory and practice, often predating modern Western biomedicine. These systems share an aim to support an innate tendency of the body toward health and can include interventions from all the other categories of CAM. Homeopathy and naturopathy are examples of alternative medical systems arising in Western culture. Homeopaths intend to stimulate the body's capacity for healing by providing minute doses of natural products. Naturopaths may use nutritional modifications, dietary supplements, homeopathic remedies, hydrotherapy, massage, and counseling to prevent illness or to rebuild health. Traditional Chinese medicine uses mind–body therapies such as tai chi and chi gong, which are meditative movement therapies, along with natural products derived from plant and animal sources, therapeutic massage, and acupuncture to facilitate and balance energy flow, which is theorized to be central to health.

According to a comprehensive report produced in 2005 by the Institute of Medicine on CAM and what is known about Americans' use of it, CAM is being integrated into conventional health care practice in hospitals and physicians' offices, some health maintenance organizations are covering selected CAM therapies, and insurance coverage for CAM is increasing. The Institute of Medicine recommended that health care should strive to be comprehensive and evidence based, with conventional medical treatments and CAM held to the same standards for demonstrating clinical effectiveness [3].

Data on the use of complementary and alternative medicine

The most reliable data on the use of CAM by the general public in the United States come from a 2004 report [4] based on the results of the 2002 National Health Interview Survey (NHIS). The NHIS, one of the major data collection systems of the National Center for Health Statistics of the Centers for Disease Control and Prevention, surveys nationally representative samples of civilian households in the United States. The 2002 NHIS included questions on the use of CAM and was administered by in-home, in-person interviews with 31,044 adults aged 18 and over, representing a response rate of 74%. Respondents were asked about their use (ever and during the past 12 months) of 27 different CAM therapies, including

10 provider-based therapies (eg, acupuncture, chiropractic, and massage therapy) and 17 CAM therapies for which a provider is not necessary (eg, natural products, special diets, megavitamin therapy, and prayer for one's own health). For therapies used during the past 12 months, respondents were queried about the health problem or condition being treated with CAM therapy and the reason or reasons for choosing CAM.

NHIH 2002 results indicated that 36% of United States adults used some form of CAM during the prior 12 months when analyses did not include prayer for health. Musculoskeletal conditions, including back pain or back problems, neck pain or neck problems, and joint pain or stiffness, were the conditions for which CAM was most often used, confirming prior studies finding chronic or recurring musculoskeletal pain linked to CAM use [5–9]. More than a quarter of those using CAM believed that conventional medicine would not help their health care problem. Consistent with earlier surveys on CAM use [5,6], the 2002 NHIS found that most CAM users also see medical doctors for conventional medical care. In addition to pain, predictors of increased CAM use included higher educational attainment, having private health insurance, living in an urban rather than rural area, having been a smoker in the past but not currently, and female gender.

Given these national data on the use of CAM by the Unites States population, it would seem by an extension of logic that there might be relatively high use of CAM by patients who have persistent facial pain because pain and female gender are predictors of CAM use, and women are at higher risk for persistent facial pain. Three published studies provide information on CAM use by clinic samples of patients who have facial pain.

Turp [10] studied prior health care use by 206 consecutive patients referred to a tertiary care facial pain clinic and found that most patients had previously consulted between one and four health care providers. Several patients had seen more than four. Chiropractors had been consulted by nearly 15% of patients, acupuncturists by 4%, and massage therapists by 2%.

Raphael and colleagues [11] indicated 22% of a sample of 63 women meeting Research Diagnostic Criteria for temporomandibular disorder (TMD) [12] but never previously treated with intraoral appliance used one or more CAM therapy for their facial pain. The following treatment modalities were classified by the investigators as CAM: acupuncture, relaxation therapy, stress management, chiropractic, transcutaneous electrical nerve stimulator, and biofeedback. Patients reporting greater interference in social functioning due to pain had used more CAM. Patients for whom an accident was the initiating event for facial pain were seven times more likely to have used CAM. Although the investigators did not raise this possibility, it may be that access to CAM therapies was affected by the onset of facial pain being linked to an accident because CAM therapies are sometimes more readily covered by insurance when provided for injuries sustained in an accident and are otherwise usually paid for out of pocket. Pain severity, pain duration, and mood did not predict CAM use. The investigators noted that the fact that the women in their sample had not previously received an intraoral splint suggested that their sample may have received fewer health care interventions than many facial pain patients seen in tertiary care centers, and therefore estimates of CAM use from this sample might underestimate CAM use by patients who have more extensive treatment histories.

DeBar and colleagues [13] surveyed 192 patients (91% female) with documented TMD meeting Research Diagnostic Criteria about CAM use. Participants had been part of pilot-phase focus groups or baseline assessment for clinical trials on CAM for facial pain. More than one third of the sample (35.9%) had used CAM for TMD, and nearly two thirds of the sample (64.1%) had used CAM for other health conditions, with more than half of these using CAM for another musculoskeletal condition (eg, back, neck, or shoulder problems). Of the 69 participants using CAM specifically for TMD, massage was the most commonly reported CAM therapy (66.7%). Chiropractic care (30.4%), biofeedback or visual imagery (39.1%), and over-the-counter herbal supplements (21.7%) were also used for TMD. Massage was reported as the most satisfactory CAM therapy for TMD, and naturopathic care, massage, and chiropractic care were most often rated very helpful for TMD. Herbal supplements and homeopathic remedies were rated among the least satisfactory and least helpful modalities used to treat TMD.

Among the most frequent reasons for using CAM for TMD in the study by DeBar and colleagues [13] was a perceived failure of conventional treatment to relieve symptoms (44.9%). Participants using CAM for TMD tended to be older, were more likely to have a history of multiple medical problems, and reported more positive psychologic functioning relative to other participants. Noting the relatively high proportion of participants in their study using CAM, the investigators suggested that it might reflect a self-selection bias because all participants were willing to take part in research on CAM. Nonetheless, the investigators noted, their list of CAM therapies was relatively narrow compared with other studies reporting lower prevalence of CAM use with more inclusive definitions of CAM, and they concluded that it is important to include systematic assessment of CAM use when providing allopathic treatment of TMD.

Scientific evaluation of complementary and alternative medicine for persistent facial pain

Published reports

To ascertain the most rigorous evaluation of completed research on CAM therapies for persistent facial pain, published peer-reviewed clinical trials randomizing patients who had facial pain to a CAM intervention or to a control or comparison group and comparing outcome on at least one

patient self-report measure of facial pain were sought in the medical literature using the PUBMED and CINAHL electronic databases. The strategy
involved pairing the word pain with facial, TMJ, TMD, and temporomandibular and with terms drawn from the literature on CAM therapies used by
facial pain patients: complementary, alternative, acupuncture, biofeedback,
relaxation, herbal, massage, chiropractic, homeopathic, and naturopathic.
Review articles were also sought in the same databases and in the Cochrane
Library. Studies were excluded if a CAM modality was administered in
combination with one or more other interventions (eg, relaxation training
or biofeedback as a component of cognitive behavioral stress management
training). Case studies were not sought.

Results

The present search strategy yielded 15 original research reports. Of these
15, eight tested biofeedback, three tested relaxation, and five tested acupuncture. (One tested biofeedback against relaxation.) Therefore, in terms of representation of the NCCAM classifications of CAM, interventions from the
mind–body interventions (biofeedback, relaxation) and alternative medical
systems (acupuncture) have been studied in controlled research available
through the current search strategy. No published results of randomized
controlled or comparison clinical trials were located testing the effects of
manipulative or body-based therapies such as chiropractic, massage, or
osteopathic manipulations, biologically based therapies such as dietary supplements or herbal remedies, or energy therapies.

Biofeedback

In a review of electromyographic (EMG) biofeedback treatment alone or
in combination with stress management training for treatment of TMD,
Crider and Glaros [14] identified six trials with either a no-treatment or placebo control. Of the six no-treatment or placebo controlled trials, three
[15–17] assessed the effects of EMG biofeedback alone on patient report
of pain. Hijzen and colleagues [15] found biofeedback to be associated
with significantly greater reduction in myofascial pain dysfunction (MPD)
pain relative to intraoral splint or no-treatment control. Dohrmann and
Laskin [16] reported reduced pain and reduced masseter EMG levels in
MPD patients who were provided instruction in EMG biofeedback (n =
16) as compared with placebo (n = 8). Dalen and colleagues [17] reported
significant reduction at follow-up in MPD pain intensity and pain duration
after participation in eight biweekly EMG sessions (n = 10) or the control
condition (n = 9). Findings from the three placebo or no-treatment control
trials therefore indicated that biofeedback training was associated with reduced pain, relative to control.

Five comparative trials were located [18–22], three of which [18–20] were
previously summarized in Crider and Glaros [14]. Olson and Malow [18]

randomly assigned MPD patients to masseter biofeedback (n = 6), frontalis biofeedback (n = 6), or frontalis biofeedback plus psychotherapy (n = 6). Relative to normative data from their patient population, the investigators reported that the three treatments were associated with reduced pain report and reduced tenderness upon examination. Frontalis biofeedback plus psychotherapy was associated with the greatest reduction in tenderness. In a sample of 30 patients, Dahlstrom and Carlsson [19] found self-report of pain to be significantly reduced at 1 month and 12 months post-treatment with EMG biofeedback training or intraoral splint, with no significant difference between treatments. Mishra and colleagues [21] compared biofeedback training (EMG and thermal), cognitive-behavioral skills training (CBST), combination biofeedback/CBST, and no-treatment control in 94 patients who had TMD who were randomly assigned to treatment. The biofeedback-only group showed the greatest improvement post-treatment, but participants in all three active treatments reported pain reduction relative to pretreatment. Combined biofeedback/CBST treatment was associated with the most improvement at 1-year follow-up. Erlandson and Poppen [22] randomized female MPD patients to three groups: Group 1 received instruction in bilateral masseter EMG biofeedback, Group 2 received bilateral masseter EMG biofeedback plus instructions on placing the jaw in a resting position, and Group 3 received bilateral masseter EMG biofeedback plus intraoral prosthetic guides. Of the patients initially reporting pain, one in four patients in Group 1 reported a decrease in pain, four of five patients in Group 2 reported a decrease in pain, and three of four patients in Group 3 reported reduced pain. Given the study design, it is difficult to make direct comparisons between groups; however, it seems that in this study EMG biofeedback was more effective in combined treatment than as a sole treatment. Funch and Gale [20] reported no between-group difference on outcomes post-treatment in patients who had chronic temporomandibular joint pain randomly assigned to biofeedback (n = 30) or relaxation training (n = 27).

To summarize the evidence from biofeedback studies, biofeedback was consistently superior to placebo or no-treatment control in terms of pain reduction in three trials. Results of comparison of biofeedback to other active treatments yielded mixed results in pain outcomes, with biofeedback alone sometimes superior to the comparison group, sometimes equivalent to comparison, and sometimes less effective than the comparison group. Participant samples were generally small in these biofeedback trials.

Relaxation

Three trials of relaxation training [20,23,24] met criteria for discussion. Additional trials incorporating relaxation training were located but are not reported here because pain was not assessed by self-report [25] or because relaxation training was provided as a component of multicomponent training [26,27]. In a comparison trial, Funch and Gale [20] found no difference on post-treatment pain report between two active treatments: relaxation training involving the use of audiotaped instructions for muscle relaxation (n = 27) and biofeedback (n = 30). Winocur and colleagues [23] evaluated the effectiveness of "hypnorelaxation" (n = 15) compared with occlusal appliance (n = 15) or minimal treatment (n = 10) for women who had masticatory myofascial pain disorder. Results indicated that both potentially active treatment groups were superior to minimal treatment with regard to muscular sensitivity on palpation, but only hypnorelaxation was significantly more effective than minimal treatment with regard to patients' self-report of pain on a visual analog scale. Sherman and colleagues [24] randomly assigned 21 patients with mixed facial pain diagnoses to a single session of stretch-based relaxation or a session of resting and found no significant group differences post-treatment on pain.

To summarize results of studies on relaxation, no placebo-controlled studies were located. Three comparison trials were located. Relaxation was equivalent to two potentially active treatments used as comparison interventions (biofeedback or resting) and was superior to occlusal appliance. As was the case with biofeedback trials, participant sample size was relatively small in studies of relaxation effects on persistent facial pain.

Acupuncture

Five qualifying trials of acupuncture for persistent facial pain were located [28–35]. In two of these, acupuncture was compared with a no-treatment control. Johansson and colleagues [28] randomly assigned 45 patients who had TMD to acupuncture, intraoral splint, or control. Pain was assessed pretreatment and at 3 months follow-up in the two treatment groups and at 2 months follow-up in the control group. Both active treatments were associated with significant improvement relative to control post-treatment. A limitation of the study results from the use of differing follow-up periods for the two treatment groups and the control group. List and colleagues [29,30] randomly assigned 110 patients who had TMD to acupuncture, intraoral splint, or wait list control. Pain diaries were completed by 96 patients, with results indicating that both active treatments were associated with significant pain reduction at post-treatment and follow-up.

Three studies compared acupuncture with another active treatment or to sham treatment. Raustia [31–33] randomly assigned 50 patients who had TMD to acupuncture or to a multimodal treatment including counseling, occlusal adjustment, splint therapy, and exercises. Immediate results slightly favored multimodal treatment; however, the two treatment groups did not differ at follow-up. Schmid-Schwap and colleagues [34] randomly assigned female patients who had TMD to needle acupuncture (n = 11) or sham laser acupuncture (n = 12). Needle acupuncture was associated with significantly greater reduction in self-reported pain immediately post-treatment; however, pain ratings were higher pretreatment in the acupuncture group.

Thus, regression to the mean cannot be ruled out. Goddard and colleagues [35] randomized 18 patients who had facial pain (15 females) to acupuncture at authentic (n = 10) versus sham (n = 8) acupuncture points. In this study, patients did not rate their clinical pain; rather, patients used visual analog scales to rate pain evoked by the maximal pressure they could tolerate from a pressure algometer applied to the masseter muscle 5 minutes before treatment and again post-treatment. Both groups showed significant reduction in their ratings of the post-treatment pressure stimulus, with no significant between-group difference, indicating that the effects on pain were not dependent upon location of needle insertion.

To summarize results of studies of acupuncture for persistent facial pain, two studies used three-group designs that permitted testing acupuncture against a control condition and comparison to an active treatment. Both studies found acupuncture to be superior to control but equivalent to the comparison treatment in terms of pain outcomes. Two studies compared acupuncture with a comparison or sham treatment and showed mixed results in terms of effects on patients' self-reported clinical pain. In one study [31–33], acupuncture was less effective than an active treatment comparison immediately post-treatment but was no different at follow-up. One study found acupuncture to be superior to sham treatment [34]. One study in patients who had facial pain using evoked facial pain rather than persistent clinical facial pain as its outcome found acupuncture to be equivalent to sham acupuncture in reduction of evoked pain. Three trials [28–33] were previously described in two published systematic reviews [36,37].

Emerging data

Two relatively large-scale, NIH-funded, randomized clinical trials have recently been completed investigating the effectiveness of CAM modalities for treatment of TMD meeting Research Diagnostic Criteria. As of this writing, results of the two studies have been submitted for publication and are under peer review. In personal communication, Nancy Vuckovic, PhD, Principal Investigator of the studies at the time of their completion, provided a description of the studies, which were supported by NCCAM through a center grant to the Oregon Center for Complementary and Alternative Medicine in Craniofacial Disorders, headquartered at the Kaiser Permanente Center for Health Research in Portland.

In Study I, participants with newly diagnosed TMD were randomized to one of five groups: (1) 10 sessions of a standardized acupuncture protocol for patients; (2) 10 sessions of a protocol allowing acupuncture treatment from a menu of acupuncture points and herbal treatment for patients diagnosed with TMD by dental criteria and also evaluated according to traditional Chinese medicine diagnosis; (3) 10 sessions of a standardized full-body massage protocol incorporating intra-oral massage; (4) 10 sessions of chiropractic treatment using a set protocol including manipulation of the full body with attention to the relationship of the pelvis to the jaw; and (5) usual care at Kaiser Permanente, which could include accessing the TMD Clinic, intraoral splints, pain medications, referral for physical therapy, stress reduction, and self-care training. Primary outcomes were pre- and post-treatment assessment of Research Diagnostic Criteria with follow-up at 3, 6, 9, and 12 months post-treatment. Secondary outcomes include assessing treatment effects on depression and assessing the relationship of social support and expectations of treatment at baseline to outcomes.

In Study II, women between 25 and 55 years of age who had TMD and comorbid conditions (eg, chronic fatigue, fibromyalgia, irritable bowel syndrome, or migraine) were randomized to one of three groups: (1) 20 sessions of traditional Chinese medicine, including acupuncture, for a total of 10.5 hours of contact over a 6-month period; (2) 10.5 hours of naturopathic care over a 9-month period; or (3) usual care the same as in Study I. This study aimed to examine a more whole-systems approach, with diagnosis and treatment undertaken within the sphere of the CAM discipline (ie, traditional Chinese medicine diagnosis, naturopathy diagnosis). Outcomes are dental outcomes related to the Research Diagnostic Criteria and the other outcomes used in Study I.

Results of these two studies, regardless of the findings, will help to move research forward in the field of CAM for persistent facial pain. Protocols were developed by experienced clinical researchers in collaboration with dental experts and experts in the CAM therapies studied, yielding an exemplary interdisciplinary effort. The study designs will help to provide valuable information about the results of these treatments used in a manner similar to how they are used clinically, with several visits over time. CAM therapies tend to be administered in the community in a highly individualized fashion, which renders them challenging to replicate in research. The protocols tested by the Oregon Center for Complementary and Alternative Medicine in Craniofacial Disorders studies, although not testing completely individualized approaches, allowed some flexibility in select treatment arms and may therefore begin to answer questions about differences between standardized versus individualized protocols for CAM treatment of facial pain. According to Dr. Vukovic, there were no adverse events resulting from the studies, with the exception of minor bruising at the point of acupuncture needle insertion, which is not unexpected.

Summary

Population-based national data suggest that greater than one third of the general adult population in the United States uses CAM. Although CAM is used for a variety of indications, musculoskeletal pain is the leading reason for CAM use. Preliminary studies of clinical samples on the use of CAM by patients who have persistent facial pain indicate that these patients use CAM therapies, including manipulative and body-based therapies, such as massage therapy and chiropractic manipulation; mind–body interventions, such as relaxation and biofeedback; biologically based therapies, such as herbal supplements; and alternative medical systems, such as homeopathy, naturopathy, and traditional Chinese medicine, in a effort to manage pain and improve health.

Initial scientific evaluation has been done on biofeedback and relaxation and on one aspect of traditional Chinese medicine (ie, acupuncture). These preliminary studies indicate superiority of the three CAM treatments relative to placebo or control and generally comparable results to other conservative treatments for persistent facial pain. Other CAM therapies in use by facial pain patients remain virtually unknown from the standpoint of controlled or comparison studies. There is a great deal of research to be done to thoroughly evaluate the safety, efficacy, and mechanisms of complementary therapies for persistent facial pain. For example, herbal and dietary supplements have become widely available and popular, and facial pain patients report their use. However, some of these products possess antiplatelet activity, hepatotoxicity, adverse interactions with central nervous system depressant drugs, and additive effects when used with opioid analgesics [38]. Fortunately, support for research on CAM has increased in recent years. To illustrate, results of two relatively large-scale, NIH-funded studies on CAM for persistent facial pain will soon be known.

We must rise to the challenge of evaluating CAM therapies so that we can best guide patients seeking relief from vexing pain, which does not always fully resolve with the approaches we use and teach in dental medicine. Additionally, we must be informed about potentially harmful CAM therapies so that we can advise patients based on unbiased evidence to help them to make informed health care decisions. In this way, we work together to best serve our patients by creating health care that is comprehensive and based upon scientific evidence of clinical effectiveness.

References

[1] National Institutes of Health National Center for Complementary and Alternative Medicine website http://nccam.nih.gov/health/whatiscam/, accessed April 1, 2006.
[2] Gremillion HA, Waxenberg LB, Myers CD, et al. Psychological considerations in the diagnosis and management of temporomandibular disorders and orofacial pain. Gen Dent 2003; 51:168–72.
[3] Institute of Medicine Committee on the Use of Complementary and Alternative Medicine by the American Public. Complementary and alternative medicine in the United States. Washington, DC: National Academies Press; 2005.
[4] Barnes PM, Powell-Griner E, McFann K, et al. Complementary and alternative medicine use among adults: United States, 2002. Advance data for vital and health statistics, no. 343. Hyattsville (MD): National Center for Health Statistics; 2004.
[5] Eisenberg DM, Kessler RC, Foster C, et al. Unconventional medicine in the United States: prevalence, costs, and patterns of use. N Engl J Med 1993;328:246–52.

[6] Eisenberg DM, Davis RB, Ettner SL, et al. Trends in alternative medicine use in the United States, 1990–1997. JAMA 1998;280:1569–75.

[7] Paramore LC. Use of alternative therapies: estimates from the Robert Wood Johnson Foundation National Access to Care survey. J Pain Symptom Manage 1997;13:83–9.

[8] Astin JA. Why patients use alternative medicine. JAMA 1998;279:1548–53.

[9] Boisset M, Fitzcharles MA. Alternative medicine use by rheumatology patients in a universal health care setting. J Rheumatol 1994;21:148–52.

[10] Turp JC, Kowalski CJ, Stohler CS. Treatment-seeking patterns of facial pain patients: many possibilities, limited satisfaction. J Orofac Pain 1998;12:61–6.

[11] Raphael KG, Klausner JJ, Nayak S, et al. Complementary and alternative therapy use by patients with myofascial temporomandibular disorders. J Orofac Pain 2003;17:36–41.

[12] Dworkin SF, LeResche L. Research diagnostic criteria for temporomandibular disorders: review, criteria, examinations and specifications, critique. J Craniomandib Disord 1992;6: 301–55.

[13] DeBar LL, Vuckovic N, Schneider J, et al. Use of complementary and alternative medicine for temporomandibular disorders. J Orofac Pain 2003;17:224–36.

[14] Crider AB, Glaros AG. A meta-analysis of EMG biofeedback treatment of temporomandibular disorders. J Orofac Pain 1999;13:29–37.

[15] Hijzen TH, Slangen JL, van Houweligen HC. Subjective, clinical and EMG effects of biofeedback and splint treatment. J Oral Rehabil 1986;13:529–39.

[16] Dohrmann RJ, Laskin DM. An evaluation of electromyographic biofeedback in the treatment of myofascial pain-dysfunction syndrome. J Am Dent Assoc 1978;96:656–62.

[17] Dalen K, Ellertsen B, Espelid I, et al. EMG feedback in the treatment of myofascial pain dysfunction syndrome. 2. Acta Odontol Scand 1986;44:279–84.

[18] Olson RE, Malow, RM. Effects of biofeedback and psychotherapy on patients with myofascial pain dysfunction who are nonresponsive to conventional treatments. Rehabil Psychol 1987;32:195–204.

[19] Dahlstrom L, Carlsson SG. Treatment of mandibular dysfunction: the clinical usefulness of biofeedback in relation to splint therapy. J Oral Rehabil 1984;11:277–84.

[20] Funch DP, Gale EN. Biofeedback and relaxation therapy for chronic temporomandibular joint pain: predicting successful outcomes. J Consult Clin Psychol 1984;52:928–35.

[21] Mishra KD, Gatchel RJ, Gardea MA. The relative efficacy of three cognitive-behavioral treatment approaches to temporomandibular disorders. J Behav Med 2000;23:293–309.

[22] Erlandson PM Jr, Poppen R. Electromyographic biofeedback and rest position training of masticatory muscles in myofascial pain-dysfunction patients. J Prosthet Dent 1989;62: 335–8.

[23] Winocur E, Gavish A, Emodi-Perlman A, et al. Hypnorelaxation as treatment for myofascial pain disorder: a comparative study. Oral Surg Oral Med Oral Pathol Oral Radiol Endod 2002;93:429–34.

[24] Sherman JJ, Carlrson CR, McCubbin JA, et al. Effects of stretch-based progressive relaxation training on the secretion of salivary immunoglobulin A in orofacial pain patients. J Orofac Pain 1997;11:115–24.

[25] Okeson JP, Kemper JT, Moody PM, et al. Evaluation of occlusal splint therapy and relaxation procedures in patients with temporomandibular disorders. J Am Dent Assoc 1983;107: 420–4.

[26] Turner JA, Mancl L, Aaron LA. Short- and long-term efficacy of brief cognitive-behavioral therapy for patients with chronic temporomandibular disorder pain: a randomized, controlled trial. Pain 2006;121:181–94.

[27] Wahlund K, List T, Larsson B. Treatment of temporomandibular disorders among adolescents: a comparison between occlusal appliance, relaxation training, and brief information. Acta Odontol Scand 2003;61:203–11.

[28] Johansson A, Wenneberg B, Wagersten C, et al. Acupuncture in treatment of facial muscular pain. Acta Odontol Scand 1991;49:153–8.

[29] List T, Helkimo M, Andersson S, et al. Acupuncture and occlusal splint therapy in the treatment of craniomandibular disorders. Part I: a comparative study. Swed Dent J 1992;16: 125–41.

[30] List T, Helkimo M. Acupuncture and occlusal splint therapy in the treatment of craniomandibular disorders. Part II: a one-year follow-up study. Acta Odontol Scand 1992;50:375–85.

[31] Raustia AM, Pohjola RT, Virtanen KK. Acupuncture compared with stomatognathic treatment for TMJ dysfunction. Part I: a randomized study. J Prosthet Dent 1985;54:581–5.

[32] Raustia AM, Pohjola RT, Virtanen KK. Acupuncture compared with stomatognathic treatment for TMJ dysfunction. Part II: components of the dysfunction index. J Prosthet Dent 1986;55:372–6.

[33] Raustia AM, Pohjola RT. Acupuncture compared with stomatognathic treatment for TMJ dysfunction. Part III: effect of treatment on mobility. J Prosthet Dent 1986;56:616–23.

[34] Schmid-Schwap M, Simma-Kletschka I, Stockner A, et al. Oral acupuncture in the therapy of craniomandibular dysfunction syndrome: a randomized controlled trial. Wien Klin Wochenschr 2006;118:36–42.

[35] Goddard G, Karibe H, McNeill C, et al. Acupuncture and sham acupuncture reduce muscle pain in myofascial pain patients. J Orofac Pain 2002;16:71–6.

[36] Ernst E, White A. Acupuncture as a treatment for temporomandibular joint dysfunction: a systematic review of randomized trials. Arch Otolaryngol Head Neck Surg 1999;125: 269–72.

[37] Rosted P. The use of acupuncture in dentistry: a review of the scientific validity of published papers. Oral Dis 1998;4:100–4.

[38] Kumar NB, Allen K, Bell H. Perioperative herbal supplement use in cancer patients: potential implications and recommendations for presurgical screening. Cancer Control 2005;12: 149–57.

THE DENTAL
CLINICS
OF NORTH AMERICA

Dent Clin N Am 51 (2007) 275–279

Index

Note: Page numbers of article titles are in **boldface** type.

A

Acupuncture, in persistent facial pain, 269–270

Analgesic systems, sex differences in, 6–8

Anticholinergic therapy, 235

Anticonvulsant drugs, in neuropathic pain, 213

Antidepressants, in temporomandibular disorders, 120–121

Arthrocentesis, in temporomandibular joint, 195–197

Arthroscopy, of temporomandibular joint, 198–200

Arthrotomy, of temporomandibular joint, 171–173

B

Benzodiazepine therapy, 238

Botulinum toxin, adverse events and side effects associated with, 250
  and experimental pain, in animals, 252
    in humans, 252–253
  cautions and contraindications to, 250–251
  consent form, 248
  for motor disorders, 239–240
  in chronic migraine, 256
  in chronic tension-type headache, 256–257
  in focal chronic orodental neuropathic pain, 257
  in focal trigeminal neuralgia, 257–258
  in orofacial pain disorders, **245–261**
  in trigeminal cephalagia, 258
  injection preparation, dosing and effect duration of, 250
  mechanism of action of, 249
  medical use of, 245–246
  myofascial trigger points and, 253–254
  off-label use of, 246
  preinjection checklist, 251
  systemic review of, 253
  temporomandibular pain and dysfunction, 254–255
  training and injection procedures for, 249–250
  US Food and Drug Administration-approved uses of, 247

Brain imaging studies, of pain, 5–6

Bruxism, 225, 226, 227–228

C

Calcium channels, voltage-gated, in pain conditions, 32–33

Carbon dioxide levels, pain and, 154

Central nervous system, pain transmission from periphery to, 46–48

Central sensitivity syndrome, 109–111

Cephalagia, trigeminal autonomic, botulinum toxin in, 258

Cervical nerves, upper, sensory innervations from, 176

Cervical spine, as origin of head and orofacial pain, 173–176
  conservative care of, 182–184
  disorders of, 161
  examination of, history taking in, 179–180
    physical examination in, 180–181
  in head and orofacial pain, 172–173
  in temporomandibular disorders, 168–179
  invasive procedures for, 181–182
  with oral appliances, in temporomandibular disorders, 171–172

Cervical traction, mechanical, 184

Cervicogenic headache, and orofacial pain, 176–177, 179

Chronic fatigue syndrome, 116

Complementary and alternative medicine,
caregories of, 263–264
data on use of, 264–266
for facial pain, scientific evaluation of,
266–268
in persistent facial pain, **263–274**

Condylotomy, modified, of
temporomandibular joint, 200–201

Counterirritation pain, 6

Cranial neuralgia, classification of, and
diagnostic criteria for, 174

D

Deafferentation pain, definition of, 211

Deep brain stimulation, in orofacial motor
disorders, 234

Demyelination, 211–212

Diffuse noxious inhibitory controls, 6–7

Disc displacement, in temporomandibular
disorders, 164–166

Diskectomy, of temporomandibular joint,
203

Dizziness, causes of, 177–178

Dopamine therapy, 238

Dysautonomia, mitral valve prolapse,
118–119

Dyskinesia(s), drug-induced, treatment of,
and dystonic extrapyrimidal reactions,
234–235
orofacial, drug-induced, 230
risk factors for, 226, 229–230
spontaneous, and dystonias, treatment
of, 235

Dystonia(s), and spontaneous dyskinesia,
treatment of, 235
oromandibular, 226, 228–229

Dystonic extrapyramidal reations,
drug-induced, 226, 230–231

E

Exercises, in temporomandibular disorders,
183

Extrapyramidal reactions, serotonergic
agents causing, 231
stimulant drugs causing, 231–232

Extrapyrimidal reactions, dystonic, and
treatment of drug-induced dyskinesia,
234–235

F

Facial pain, classification of, and diagnostic
criteria for, 174
migraine and, 131
persistent, complementary and
alternative medicine for, **263–274**
persistent idiopathic, 45

Fatigue, as symptom of pain, 150

Fibromyalgia, 115–116

G

G-protein-coupled receptors, 24–25

Gamma-aminobutyric acid receptor agonist
therapy, 235–238

Gate Control of pain, and pain modulation,
48, 49

Glial activation, and central sensitization,
54

Glial influences on pain, 52–53

H

Hansen's disease, 146

Head, and orofacial pain, cervical spine
considerations in, 172–173
of cervical spine origin, 173–176

Headache, neuromuscular disorders and, 56
teeth and, 130–131
temporomandibular disorders and,
129–144
tension-type, botulinum toxin in,
256–257
treatment of, targeting
temporomandibular disorders,
136–140

Headache disorders, classification of, and
diagnostic criteria for, 174

Heart rate, variability of, as measure of
health, 152–153

Herpes zoster virus, neuralgia following,
219–221
treatment of, 220–221

Hypermobility, in temporomandibular
disorders, 163–164

Hyperprolactinemia, 117–118

Hypothalamic-pituitary-adrenal axis,
111–113, 153–154
and sleep, 113–115

Hypothyroidism, 119

I

Inflammation, in temporomandibular disorders, 163

Ion channels, voltage-gated, 25

Irritable bowel syndrome, 116–117

J

Joint intracapsular disorders, diagnostic and nonsurgical management considerations in, **85–103**

L

Leprosy, 146

M

MAP kinase cascades, 49, 50

Mastication, muscles of, orofacial pain and, 154

Masticatory muscle pain, 167–168

Menstrual migraine, 119–120

Microvascular decompression, in orofacial motor disorders, 233–234

Migraine, 129
  chronic, botulinum toxin in, 256–257
  facial pain and, 131
  menstrual, 119–120
  triggering factors in, 129

Mitral valve prolapse dysautonomia, 118–119

Motor disorders, hyperkinetic, medications for management of, 236–237

Motor suppressive medications, 235–240

Multiple chemical sensitivity syndrome, 117

Muscle spasm, 61–62

Myalgia disorders, masticatory, diagnostic criteria for, 62

Myectomy, in orofacial motor disorders, 234

Myofascial pain, 53–55, 61
  temporomandibular disorders and, 134–136

Myofascial trigger points, botulinum toxin and, 253–254

Myositis, 61

N

N-methyl-D-aspartate receptor, 50

Neck pain, in temporomandibular disorders, 168

Neuralgia, post-herpetic, 219–221
  treatment of, 220–221
  trigeminal. See *Trigeminal neuralgia.*

Neuromuscular disorders, headache and, 56

Neuronal receptors, and drugs modulating odontogenic pain, 25, 26–27

Neurons, second-order, 47, 48

Neuropathic pain, in orofacial region, 56–57

O

Occipital nerve, 175

Odontalgia, atypical, and headache, 130

Odontogenic pain, drugs modulating, neuronal receptors and, 25, 26–27
  genetic analysis of, 19
  molecular approaches to, 19
  peripheral mechanisms of, **19–44**

Opiod analgesia, sex differences in, 7

Oral motor disorders, **225–243**
  four most common, 225–227

Orofacial motor disorder(s), deep brain stimulation in, 234
  differential diagnosis of, 232
  interventional approaches to, 233
  medical treatment strategy in, 233
  myectomy in, 234
  pallidotomy in, 234
  surgical microvascular decompression in, 233–234
  treatment of, 232–233

Orofacial pain disorder(s), botulinum toxin in, **245–261**

Orofacial pain(s), biological factors contributing to, 148–149
  central mechanisms of, **45–59**
  epidemiology of, 1–2
    and gender differences in, **1–18**
  excitory factors in, 149–150
  features of, biopsychosocial model and, 148–154
  gender differences in, 2
  impact of central sensitization on, and temporomandibular disorders, 53–57
  importance of pain in region, 149
  laboratory models of, 4

Orofacial pain(s) (*continued*)
management of, biobehavioral
approaches to, 155–157
neuropathic, **209–224**
adjuvant drugs used in, 213, 214
clinical features association with,
211
pathophysiology of, 210–214
personality disorders and, 148
psychological factors associated with,
145–160
referrals in, 147
temporomandibular disorders and,
disorders associated with, 105
trauma exposure and, 147
Oromandibular dystonia, 226,
228–229

P

Pain, brain imaging studies of, 5–6
counterirritation, 6
definition of, 45
diagnosis and manaagement of,
molecular model of, 35–36
experimental, responses to, clinical
relevance of, 8–9
sex differences in response to,
animal research in, 3
human research in, 3–4
experimental studies of, future
directions in, 11–12
facial, migraine and, 131
persistent, complementary and
alternative medicine for,
263–274
persistent idiopathic, 45
fatigue as symptom of, 150
glial inflences on, 52–53
myofascial. See *Myofascial pain.*
neuropathic, definition of, 210
nociceptive, 210
nonpharmacologic treatment of,
responses to, 9
orofacial. See *Orofacial pain(s).*
perception of, pretreatment
expectations and, 11
sex differences in, mechanisms
underlying, 9–11
processing, central, and central
sensitization, 48–51
sensitivity to, factors reducing, 150
sleep variables and, 151
temporal summation of, 4–5
unremitting, as stressor, 151–152
Pain-modulating circuits, 51–52
Pallidotomy, in orofacial motor disorders,
234

Peptides, in tooth pulp, 22
trigeminal system, 22
Personality disorders, orofacial pain and,
148
Physical therapists, temporomandibular
disorders and, 161
Posttraumatic stress disorder, 147–148
Potassium channels, voltage-gated, in pain
conditions, 31–32
Psychiatric disorders, orofacial pain and,
147
Psychological factors, associated with
orofacial pain, **145–160**

R

Relaxation training, in persistent facial
pain, 268–269

S

Sensory neurons, classes of, 22
receptors and ion channels in, 23–24
Sensory system, afferent, 46–48
Serotonergic agents, causing extrapyramidal
reactions, 231
Skeletal muscle relaxants, 238–239
Sleep variables, pain and, 151
Sodium channels, voltage-gated, in pain
conditions, 29–31
Stress-related disorders, insufficient
glucocorticoid signaling in, 114

T

Temporomandibular disorders, 45
acute, symptoms related to, 106, 107
acute to chronic pain in, time course
of, 105, 106
and head and orofacial pain, cervical
spine considerations in, 168–179
and headache, **129–144**
epidemiology of, 132
etiology of, 131–132
nonsurgical treatment of,
137–140
surgical treatment of, 140
and myofascial pain, 134–136
and neck pain, 168
and orofacial pain, disorders
associated with, 105
antidepressants in, 120–121
arthrogenous, 163–167

cervical spine and, 168–179
cervical spine considerations in, 169–170
chronic, symptoms related to, 106, 107
classsification of, 115
clinical management of, 121
common, 162
conditions with symptoms common to, 115–117
disc displacement in, 164–166
evaluation of, 121–122
features associated with, **105–127**
fibrous adhesions in, 166–167
head and orofacial pain in, **161–193**
headache treatment targeting, 136–140
historical background of, 108–109
hypermobility in, 163–164
inflammation in, 163
myogenous, 167–168
  clinical presentation of, 63–66
  cognitive-behavioral therapy in, 73–74
  comorbid conditions and, 65–66
  control of contributing factors in, 78
  diagnostic and management considerations in, **61–83**
  diagnostic tests in, 67
  etiology and epidemiology of, 66
  limited range of motion in, 63–64
  muscle exercises in, 74–75
  muscle therapy in, 75–76
  muscle weakness in, 63, 64
  orthopedic intraoral splints in, 71–73
  pain clinic team management in, 78–80
  pain in, 63
  pathophysiology of, 66–67
  pharmacotherapy in, 76–78
  self-care in, 69, 71
  treatment of, 68–80
physical therapists and, 161
physical therapy management of, 161
studies of, 122–125

Temporomandibular joint, anatomy of, 85–87
anterior positioning appliance, 93
arthrocentesis in, 195–197
arthroscopy of, 198–200
disc derangement disorders of, 133

disc displacement with reduction, 89–91, 133–134
  treatment of, 93–96
disc displacement without reduction, 91, 133–134
  treatment of, 97–99
diskectomy of, 203
inflammatory conditions of, 132–133
intracapsular disorders of, 89–99
  nonsurgical management of, 91–93
  supportive therapies in, 96–97, 99
modified condylotomy of, 200–201
normal function of, 87–89
pain in, 55–56
replacement of, 204–206
surgery of, arthrotomy in, 171–173
  for internal derangement, **195–208**
  indications for, 197–198
  open joint, 171–173

Tinnitus, subjective, and secondary otalgia, 178–179

Tooth pulp, composition of, 20–22

Tooth (Teeth), and headache, 130–131
innervation of, 22

Toothache, atypical odontalgia/non-odontogenic, 218–219
study of peripheral pain mechanisms and, 20

Transient receptor potential channels, in transduction of sensory stimuli, 33–35

Trigeminal deafferentation, 130–131

Trigeminal neuralgia, botulinum toxin in, 257–258
incidence of, 215
mechanisms of, 216, 218
pre-trigeminal neuralgia before, 216
secondary to dental treatments, 217–218
treatment of, 216–217, 218
trigger zones of, 215

Trigeminal nucleus caudalis, 46, 47

Trigeminal pain, 145

Trigeminocervical nucleus, 174–175

Tryptase, release of, 23

Moving?

Make sure your subscription moves with you!

To notify us of your new address, find your **Clinics Account Number** (located on your mailing label above your name), and contact customer service at:

E-mail: elspcs@elsevier.com

800-654-2452 (subscribers in the U.S. & Canada)
407-345-4000 (subscribers outside of the U.S. & Canada)

Fax number: 407-363-9661

Elsevier Periodicals Customer Service
6277 Sea Harbor Drive
Orlando, FL 32887-4800

*To ensure uninterrupted delivery of your subscription, please notify us at least 4 weeks in advance of move.

ELSEVIER